MW00837329

Introduction to

Speech Sound Disorders

Introduction to
Speech Sound Disorders

Françoise Brosseau-Lapré, PhD, CCC-SLP, S-LP(C)
Susan Rvachew, PhD, S-LP(C)

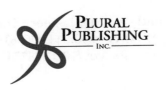

PLURAL
PUBLISHING
INC.

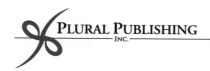

PLURAL PUBLISHING
INC.

5521 Ruffin Road
San Diego, CA 92123

e-mail: information@pluralpublishing.com
Website: http://www.pluralpublishing.com

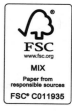

FSC
www.fsc.org
MIX
Paper from
responsible sources
FSC® C011935

Copyright © 2020 by Plural Publishing, Inc.

Typeset in 10.5/13 Palatino by Flanagan's Publishing Services, Inc.
Printed in the United States of America by McNaughton & Gunn, Inc.

All rights, including that of translation, reserved. No part of this publication may be reproduced, stored in a retrieval system, or transmitted in any form or by any means, electronic, mechanical, recording, or otherwise, including photocopying, recording, taping, Web distribution, or information storage and retrieval systems without the prior written consent of the publisher.

For permission to use material from this text, contact us by
Telephone: (866) 758-7251
Fax: (888) 758-7255
e-mail: permissions@pluralpublishing.com

Every attempt has been made to contact the copyright holders for material originally printed in another source. If any have been inadvertently overlooked, the publishers will gladly make the necessary arrangements at the first opportunity.

Library of Congress Cataloging-in-Publication Data

Names: Brosseau-Laprâe, Franðcoise, author. | Rvachew, Susan, author.
Title: Introduction to speech sound disorders / Francoise Brosseau-Lapre, Susan Rvachew.
Description: San Diego, CA : Plural Publishing, [2020] | Includes bibliographical references and index.
Identifiers: LCCN 2018028734| ISBN 9781597568036 (alk. paper) | ISBN 1597568031 (alk. paper)
Subjects: | MESH: Speech Sound Disorder | Speech Perception | Phonetics
Classification: LCC RC424.7 | NLM WL 340.2 | DDC 616.85/5--dc23
LC record available at https://lccn.loc.gov/2018028734

CONTENTS

Preface   *ix*
Reviewers   *xi*

1 Concepts in Phonetics and Phonology   1

1.1 Phonetic Concepts   2
   1.1.1 Articulatory Phonetics   3
1.2 Describing Articulatory Knowledge   11
   1.2.1 International Phonetic Alphabet   11
   1.2.2 Broad and Narrow Transcription of Speech   15
   1.2.3 Visual Analysis of Articulation   18
1.3 Describing Perceptual Knowledge   20
   1.3.1 Continuous versus Discrete Nature of Speech Information 20
   1.3.2 Categorical Perception   22
1.4 Phonological Concepts   26
   1.4.1 Phones, Phonemes, and Allophones   26
   1.4.2 Phonotactic Rules   27
   1.4.3 Nonlinear Phonology   28
   1.4.4 Prosody   29
   1.4.5 Syllabifying Words   30
   1.4.6 Consonant Features in Nonlinear Phonology   32
   1.4.7 Phonological Processes   36

2 Phonological Development   41

2.1 Speech Perception Development   42
   2.1.1 Infants   42
   2.1.2 Toddlers   45
   2.1.3 Preschoolers   46
   2.1.4 School-Age Children   49
2.2 Early Speech Production Development   50
   2.2.1 Prelinguistic Vocal Development   50
   2.2.2 First Words   53

2.3 Phonological Development   57
    2.3.1 Phoneme Acquisition Norms   58
    2.3.2 Phonological Process Norms   63
    2.3.3 Acquisition of Prosodic Units   67

3 Assessment   79

3.1 Purposes of Evaluation   80
    3.1.1 Screening Assessment   80
    3.1.2 Diagnostic Assessments   81
3.2 Types of Measurement Tools   82
    3.2.1 Standardized versus Informal Measurement Tools   82
    3.2.2 Norm-Referenced versus Criterion-Referenced Measurement Tools   83
    3.2.3 Static versus Dynamic Measurement Tools   85
3.3 Planning the Assessment   86
    3.3.1 Referral   86
    3.3.2 Case History   87
3.4 Components of the Speech Assessment   90
    3.4.1 Norm-Referenced Single-Word Articulation/Phonology Test   91
    3.4.2 Stimulability Testing   96
    3.4.3 Oral Mechanism Examination   96
    3.4.4 Continuous Speech Sample   102
    3.4.5 Hearing Screening   105
    3.4.6 Inconsistency and Variability Assessment   105
    3.4.7 Intelligibility   106
    3.4.8 Participation   109
    3.4.9 Language Screen or Test   110
    3.4.10 Phonological Processing   111
3.5 Considerations for Dialect Speakers, Children Speaking English   117
    as a Second Language, and Multilingual Children

4 Diagnosis   121

4.1 Classification of Speech Sound Disorders   122
4.2 Linguistic Classification of Speech Sound Disorders   125
    4.2.1 Phonetic versus Phonemic Disorder   125
    4.2.2 Model for Differential Diagnosis   126
4.3 Speech Disorders Classification System   131
    4.3.1 Speech Delay   132
    4.3.2 Speech Errors   134
    4.3.3 Motor Speech Disorders   134
4.4 Psycholinguistic Approach   136
    4.4.1 Speech Perception   137
    4.4.2 Phonological Awareness   138
    4.4.3 Nonword Repetition   138

4.4.4 Multisyllable Repetition 139
4.4.5 Undifferentiated Lingual Gestures 139
4.4.6 Tongue Strength 140
4.5 Epidemiology of SSD 141
4.5.1 Prevalence of SSD 142
4.5.2 Comorbidity 144
4.5.3 Short- and Long-Term Outcomes 145

5 Treatment Planning **151**

5.1 Deciding Whether to Provide an Intervention 152
5.1.1 Norm-Referenced Approach 152
5.1.2 Medical Approach 155
5.1.3 International Classification of Functioning, Disability, and 156
Health Framework
5.1.4 Recommended Protocol for Deciding When to Treat 157
5.2 Service Delivery Options 160
5.2.1 Intensity of Intervention 161
5.2.2 Intervention Agents 164
5.3 Intervention Goals 165
5.3.1 Types of Goals 166
5.3.2 Goal Attack Strategies 169
5.3.3 Selecting Goals 169
5.4 Monitoring Treatment Progress 175
5.4.1 Instructional Objectives 175
5.4.2 Generalization 178
5.4.3 Evidence-Based Practice 180

6 Input-Oriented Approaches **183**

6.1 Rationale for the Input-Oriented Approach 184
6.2 Focused Stimulation 184
6.3 Ear Training 189
6.4 Dialogic Reading 194

7 Output-Oriented Approaches **199**

7.1 Rationale for the Output-Oriented Approach 200
7.2 Vocal Play 200
7.3 Fundamentals of the Sensorimotor Approach 203
7.3.1 Nonsense Syllable Drills 204
7.3.2 Sensorimotor Therapy Procedures 207
7.4 Traditional Articulation Therapy 216
7.4.1 Ear Training 216
7.4.2 Establishment 217

7.4.3 Stabilization of New Phonemes   221
7.4.4 Transfer and Maintenance   226

8 Phonological Approaches   233

8.1 Rationale for a Phonological Approach   234
8.2 Word-Based Phonology: Core Vocabulary Approach   236
8.3 Phonological Patterns: Cycles Remediation Approach   244
8.4 Meaningful Minimal Pairs Procedure   248
8.5 Metaphonological Knowledge   252
     8.5.1 Speech Therapy Procedures That Promote Phonological   254
            Awareness
     8.5.2 Structured Emergent Literacy Interventions   257
     8.5.3 Reading and Spelling Interventions   259
8.6 Conclusion   261

References   *265*
Index   *285*

PREFACE

The motivation and inspiration for *Introduction to Speech Sound Disorders* comes from our work as pediatric speech-language pathologists, as instructors and mentors of students in communication sciences and disorders, and as researchers in the assessment and treatment of speech sound disorders. This comprehensive textbook was written for undergraduate students in speech, language, and hearing sciences as well as their instructors. Children with speech sound disorders form the largest part of the speech-language pathologist caseload in child-focused settings. A course on speech sound disorders is often among the first courses with a clinic focus offered in the curriculum of programs in our discipline. However, this does not mean that speech sound disorders is an easy subject, or that treating children with speech sound disorders is easy to do—in fact, phonological development is a complex process, speech sound disorders are varied and challenging, and competent treatment of children requires a broad range of domain-specific and domain-general skills.

With this book, we aimed to introduce undergraduate students to foundational concepts and procedures that will prepare students for graduate level study of speech sound disorders and early supervised clinical practice with children. The text and associated companion website are intended to support new and experienced instructors as they strive to facilitate novice-level clinical competencies in their speech-language pathology students. The book is organized in a coherent manner to ensure that all new terms are defined. Furthermore, important concepts are reintroduced repeatedly in new contexts to enrich learning. Practice activities are provided in each chapter to encourage interactive learning. The flow of the chapters was carefully developed to ensure that students can build on previous knowledge and proceed from introduction to practice.

One challenge for instructors of courses on speech sound disorders is the varied range of knowledge that students bring to this course—some will remember all concepts covered in their prerequisite phonetics course and speech and hearing science course, and some students will have forgotten most of the information they learned one or two years earlier. For this reason, Chapter 1 defines the major concepts and constructs in phonetics and phonology currently framing the study of speech sound disorders in children that we wish every undergraduate student remembered. This chapter can be covered in the course or not—it could be assigned as independent work for students who need to review this material, and the instructor could begin the course with

Chapter 2. The second chapter provides a thorough description of typical and atypical development of speech perception and speech production in infants, toddlers, preschoolers, and school-age children. Subsequent chapters cover assessment, interpretation and diagnosis, treatment planning, and the selection and implementation of an appropriate intervention. The last chapters of the book describe input-oriented, output-oriented, and phonological approaches. Detailed examples, illustrations, tables, and figures increase comprehension throughout each chapter. Key point boxes encourage review of important concepts at the end of each section.

It is our hope that this book will raise the standard for undergraduate instruction in the field of speech sound disorders and that we will inspire students to pursue careers dedicated to improving the communication abilities of children. Our lives have been immeasurably enriched by our many years of service to children with speech and language disorders, to whom we dedicate this book. We also thank our families for all the support they provided to us throughout the process of writing our second book together: Françoise's husband Ray and her daughters Sophie, Laura, and Catherine and Susan's husband Ken Bott and her daughter, Vivian Bott.

REVIEWERS

Plural Publishing, Inc. and the authors would like to thank the following reviewers for taking the time to provide their valuable feedback during the development process:

Christina M. Hagedorn, PhD, TSSLD, CCC-SLP
Assistant Professor
College of Staten Island–City University of New York
The CUNY Graduate Center–City University of New York
New York, New York

Leisa Harmon, MS, CCC-SLP
Assistant Professor/Externship Coordinator
Communication Disorders
Minot State University
Minot, North Dakota

AnnMarie C. Knight, PhD, CCC-SLP
Assistant Professor
Speech-Language Pathology
Columbia College
Columbia, South Carolina

Carol L. Koch, EdD, CCC-SLP
Professor and Graduate Program Director
Communication Sciences and Disorders
Samford University
Birmingham, Alabama

Jennifer M. D. Kremkow, PhD, CCC-SLP
Assistant Professor
Department of Communication Sciences and Disorders
Elmhurst College
Elmhurst, Illinois

Sue Ann S. Lee, PhD, CCC-SLP
Associate Professor
Department of Speech, Language & Hearing Sciences
Texas Tech University Health Sciences Center
Lubbock, Texas

Marcella McCollum, MA, CCC-SLP
Clinical Faculty, Lecturer
Communicative Disorders and Sciences
San Jose Sate University
San Jose, California

Keri Parchman-Gonzalez, MA, CCC-SLP
Clinical Assistant Professor
Department of Communication Sciences and Disorders
The University of Texas Rio Grande Valley
Edinburg, Texas

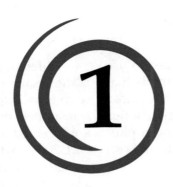

Concepts in Phonetics and Phonology

Learning Objectives

- Explain the difference between phonetics and phonology.
- Determine the phonetic repertoire from the transcription of a child's speech sample.
- Evaluate the advantages and disadvantages of transcription to describe articulatory knowledge.
- Define categorical perception and differentiate identification and discrimination tests of phoneme perception.

- Define phoneme, allophone, and phonotactic rule.
- Describe the three primary components of prosody and identify words with trochaic and iambic prosodic patterns.
- Diagram the internal components of syllables (onset, nucleus, coda).
- Identify common patterns of phonological error in child speech.

There is great power in being able to communicate effectively, which requires at a minimum being understood by our communication partner. However, the value of producing speech accurately is often taken for granted. Most of us use speech to communicate, without difficulties, and do not reflect on the way in which speech sounds are produced and combined to produce language. Speech-language pathologists (SLPs) must be able to describe the child's ability to produce speech sounds clearly, perceive speech sounds accurately, and combine speech sounds into words that other listeners will understand. Although the child's knowledge of these aspects of phonetics and phonology is implicit, the SLP's knowledge must be explicit. That is, the SLP must not only be able to say a word; he or she must be able to explain why that is the appropriate word to use in that context, describe the sounds that make up the word, and show how those sounds are produced. The first part of this chapter presents basic concepts in phonetics, and the second portion focuses on basic concepts in phonology.

1.1 PHONETIC CONCEPTS

Phonetics is concerned with the physical characteristics of speech sounds as produced by the speaker to transmit meaning and as received by the listener to understand what was said (Ohala, 1999). A **phone** is the smallest unit of speech; any sound that is used for speech in any of the languages of the world is a phone. Phonetics is therefore the study of speech sounds, or the study of phones. By convention, speech sounds that are produced by a speaker (phones) are represented between square brackets [ ]. These square brackets are differentiated from slashes / /, which are used to identify **phonemes**, a more abstract representation of speech sounds that will be discussed in section 1.4.

Different tools and scientific specializations are required to study speech sounds as they are produced, as they are transmitted through the air, and as they are received by the listener (Pierrehumbert, 2003). **Articulatory phonetics** is concerned with the way that speech sounds are produced with the articulators. **Articulators** are the parts of the human body that are involved in speech production, as will be described further in this chapter. **Acoustic phonetics** is the study of speech sounds as transmitted through the air in the form of sound waves. Acoustic phonetics may also be concerned with the relationship between the acoustic properties of sound waves and the way that the listener perceives different speech sounds. This process is called **phonetic encoding**. Figure 1–1 presents a simple schema of the speaking and listening process as related to these branches of phonetics. In the figure, the speaker wants to transmit a message about the cat. In order to do so, the speaker must access a semantic representation ("cat") that contains information about the meaning of this word and a phonological representation (/kæt/), shown in the figure as a series of pho-

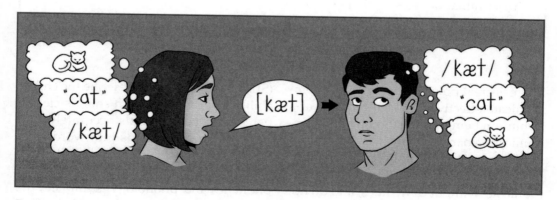

Figure 1–1. *Phonetics is concerned with the production, transmission, and encoding of speech sounds (see text for explanation). Used with permission from Ellen Graham-Platt.*

nemes for convenience, but actually containing more abstract information about the phonology of this word, as will be discussed in more detail later in this chapter. Once having accessed these abstract representations, the speaker retrieves and sequences **articulatory-phonetic representations** [k], [æ], [t] and sends the corresponding motor commands to the articulators to produce the word. The acoustic signal is transmitted through air and reaches the listener's outer ears; the eardrum vibrates; the vibrations are carried through the middle ear to the inner ear, and the cochlea provides auditory input to the central auditory system in the brain. The listener must now reverse the speaker's process to abstract the sequence of sounds ([kæt]), this time in the form of an **acoustic-phonetic representation**, and link the result to the corresponding phonological (/kæt/) and semantic ("cat") representations to understand the speaker's intended meaning.

1.1.1 Articulatory Phonetics

Articulatory phonetics focuses on how speech sounds are produced and how these sounds can be classified based on aspects of their production. Articulation usually refers more broadly to the general production of speech by a talker, such as whether the individual articulates speech sounds clearly and precisely or mumbles.

Three physiological subsystems contribute to speech production: the respiratory system, the phonatory system, and the articulatory/resonating system. Figure 1–2 shows a simplified schema of these three subsystems. First, the respiratory system provides airflow, the required energy source to produce speech sounds.

Second, the larynx (also called "voice box") is the main component of the phonatory system. The vocal folds are situated in the larynx and vibrate very rapidly, setting the airflow into vibration, creating sound. Third, the articulatory/resonating system is composed of the pharyngeal, oral, and nasal cavities. These three cavities form the vocal tract. The cavities of the vocal tract resonate the vibrating sound waves as they pass through from the larynx to the outside air. Specifically, when the speaker varies the size and shape of the vocal tract, the sound waves are modified, to create all the vowels and consonants (Kent, 1997). The human vocal tract is shown in Figure 1–3. The shape and size of the vocal tract is primarily modified by movements of the tongue, although the lips, teeth, hard palate, and velum also impact speech production.

Practice 1–1

Articulators are the parts of the body that you move to produce speech. Produce the words "key," "me," "see," "bee," and "boot." Notice that changes in the larynx and in the manner of airflow through the vocal tract also result in different speech sounds. Try to sense how changes in the position of the tongue and the lips impact speech production. The shape of your lips when saying [b] in "bee" and "boot" were probably different because of **co-articulation**.

While producing speech, the stages of respiration, phonation, and articulation do not each have a clear and distinct beginning. Speech is continuous, and the

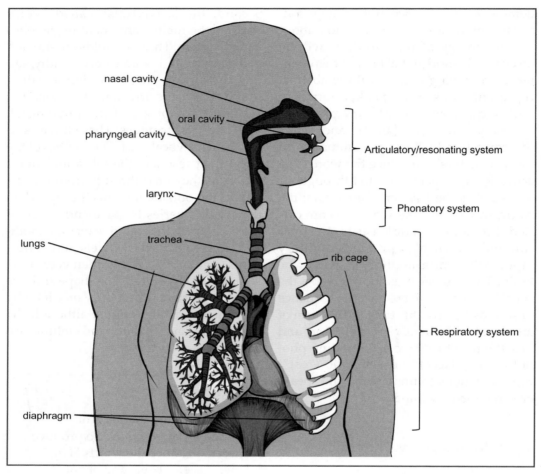

Figure 1–2. *Simplified schema of the speech production system. Used with permission from Ellen Graham-Platt.*

articulators are in constant motion when the air is flowing. **Co-articulation** occurs when articulators are moving at the same time to produce two different but overlapping phones. In the words "bee" and "sheep" the lips will be spread even before speaking, whereas the lips will be rounded at the beginning of the words "boot" and "shoe," anticipating the upcoming vowels in these words. **Assimilation** refers to the articulatory changes that occur when one phone becomes more like an adjacent

(neighboring) phone or another phone in the word which is not directly adjacent. Assimilation is the reason that the word "pumpkin" is not pronounced the way it is spelled: the [k] at the beginning of the second syllable makes it easier to end the first syllable with the tongue raised at the back of the mouth. In normal speech production, the movement of the articulators will be modified depending on preceding or following phones to reduce effort and increase efficiency of speech

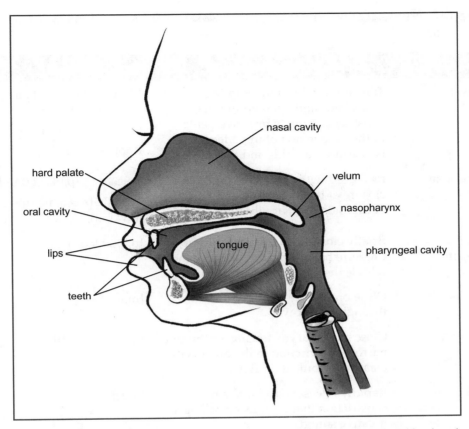

Figure 1–3. *The adult human vocal tract with articulators labeled. Used with permission from Ellen Graham-Platt.*

production. Therefore, co-articulation and assimilation occur very frequently in adult and child speech.

Given the importance of articulatory phonetics to the competent practice of speech-language pathology, a brief overview of the articulatory characteristics of English vowels and consonants is provided here. Consultation with a detailed phonetics text is advised for all SLPs, however (e.g., Shriberg & Kent, 2013; Small, 2016). Phone classes are first determined by **manner of articulation**, that is, the manner or type of constriction that is made in the vocal tract. Phone classes are

further distinguished by **place of articulation**, that is, the location of the constriction in the vocal tract. Finally, phones may be **voiced** or **voiceless**, in other words, produced with or without vibration of the vocal folds.

Beginning with the manner classes, summarized in Table 1–1, **vowels** are produced with an open vocal tract. Vocal fold vibration is usually maintained throughout the production of the sound, but otherwise the airflow through the vocal folds to the lips is mostly unblocked. In English the airflow is directed through the oral cavity during most vowels, although there

Table 1–1. *Articulatory Characteristics of Major Classes of Phones in English by Manner of Articulation*

Manner Class	Articulatory Characteristic	English Phones
Vowels	Transmit air through vibrating vocal folds and open vocal tract; constrictions made by movements of the tongue do not impede airflow between vocal folds and lips.	Monophthongs: [i,ɪ,ʊ,u,e,o, ɛ,ə,ʌ,ɔ,æ,a,ɑ] Diphthongs: [aɪ,aʊ,ɔɪ,oʊ,eɪ] Rhotics: [ɚ,ɝ]
Consonants	Produced with partial or complete closure of the vocal tract and with the vocal folds open or vibrating.	Voiceless: [p,t,k,ʔ,f,θ,s,ʃ,tʃ,h] Voiced: [b,d,g,m,n,ŋ,v,ð,z,ʒ, dʒ,w,j,ɹ,l]
Plosives (stops)	Briefly close vocal tract to build up air pressure behind the constriction; then release the pressure in the oral cavity.	[p,b,t,d,k,g,ʔ]
Nasals	Close oral cavity but permit airflow through nasal cavity.	[m,n,ŋ]
Fricatives	Close nasopharynx forcing air through narrow constriction in the oral cavity, creating turbulent air flow.	[f,v,θ,ð,s,z,ʃ,ʒ,h]
Affricates	Rapidly release a stop into a narrow constriction that permits a prolonged fricative sound.	[tʃ,dʒ]
Approximants	Approximate the articulators more closely than in the case of vowels but without creating a constriction narrow enough to produce turbulent noise.	Glides: [w,j] Liquids: [ɹ,l]

may sometimes be nasal airflow due to assimilation. Oral airflow is accomplished by raising the velum to close the passage between the pharyngeal and nasal cavities. This passage, shown in Figure 1–3, is called the nasopharynx or the velopharyngeal port. The position of the lips impacts the length of the vocal tract—retracting the lips shortens the tract, while rounding and protruding them lengthens the tract. The position of the tongue will modify the size of the pharyngeal cavity (shown in Figure 1–3), such that the pharyngeal cav-

ity will enlarge when the tongue is moved forward, and diminish when the tongue is moved toward the rear of the mouth. Each shape of the vocal tract will have different resonance characteristics, resulting in the production of a different vowel. For example, the vowel in "bee" is produced with a constriction near the front of the mouth which shapes the vocal tract into two parts—a large back cavity joined to a small front cavity. In contrast, the vowel in the word "boot" is produced with a constriction near the back of the mouth so that the front and back cavities are both large. The front cavity can be made larger still by lowering the jaw, as in words like "bad" and "bought." When the configuration of the vocal tract changes during the production of the vowel, there is a change in the resonance quality within the same vowel, and a **diphthong** is produced, as in the word "bye" (Ladefoged & Johnson, 2010).

As opposed to the relatively open vocal tract configuration for vowels, **consonants** are characterized by constriction in the oral and/or pharyngeal cavities. For certain consonants, the vocal tract will be completely closed for a moment. For others, the airflow will encounter obstacles, resulting in a partial closure of the vocal tract. In English many but not all consonants are produced in two forms, the **voiced** form and the **voiceless** form, with pairs at the same place of articulation known as **cognates**.

Practice 1–2

Place your fingers over your "Adam's apple" on the front of your neck and slowly say the sound [p] with a puff of air; then slowly say the sound [b]. You should notice vibration on your fingers during the second sound that was absent during the first sound. Take care to say [p] and not [pa] and compare with [b] and not [ba] because the vocal folds will vibrate during the vowel [a], making it hard to differentiate the voicing characteristics of the two consonants. Try this again with prolonged production of [s] and [z], noticing the lack and presence of vibration during the production of these **voiceless** and **voiced cognates**.

Plosives are produced with a complete but brief interruption of the airflow through the vocal cavity, which is why these phones are also called stops. Closure of the nasopharynx is essential so that air cannot escape through the nose. At the same time, a second closure is created with the tongue or lips in the oral cavity, which creates a build-up of air pressure behind the constriction. When this pressure is suddenly released, an audible burst of air may result that is called **aspiration**.

Nasals are sometimes referred to as nasal stops because their production requires a constriction to close the oral cavity. However, during the production of nasals the velopharynx remains open, allowing sound to enter and escape the nasal cavity. This also lengthens the vocal tract, and changes the resonance of these sounds.

In contrast to stops, **fricatives** are produced with a partial rather than complete closure of the vocal tract. When the air passes through the narrow constriction in the vocal tract, turbulence is created, resulting in a friction noise. Fricatives also require closure of the velopharyngeal port to prevent nasal air escape. The lack of complete interruption of the airflow means that fricative sounds can be prolonged (such as the sound [s] that can be produced continuously for a few seconds, as in "ssssssssss"). A related phone class comprises the **affricates**, which combine characteristics of a plosive and a fricative sound. Initially, the oral cavity is sealed and air pressure builds behind the tongue. The tongue then quickly releases contact with the palate to create a constricted opening that permits a prolonged fricative sound to follow the release of the stop.

Approximants are produced by approximating the articulators more closely than in the case of vowels but without creating a constriction narrow enough to produce turbulent noise. There are two types of approximants, the glides and the liquids. **Glides** are produced with less constriction than during production of a liquid but more than in the production of vowels. Glides are sometimes called semi-vowels, since their production initially requires a slight constriction before transitioning into a more vowel-like open vocal tract. **Liquids** are more consonant-like than the glides but they are continuous in the manner of approximants. During their production there is some constriction in the vocal tract, but the oral cavity is fairly open, and the velopharynx closed. In English, one liquid is a **rhotic**, specifically the sound at the beginning of the word "row" and the end of the word "bar." This phone can be pronounced with different tongue configurations, as shown in Figure 1–4. The other liquid, specifically the phone at the beginning of the word "low" and the end of the word "ball," is called a **lateral** because air escapes around the sides of the tongue when the tongue tip is held at the top of the mouth near the alveolar ridge. The liquids /l/ and /ɹ/ may be produced with the tongue tip in a **retroflex** position in which the tongue tip is curled back, but this articulatory gesture is not required to achieve the correct sound.

Practice 1–3

Compare your tongue posture for liquid consonants in the words "row" versus "low" and in "light" versus "pull." How do you shape your tongue when you say the liquid sounds in these words? Is the tongue tip curled back? Is the tongue body more forward or more back in your oral cavity?

Phones that are differentiated by manner of articulation are also differentiated by the location of the constriction in the vocal tract, that is, by place of articulation. The different places of constriction are shown in Figure 1–5 and described in Table 1–2. Not all possible places of articulation are used by all languages. Furthermore, within one language such as English, not all places of articulation are used within every manner class.

Moving from the front of the vocal tract and working back, the first place of articulation in English is **bilabial**, meaning sounds that are produced by putting the upper and lower lip together. Sometimes these phones, which include plosives, nasals, and a glide, are referred to simply as labial. In the fricative class there are **labiodental** phones, produced by placing the top teeth on the lower lip.

Moving to phones that are produced with constrictions of the tongue tip or blade, **dental** phones are produced by placing the tongue tip between the front teeth, and are thus also called interdental. In English the only interdental phones are fricatives. **Alveolar** sounds are produced by putting the tongue tip up against the alveolar ridge, the bumpy area just behind the upper front teeth. However, these sounds can be produced by placing the tongue tip against the top or bottom teeth as well. In English the alveolar class includes stops, nasals, fricatives, and approximants. **Post-alveolar** sounds in English are fricatives and are therefore produced by bringing the tongue blade close to the area of the palate that is just behind the alveolar ridge. There are no palatal fricatives in English to contrast with the post-alveolar fricatives and therefore the articulatory placement of the tongue during the production of these sounds can be quite variable—the tongue might be

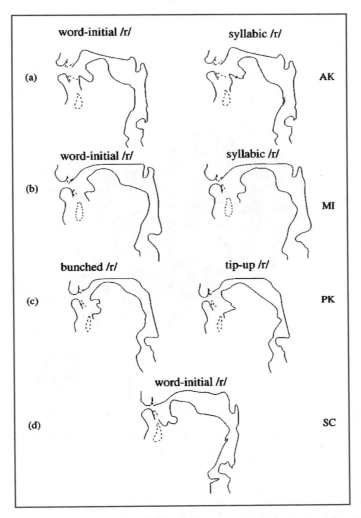

Figure 1–4. *Sagittal profiles of the vocal tract during production of [ɹ] by four different adult talkers. Source: Alwan, Narayanan, and Haker (1997). Toward articulatory-acoustic models for liquid approximants based on MRI and EPG data. Part II. The rhotics. Journal of the Acoustical Society of America by the Acoustical Society of America, 101, Figure 1, p. 1079. Reproduced with permission from the American Institute of Physics for the Acoustical Society of America.*

placed in the post-alveolar region or fully in the palatal region (where the hard palate rises behind the alveolar ridge, in the middle of the mouth). English contains two post-alveolar affricates as well.

The tongue body or dorsum is brought into contact with the velum to produce the **velar** phones, which include two stops and a nasal. The liquid [w] also has a velar constriction and is

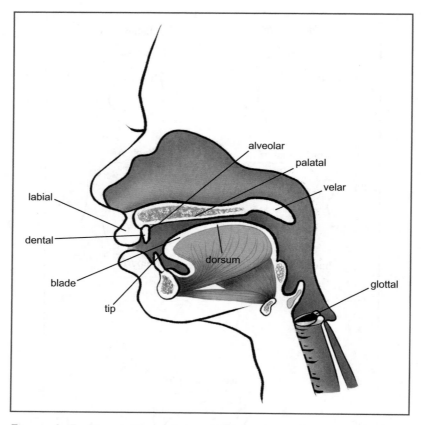

Figure 1–5. *Places of constriction of the vocal tract for consonant articulation. Used with permission from Ellen Graham-Platt.*

therefore properly classed as a bilabial-velar approximant, although it is put with the bilabials on Table 1–2 for convenience and due to the prominent labial constriction. Moving farther back in the vocal tract, one sound is produced with an obligatory constriction in the pharyngeal cavity, specifically the rhotic "r": as shown in Figure 1–4, there are three constrictions involved in this phone—one in the pharyngeal cavity, one in the oral cavity in the alveolar or palatal region, and one at the lips. This phone is not classed as a pharyngeal phone, however, in English but rather as an alveolar approximant. Two sounds are produced via constrictions in the larynx: a **glottal** stop in which full closure of the vocal folds results in a build-up of pressure behind them that is released with a "pop" upon opening; and a glottal fricative [h] that is considered by many linguists to be a glide because the constriction is wide and closes into a vowel that is continuous with the [h] by sharing the same vocal tract configuration (Bernhardt & Stemberger, 2000). Both of these glottal sounds are voiceless.

Table 1–2. *Articulatory Characteristics of Major Classes of Phones in English by Place of Articulation*

Place Class	Articulatory Characteristic	English Phones
Bilabial (Labial)	Produced by putting the upper and lower lip together.	[p,b,m,w]
Labiodental	Produced by placing the top teeth on the lower lip.	[f,v]
(Inter)dental	Produced by placing the tongue tip between the front teeth.	[θ,ð]
Alveolar	Usually produced by placing the tongue tip on or near the alveolar ridge, although sometimes against the upper or lower front teeth.	[t,d,n,s,z,ɹ,l]
Post-alveolar	Usually produced by placing the tongue blade just behind the alveolar ridge or sometimes farther back in the palatal region.	[ʃ,ʒ,tʃ,dʒ,j]
Velar	Produced by bringing the tongue dorsum into contact with the velum or the back part of the palate.	[k,g,ŋ]
Glottal	Produced by closing or constricting the vocal folds.	[ʔ,h]

Note. Voiceless cognates are always shown first followed by the voiced cognate when both members of the pair are produced at a given place of articulation.

Box 1–1. Articulatory Phonetics: Key Points

- Phonetics is the study of speech sounds.
- A phone is the smallest unit of speech.
- Articulatory phonetics is the study of speech sounds as they are spoken.
- Vowels are characterized by an open vocal tract.
- Consonants are characterized by constriction in the oral and/or pharyngeal cavities.

1.2 DESCRIBING ARTICULATORY KNOWLEDGE

1.2.1 International Phonetic Alphabet

The International Phonetic Alphabet (IPA) contains symbols which can be used by a trained listener to transcribe the speech produced by a speaker of any of the world's languages. Figure 1–6 presents the IPA chart. The chart includes symbols for consonants, vowels, suprasegmental features, diacritics, and tones and word accents. Most of the examples contained in

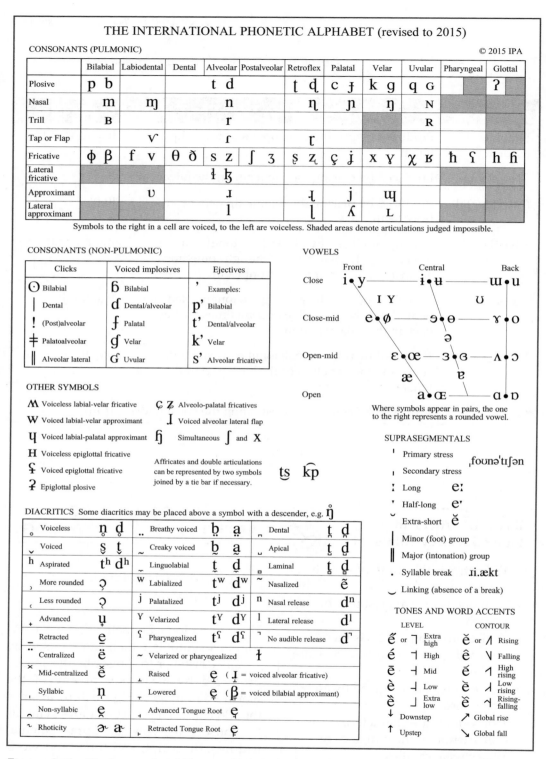

Figure 1–6. *The International Phonetic Alphabet. Source: IPA Chart, http://www.internationalpho neticassociation.org/content/ipa-chart, available under a Creative Commons Attribution-Sharealike 3.0 Unported License. Copyright © 2015 International Phonetic Association.*

this textbook will involve General American English produced by children, and therefore typically producing pulmonic consonants and vowels (meaning that speech is produced while pushing air out of the lungs). Specific diacritics that are commonly used to transcribe the speech produced by children with speech sound disorders (SSDs) will be introduced: many of these are found on the IPA chart, but when children have severe disorders or unusual articulatory systems it is sometimes necessary to use special symbol sets that were developed for clinical use (e.g., see Shriberg & Kent, 2013). Each symbol in the IPA chart represents a single phone or speech sound; organized according to

manner, place, and voicing as defined in the previous section and in Tables 1–1 and 1–2. The symbols that pertain to General American English have been highlighted in Tables 1–1 and 1–2, and examples of words containing these English vowels and consonants are presented in Table 1–3, keeping in mind that there may be some differences in pronunciation due to regional variations in English dialect.

In some cases the symbols are the same as those that might be used when writing a word with traditional orthography, especially in relation to consonants: for example, the word "sit" has an alveolar fricative at the beginning, /s/, and an alveolar stop at the end, /t/, and both of

Table 1–3. *Examples of Words Containing the Vowels and Consonants of General American English*

[i]	"beet" → [bit]	[h]	"hat" → [hæt]	[f]	"foot" → [fʊt]
[ɪ]	"bit" → [bɪt]	[w]	"web" → [wɛb]	[v]	"vase" → [veɪs]
[ʊ]	"put" → [pʊt]	[j]	"yes" → [jɛs]	[θ]	"thumb" → [θʌm]
[u]	"boot" → [but]	[ɹ]	"red" → [ɹɛd]	[ð]	"this" → [ðɪs]
[e]	"bake" → [bek] or [beɪk]	[l]	"leaf" → [lif]	[s]	"soap" → [sop]
[ɛ]	"bet" → [bɛt]	[m]	"moon" → [mun]	[z]	"zoo" → [zu]
[ə]	"the" → [ðə]	[n]	"nut" → [nʌt]	[ʃ]	"ship" → [ʃɪp]
[o]	"boat" → [bot] or [boʊt]	[p]	"pig" → [pɪg]	[ʒ]	"beige" → [beɪʒ]
[ʌ]	"but" → [bʌt]	[b]	"boy" → [bɔɪ]	[tʃ]	"chin" → [tʃɪn]
[ɔ]	"bought" → [bɔt]	[t]	"toy" → [tɔɪ]	[dʒ]	"jump" → [dʒʌmp]
[æ]	"bat" → [bæt]	[d]	"door" → [dɔɹ]		
[a]	"father" → [faðɚ]	[k]	"cup" → [kʌp]		
[ɑ]	"hot" → [hɑt]	[g]	"go" → [go]		
[ɚ]	"father" → [faðɚ]	[p]	"pig" → [pɪg]		
[ɝ]	"bird" → [bɝd]				

these sounds are represented with IPA symbols that are the same as the printed letters. There are more consonant symbols than there are letters, so that consonant sounds across all the different languages of the world can be represented. Consider the case of Spanish, which has an alveolar trill [r] in the phonetic repertoire (see https://www.asha.org/upload edFiles/practice/multicultural/Spanish PhonemicInventory.pdf). For example, in the word "ropa" (clothing) → [ropa], the first sound is produced by vibrating the tongue tip against the alveolar ridge to produce what is sometimes called a "rolling r." Notice that the IPA symbol for the alveolar trill [r] is the same as the letter that goes at the beginning of words such as "red" or "robin." However, this sound at the beginning of these English words is not a trill; it is an approximant for which the IPA symbol is [ɹ]. It is possible that the SLP might assess a child who speaks Spanish and English and produces both the alveolar trill [r] (with a vibrating tongue) and the alveolar approximant [ɹ] (with a smooth tongue glide). For this reason it is necessary to differentiate these distinct phones by using the correct IPA symbols, as we do throughout this book. However, several of the articulation tests that are discussed in Chapter 3 use the "r" to refer to the English alveolar approximant. The use of this symbol is context specific and the SLP will need to be aware of the context when it appears on tests and in reports in order to interpret its meaning.

The vowel chart in Figure 1–6 is often referred to as the vowel quadrilateral or the vowel parallelogram. The vowels in the middle are referred to as central vowels (i.e., [ə] is the most central vowel) and the most extreme vowels in the space are on the corners (i.e., in English [i,u,a,ɑ]). The vowels are organized by place of constriction so that vowels with front constrictions are on the left and vowels with back constrictions are on the right. Further organization reflects jaw height, with close vowels at the top involving a high jaw position and open vowels at the bottom involving a low jaw position. The presence or absence of lip rounding distinguishes pairs of vowels that share placement of the primary constriction and degree of opening of the vocal tract. The English vowels which are rounded are [u,o,ɔ]. Vowels are also often described as being either tense or lax (Shriberg & Kent, 2003). Tense vowels are presumably produced with more muscular activity than lax vowels but this description has not been confirmed as a consistent characteristic in instrumental studies (Raphael & Bell-Berti, 1975). In English, the tense vowels [i,e,u,o] and their respective lax vowel cognates [ɪ,ɛ,ʊ,ɔ] are more consistently differentiated by duration and spectral characteristics. The r-colored vowels (i.e., rhotics [ɝ,ɚ]) are not represented per se on the vowel quadrilateral on the IPA chart; the symbol for rhoticity is found in the diacritic section. Both vowels are central, mid, and generally rounded; the first one is tense and the second is lax. The example words shown in the first column of Table 1–3 give a rough approximation of how these vowels are pronounced. Notice again that there is some overlap between printed letters and vowel symbols but the relationship is not perfect. The pronunciation of vowels in printed words often depends on extra letters: for example "sit" is pronounced as [sɪt] with a lax vowel and "seat" is pronounced with the tense vowel [sit] and "site" is pronounced as [saɪt] with a diphthong as indicated by the optional tie bar over the two phones that make up this sound. Certain websites and digital apps provide more information in the form of linked audio files, diagrams and videos that relate the sound of the phone to its articulatory characteristics (e.g., IPA Phonetics; Esling, 2015).

The transcription of vowels can be difficult: since the tongue and the lips do not establish contact with one another, there can be considerable variation in the exact placement of the articulators each time they are produced. The differences between one vowel and another can be subtle and there may be large "gray" areas between them. Therefore, words like "can" and "kin" often sound similar even when produced by the same speaker. It is also important to remember that every English speaker uses a **dialect** of the language, which refers to a varied form of English shared by speakers of the same geographical region, ethnic group, or social class. Different dialects use different sets of vowels so that the word "bought" may be pronounced as [bɔt] on the east coast of the United States but as [bɑt] in more westerly regions. No dialect is superior to another; nonetheless, General American English, the "standard" dialect of English in North America, is typically promoted in the educational system (Adler, 1984). Speakers also use different registers of their dialect depending on their audience, topic of conversation, and social setting, as for example, a formal register during an interview for employment but an informal register with friends. The Atlas of North American English (Labov, Ash, & Boberg, 2006) describes the pronunciation and vowel systems of English dialects in the United States and Canada and maps their ongoing sound changes.

The pulmonic consonants are shown at the top of Figure 1–6 in a table that is organized by manner of articulation (in rows) and by place of articulation (in columns). There are many more phones

shown on this table than on Tables 1–1 and 1–2 because English does not include all the possible consonants that are used in the world's languages. It is useful to have access to these extra symbols, however, because sometimes children who are learning language or people who have a speech disorder will use sounds that do not typically occur in their native language. For example, a toddler may attempt to say the sound [b] with an imprecise lip closing gesture, resulting in a bilabial fricative, in which case you would transcribe the sound that the toddler said with the symbol [β]. Sometimes the diacritics shown on Figure 1–6 are also helpful to transcribe exactly what the child said. If, for example, the toddler also nasalized the vowel in the word "bean," a diacritic would be added to indicate this additional imprecision, "bean" → [β̃in].

1.2.2 Broad and Narrow Transcription of Speech

IPA symbols can be used by a trained listener to create a **broad transcription** of speech. The speech should be transcribed as it was heard, and not as it is expected to be heard. In other words, speakers may produce words differently than what you expect based on the dictionary pronunciation guide of the word. For example, if you are speaking in front of your classroom, you may produce the utterance "Good morning, everyone" as [ɡʊd ˈmɔrnɪŋ ˈɛvɹiˌwʌn], but produce the same utterance as [ɡʊʔ ˈmɔːnɪn ˈɛβiˌwʌn] when seeing your friends at breakfast. Across and within adult speakers, there is variation in pronunciation depending on the social context and audience. Children with speech abilities that are within normal limits for their age, as well as children with SSD, also frequently pronounce words differently than adults. IPA symbols that are not typically used in the dictionary pronunciation guide of English words may be used to describe the speech of all speakers. For example, in the second pronunciation of "good morning, everyone" the **glottal stop** [ʔ] was produced. In typical adult speech, the glottal stop can replace some plosive sounds, as in the example provided. Some children with SSD replace many consonants with glottal stops, more so than is expected for same-aged children. Children also sometimes produce the **lateral fricative** [ɬ] in place of [s, z]: this is called a lateral lisp because the airflow escapes laterally into the cheeks instead of along the central groove in the middle of the tongue.

The diacritic symbols of the IPA chart can be used to create a **narrow transcription** of speech, providing additional phonetic detail about the sounds that were produced. Consider for example, the varied articulatory characteristics of the [t] in [tʰek ðə plæstɪk fʊtˈbal aʊɾəv ðə bæθtʰʌb] ("Take the plastic football out of the bathtub"). Diacritics are shown in the middle of Figure 1–6 (see also Ball, Müller, & Rutter, 2010).

There are several advantages in using phonetic transcription to describe articulatory knowledge. First, little or no technology is required for a trained listener to transcribe a talker's articulatory performance. It is therefore possible to interact more naturally with a child, such as while reading a book or playing with toys —these are like real-life activities the child engages in, adding **ecological validity** to your observations of the child's speech. Using phonetic transcription is also inexpensive. Another advantage of transcription is that you can learn to extract the phonetic repertoire from the transcription of the speaker's speech.

A **phonetic repertoire** is an inventory of the phones produced by the child. In clinical practice, the phonetic repertoire is usually derived from a broad transcription of the speech sample. The vowel and consonant inventories are organized in a manner similar to the IPA chart. By convention, a phone that was produced only once appears between parentheses. All the phones produced by the child are included, even if they are not part of the vowel and consonant inventory of the specific language(s) the child is learning. Demonstration 1–1 shows the phonetic inventory (consonants and vowels) derived from a short speech sample, recorded from an 18-month-old child who was in the single word stage of vocal development. Notice that phones are listed in the inventory even if they are not used correctly. Furthermore, the use of non-English phones, by this child growing up in a monolingual English-speaking family, is noted with the appearance of bilabial and velar fricatives [β,x] probably reflecting imprecise articulation of the intended stops.

Practice 1–4

Find a partner in your class and ask him or her, "What was the most important point you learned in class today? Tell me in one sentence." Transcribe your partner's answer using IPA symbols to create a **broad transcription**. Organize the phones that your partner used in a chart to show the **phonetic repertoire**, one chart for consonants, one for vowels. Notice that your partner's sentence is too short to have a complete picture of the phonetic repertoire. In clinical practice you would try to transcribe 100 words.

Phonetic Inventory Derived from Broad Phonetic Transcription

of a Speech Sample

A. Gloss and transcription of speech sample

"apple"	[æpə], [æbo]
"ball"	[bo]
"bubble"	[bʌpɔ]
"bus"	[bɛ]
"Coco"	[kɔxo], [kogɔ], [gɔgo]
"Dito"	[dɪdo], [dido], [dædo]
"grapes"	[bʊə]
"hello"	[hajo]
"home"	[həm]
"key"	[gi]
"moomoo"	[mʌːmʌ], [mumʊ]
"onion"	[hajʌ], [anjʌ], [æːjæ]
"seesaw"	[isa]
"teevee"	[βi], [ti]

Orthographic transcription (gloss) and broad phonetic transcription of the child's free speech sample.

B. Consonant repertoire

p b	t d	k g	
m	(n)	ŋ	
(β)	(s)	(x)	h
	j		

Consonant repertoire includes native and non-native consonant phones produced by the child.

C. Vowel repertoire

i ɪ u
ə o
(ɛ) ʌ ɔ
æ a

Phones that appear only once are in parentheses.

Phones are organized by place and manner of articulation.

1.2.3 Visual Analysis of Articulation

The phonetic transcription and phonetic repertoire shown in the previous section describe the child's articulatory knowledge. However, phonetic transcription is an abstract representation of the sounds that the listener hears. Human speech perception is biased, and transcription of the same speech sample by different listeners will most likely vary depending on the listener's experience with transcription and language background. Transcription also requires that sounds be represented as discrete symbols, even though the boundaries between one phone category and another are not sharp. The movements of the articulators are continuous, and overlap in time due to co-articulation. Various technologies can be used to visualize the articulators during normal speech, and to diagnose and treat SSD. Tools to visualize the vocal tract include X-ray (e.g., Delattre & Freeman, 1968), ultrasound (e.g., Preston et al., 2017), and magnetic resonance imaging (e.g., Alwan, Narayanan, & Haker, 1997).

Studies using visual technologies have revealed the many-to-one relationship between articulatory gestures and phonetic categories. Every time a consonant is produced, the articulatory gestures of the speaker will be somewhat different because the sounds that come before and after impact the exact articulatory gestures that are used. Different speakers have slight alterations in the shape of their vocal tracts as well that influence the exact form of the articulatory gestures that are used to produce speech sounds. Different speakers, or the same speaker, can use different articulatory gestures to achieve the same acoustic effects, however—as is shown in Figure 1–4. Many tongue positions all result in the sound [ɹ]. This phenomenon is known as **motor equivalence.** When moving from one phoneme to the next, talkers use combinations of articulatory gestures that require the least effort to be understood.

Practice 1–5

Say the words "see" and "Sue"; pay attention to lip and tongue placement when you produce the sound /s/ in these two contexts. Was your tongue tip in the same place at the beginning of both words? When did you begin to round your lips for the [u] sound in the word "Sue"? Even though the lip and tongue gestures are slightly different when you start the words "see" and "Sue," the sound at the beginning of the words is [s]. This is called **motor equivalence.** Try this again with the words "she" and "shoe."

Technologies that permit visualization of the articulatory gestures during speech production are especially helpful to understand why some individuals are not producing speech accurately. Some technologies may be useful for diagnosis and intervention purposes. **Electropalatography (EPG)** provides information about patterns of tongue contact with the palate during speech production. A series of electrodes are embedded inside a pseudopalate. Typically, the pseudopalate is custom made for each user's hard palate (e.g., McLeod & Singh, 2009), an expensive process. The EPG data are transmitted from the electrodes to a computer that displays the pattern of contacts over time. EPG has been used to investigate co-articulation in normal articulation (e.g., Gibbon, 1999) as well as atypical articulation in children with SSD. Figure 1–7 shows the EPG display of tongue contact during production of the alveolar and velar stops.

Ultrasound visual feedback is less expensive and more portable than EPG. An ultrasound probe is placed under the chin of the speaker, who can see the visual display of his or her tongue shape on a computer. Only the surface of the tongue is revealed by ultrasound (Bernhardt, Gick, Bacsfalvi, & Adler-Bock, 2005; Preston, Brick, & Landi, 2013). Several studies are currently investigating the efficacy of ultrasound visual feedback in speech therapy. Figure 1–8 illustrates speech therapy with ultrasound: the SLP is holding the ultrasound transducer under the child's chin while real-time images of his tongue are projected on the computer screen.

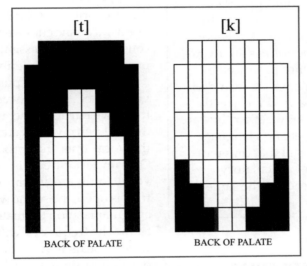

Figure 1–7. *EPG display of tongue contact (in black) during the production of [t], [k]. Used with permission from F. Brosseau-Lapré.*

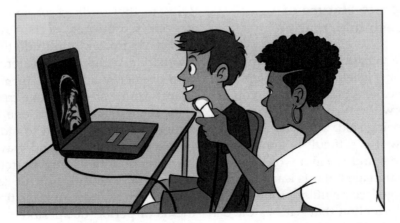

Figure 1–8. *Ultrasound visual feedback during speech therapy. Used with permission from Ellen Graham-Platt.*

Box 1–2. Describing Articulatory Knowledge: Key Points

- The International Phonetic Alphabet contains symbols to transcribe the consonants and vowels produced by a speaker of any of the world's languages.
- Phonetic transcription requires little technology and provides an abstract representation of the speaker's articulatory knowledge.
- A phonetic repertoire is an inventory of the phones produced by the speaker. Phones are included even if they are used incorrectly and regardless of whether they are found in the speaker's language.
- Visual tools reveal that different combinations of articulatory gestures can produce the same sound.

1.3 DESCRIBING PERCEPTUAL KNOWLEDGE

1.3.1 Continuous versus Discrete Nature of Speech Information

If you have visited a foreign country, or found yourself listening to a conversation between speakers of a language you are not familiar with, you may have wondered what was being said. You may also have noticed how it is difficult to know when a word starts, and when a word ends in this other language. Infants learning their own language face a similar problem. The acoustic information that reaches the ear of the listener is largely continuous. The

ability to perceive what is being said, called speech perception, requires the construction of a sound-based representation of speech from the input, in other words an **acoustic-phonetic representation**. Traditionally, theorists believed that the listener was abstracting a string of speech sounds, ordered linearly, from the speech they heard. In this case, it was assumed that the speech input must contain **acoustic cues** that would correspond to natural categories of speech sounds. In other words, acoustic cues were hypothesized to consist of units of essential acoustic information that would define speech sounds.

When sound is pushed through the vocal tract, soundwaves are produced that have particular acoustic qualities that may be perceived as cues to the shape of the vocal tract that produced the sound. One important cue is periodicity: if the vocal folds are vibrating and the vocal tract is open, the soundwave will repeat in a regular fashion to create a **periodic** wave form. The **frequency** with which a soundwave repeats may be high (many repeats per unit of time) or low (few repeats per unit of time), with these sounds perceived as high or low pitch. Speech sounds are complex, being composed of many waves of different frequencies. **Amplitude** pertains to the loudness of sounds. When speech is produced, certain frequencies will have greater amplitude than others: those frequencies with greater concentration of energy are called **formants**. Formants can be steady at one frequency or they can transition from one frequency to another. Some speech sounds are **aperiodic** in that their sound waves do not have regular repeating patterns in the waveform. The **duration** of certain elements such as formant transitions or segments of period or aperiodic energy are important cues to phoneme identity. The acoustic characteristics of speech can be visualized with acoustic analysis software that produces a **waveform display** or a **spectrogram** of sound energy.

The acoustic correlates of some distinctive features can be seen in Figure 1–9, which presents an acoustic waveform of the phrase "Nice weather today." The top of the figure is a broad band spectrogram which shows changes in the relative concentration of energy at different frequencies over time. Frequency is shown on the *y*-axis, time on the *x*-axis, and relative amplitude of the frequency is represented by the intensity of the gray scale. The dark bars indicating the formants are at different frequency locations in each syllable, reflecting the different vowels. The formant transition at the beginning of [wɛ] is long but the formant transition at the beginning of [de] is short. The waveform display is shown at the bottom of the figure and provides some information about major sound classes. For example, in the word "nice" /naɪs/ the highest amplitude peak is associated with the vowel [aɪ]. The aperiodic segment of the waveform associated with the fricative [s] is much longer in duration than the aperiodic segment of the waveform associated with the stop [t]. Acoustic cues to any given phoneme bundle together to differentiate the phoneme from others. For instance, the cues that correspond to the [d] at the beginning of [de] include the release burst (short segment of aperiodic energy) followed by the brief formant transition. The cues to [t] are similar except that the release burst is longer and aperiodic. The cues that correspond to the [s] at the end of [naɪs] include an even longer segment of aperiodic noise with energy concentrated in the higher frequencies.

Voicing is signaled by the presence of a regularly repeating pattern in the

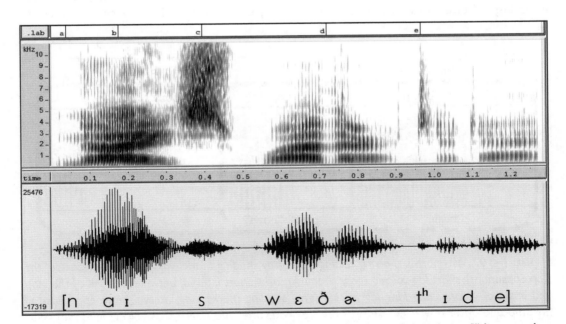

Figure 1–9. *Spectrogram (top) and waveform (bottom) displays of the phrase "Nice weather today" [naɪs wɛðɚ tʰɪde] spoken by a male talker. See text for details. Used with permission from Susan Rvachew.*

waveform and by evenly spaced striations in the spectrogram, both indicating the vibration of the vocal folds, as clearly visible in the vocalic portions of the phrase illustrated in Figure 1–9. The difference between voiced and voiceless consonants is determined by the timing of voicing relative to the release burst. This cue is called **voice-onset time (VOT)**. Voicing can begin before the release burst (voicing lead), shortly after the release burst (short lag voicing), or significantly after the release burst, usually accompanied by aspiration (long lag voicing). We are used to thinking of the feature [voice] in binary terms such that [p] is voiceless and [b] is voiced, but the underlying acoustic cue to these categories is continuous in nature. Furthermore, the way in which the continuum of potential VOT values is organized into categories differs by language group, as shown in Figure 1–10 for English and French. In English, /p/ is produced with long lag voicing and /b/ is produced

with short lag voicing. The voicing contrast in French is rather different: the /b/ is produced with voicing lead and the /p/ is produced with short lag voicing.

To determine the utility of any proposed features of speech sounds and their associated acoustic cues, it is necessary to investigate the responses of listeners to speech input. The speech input can be structured in a way to highlight the acoustic-phonetic information that is presumed to constitute an acoustic cue. By doing so, researchers can study how listeners perceive the continuous speech input.

1.3.2 Categorical Perception

Categorical perception occurs when a listener designates a group of stimuli that are physically different as belonging to the same category (Diehl, Lotto, & Holt, 2004). Therefore, a test of categorical perception involves **identification**: the lis-

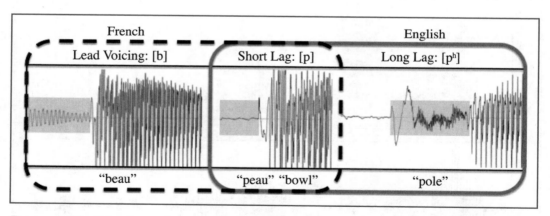

Figure 1–10. *Waveforms showing voicing lead (gray shading marks voicing before release of the stop consonant), short lag voicing (gray shading marks short interval between release of the stop and onset of voicing) and long lag voicing (gray shading marks long interval between release of the stop and onset of voicing). The [b] and [p] categories are realized as voicing lead and short lag voicing in French, whereas the same categories are realized as short lag voicing and long lag voicing in English. Used with permission from Andrea MacLeod.*

tener is asked to identify or label the category that each stimulus belongs to. For example, you might listen to a recording of a person saying the words in order: "seat, seat, sheet, seat, sheet, sheet." After each word you point to a picture to indicate which word you heard. You should notice a relatively high frequency fricative sound at the beginning of the first, second, and third words that will help you to identify these words as corresponding to the picture of the chair (something to sit on). You would point to the same picture for each of these three words even if they were not produced exactly the same, which is possible because there is always some variability in tongue placement while speaking. If the first "seat" is said with the tongue tip near the teeth and the second "seat" is said with the tongue tip farther back along the alveolar ridge, the words will not be identical but both will have a high frequency fricative sound that is heard as [s] at the beginning. If the tongue is pulled too far back into the oral cavity, however, a [ʃ] will result, causing you to point to the bedding when you identify the word "sheet."

Usually, the stimuli that belong to the same category are hard to discriminate, even though they are not physically the same. For this reason, a **discrimination** test is also an important part of determining which sounds are perceived categorically. Consider again the recordings of the words "seat, seat, sheet, seat, sheet, sheet." If you were asked to listen to the second word followed by the fifth word, "seat—sheet" and then indicate if these words are the same or different, it would probably be easy to say that they sound different. This is an example of across-category discrimination. However, if you were asked to listen to the first word fol-

lowed by the second word, "seat—seat" and then indicate if these words are the same or different, it would probably be hard to say that they sound different. This is an example of within-category discrimination in which the two words are acoustically slightly different even though they are made up of speech sounds that belong to the same category. Within-category discrimination of consonants is more difficult than within-category discrimination of vowels, and therefore perception of consonants is more categorical than the perception of vowels.

Speech stimuli are not the only stimuli that are perceived categorically, however. Demonstration 1–2 illustrates a set of visual stimuli, specifically circles and squares printed by a 5-year-old girl. None of them are the same, although some of them are more alike than others. The identification responses provided by five adults who viewed these stimuli show that they were perceived categorically. The adults were shown one shape at a time in random order and asked to identify them as either a "square" or a "circle." Shapes 1 to 3 were consistently identified as "square" and shapes 5 to 7 as "circle." Half of the ratings for shape 4 were "square." The adults were then shown pairs of two images generated by a computer that differed in equal angle amounts, and asked whether the two shapes were the same, or different. Remember that a square has four sides of equal length and 90-degree angles. The discrimination responses shown in the demonstration vary along the continuum of stimuli; close to 90 degrees, discrimination is poor. In other words, within shapes that are rated consistently as a "square," it is very difficult to notice that the two shapes are in fact slightly different if they

Demonstration 1–2

Categorical Perception of Circles and Squares

A. Shapes printed by a 5-year-old girl when asked to draw squares and circles.

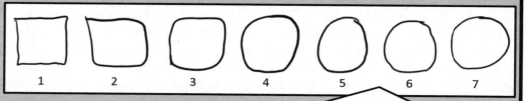

The shapes were ordered based on their angles and lengths of the sides.

B. Adults were shown each shape one at a time in random order and asked to identify each shape as a square or a circle.

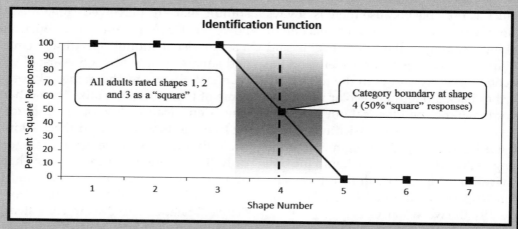

C. Adults were shown pairs of shapes differing by equal amounts and asked if they were "same" or "different."

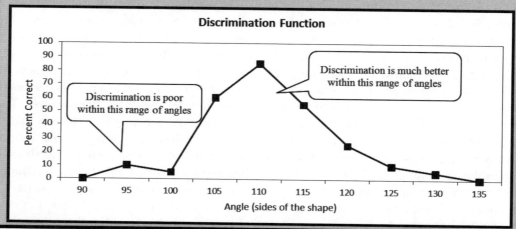

vary by 10 degrees. Closer to the boundary of ambiguous shapes that are rated inconsistently as "square," it is easier to discriminate both shapes as different.

Practice 1–6

Categorical perception is not limited to auditory stimuli. Your class can categorize shades of "red" and "orange" by collecting a set of items from among your members that represent a range of shades along this color dimension. Ask every student in your class to label each object as "red" or "orange." Sum the "red" votes for each object and then organize them in a row by the number of "red" votes from most to least. Probably some shades will be labeled as "red" by everyone. Other shades might be labeled "red" by some students but "orange" by others. The shades that are ambiguous, yielding "red" labels from approximately 50% of the class, are at the boundary between the "red" and "orange" categories. Do all the items labeled "red" look to be exactly the same color? If not, you are able to discriminate different shades of red. Speech sounds that belong to the same category are more difficult to discriminate than colors.

Early speech perception studies presented listeners with syllables or words selected to represent each feature contrast that the researchers wanted to investigate. Miller and Nicely (1955) used a speech perception identification task and presented adults with recordings of consonant-vowel (CV) syllables. All the syllables consisted of one of 16 consonants combined with the vowel [ɑ]. The listeners heard these syllables in noise, and were asked to write down what they heard. With children, an adaptation of an identification task would be to ask them to point to a picture that matches what they heard. For example, Waldman, Singh, and Hayden (1978) presented children with four pictures: "lake," "make," "rake," and "wake." The examiner produced a word and asked the child to point to what was said.

Discrimination tasks require the listener to indicate whether two stimuli are the same or different (Graham & House, 1971). Other examples of discrimination tasks include an oddity task in which the listener hears three or more stimuli and is required to indicate which one is different from the others. In the ABX task, the listener judges which of the first two is the same as the third (Singh & Becker, 1972).

Early on, researchers developed speech identification and discrimination studies to attempt to predict how listeners would categorize stimuli based on the number of different features between two stimuli. The results were more complicated than anticipated. For instance, Miller and Nicely (1955) found that listener confusions were not always predicted by the features in the stimuli as expected: for example, the researchers expected listeners to confuse [f] and [v] because these two phones differ by one feature (voice); instead, listeners misidentified target [f] as [θ], even though these phones differ by two features ([θ] is produced at a different place of articulation and it is less "hissy" or **strident** than [f]). One difficulty with these early studies is that they used natural speech, generally produced by a single adult speaker. Therefore, the different stimuli did not control for the continuous and interacting nature of the various acoustic cues to speech contrasts. When testing a child's speech perception skills, the speech stimuli should be varied enough to reveal which acoustic cues the child is attending to when identifying and discriminating the speech sound contrast. For example, the /s/-/θ/ contrast is differentiated by duration (/s/ is longer than /θ/) and amplitude (/s/ is louder and more strident than /θ/) as well as some frequency cues. A child may indicate that "sink" and "think" sound different but make this judgment on the basis of the duration cue alone without having any knowledge of the amplitude and frequency cues that are essential to learning the production of these sounds. Each language learner must discover a strategy for abstracting phones from the input that is adapted to the language or languages being learned. Assessing perceptual knowledge requires sophisticated tools that reveal the listener's perceptual strategies for understanding speech in ideal and challenging environments.

Practice 1–7

With a partner in your class, describe or demonstrate how you would assess the categorical perception of the voiced and voiceless cognates /t/ and /d/. Remember to include an identification task and a discrimination task. Remember that everyone perceives voiced and voiceless speech sounds a little bit differently, depending on their language experiences. Your classmate may not perceive the speech stimuli that you produce in the way that you expect.

Box 1–3. Describing Perceptual Knowledge: Key Points

- Categorical perception occurs when a listener designates a group of stimuli that are physically different as belonging to the same category.
- Identification tasks require the listener to identify or label the category that each stimulus belongs to.
- Discrimination tasks require the listener to indicate whether two stimuli are the same or different.

1.4 PHONOLOGICAL CONCEPTS

1.4.1 Phones, Phonemes, and Allophones

Phonology is the study of the sound system of languages: specifically, for any given language, the linguist describes the speech sounds that are used and identifies the rules that govern how they are combined into words. (Ladefoged & Johnson, 2010). The **phoneme** is the smallest unit of sound in a specific language that distinguishes the meaning of one word from another. Phonemes are represented with IPA symbols placed between slashes: / /. Remember that a **phone** is the speech sound produced by the talker independently of the specific language(s) the speaker is learning; a phone is defined by the articulatory characteristics of the sound. Recall also that phones are represented with IPA symbols placed between squared brackets: [ ]. In contrast, a **pho-**

neme is language dependent and is the mental image of the sound we intend to produce. When two words have different meanings and differ by only one phoneme, they are called **minimal pairs** (Barlow & Gierut, 2002). For example, "mud"→ [mʌd] and "mug"→ [mʌg] are minimal pairs—the difference between the phones [d] and [g] is enough to change the meaning of the word. Therefore, in English, /d/ and /g/ are phonemes. Some words differ only based on the presence/absence of a phoneme, such as "arm" → [ɑɹm] and "farm" →[fɑɹm]. In this case, these two words are considered **near minimal pairs**.

Remember that we do not articulate phones in an identical manner every time we produce them. Depending on the phonetic context, there will be subtle differences in how a specific phone is produced. **Allophones** are phones that are slightly different from one another but belong to the same phoneme category. Recall the diacritic symbols which can be used to derive a narrow transcription of the phones. In the sentence "Take the plastic football out of the bathtub," /t/ was produced as [tʰ], [t], [tˀ], and [t̪].

One way to identify allophones of the same phoneme is to look for phones that are in **complementary distribution**: this means that the phones never occur in the same context. For example, in English, the stops are always aspirated at the beginning of words, "take" → [tʰeɪk]. When stops are combined with "s" to form a consonant cluster, the stop is no longer aspirated, "steak" → [steɪk]. The predictable appearance of the aspirated phone in the word-initial context and the unaspirated phone in the cluster context means that [tʰ] and [t] are allophones of the phoneme /t/. These productions of /t/ are allophones, since they do not signal a change of meaning.

Practice 1–8

Find three pairs of words in English that differ by two phones, such as "pea"/"bee" ([p]-[b]), in other words, three **minimal pairs**. List the two phones by which these word pairs differ: these are **phonemes** in English.

1.4.2 Phonotactic Rules

All languages combine sounds to form words according to certain rules. **Phonotactics is the description of the permitted sequences of consonants and vowels in a language.** In English, consonant-vowel combinations (CV, ex. "bee"/bi/), vowel-consonant (VC, ex. "up"/ʌp/) and consonant-vowel-consonant (CVC, ex. "bike" /baɪk/) are permissible. More complex structures are also allowed, such as CCV (ex. "ski"/ski/), CCCVC (ex. "street" /stɹit/), and CVCCC (ex. "farms"/fɑɹmz/). However, it is not possible to have CCCCV or VCCCC. Some syllable structures allowed in one language may not be permissible in another. For example, many languages do not allow any consonant clusters, whereas others allow as many as five or six consonants in a row.

In addition to rules specifying which syllable structures are allowed in a language, there are rules regarding the specific consonant and vowels that can be combined, and the order in which they may be combined. Consider the word "psychology"—in English, the sequence [ps] as a word-initial consonant cluster is not allowed and therefore we pronounce the word as [saɪˈkɑlədʒi], omitting the initial /p/. In French, however, the initial consonant cluster [ps] is permissible and therefore the word is pronounced [psikolo'ʒi]. Rules governing the sound sequences that may occur in a language have the effect of constraining the specific phones that may appear in certain word positions. Continuing with the example of consonant sequences, liquids and glides can occur in the second position but never in the first position in the sequence (that is, [blid] but not [lbid]). Certain phonemes may occur only in certain syllable positions, such as /ŋ/, which may occur after the vowel but not before it (that is, [taŋ] but not [ŋat]).

1.4.3 Nonlinear Phonology

Phonotactic rules describe constraints on syllable structure in terms of linear sequences of phonemes. These constraints are more adequately described by a hierarchical representation of phonological units in which subsyllabic units are nested within syllables, syllables are nested within words, and words are nested within the larger units that we use to organize our utterances. This nonlinear hierarchy of phonological units is described in detail in other sources (Bernhardt & Stemberger, 1998; O'Grady & Dobrovolsky, 1997; Rvachew & Brosseau-Lapré, 2018; Shattuck-Huffnagel & Turk, 1996). Here we will focus on the most basic unit, the syllable.

The hierarchical organization of the syllable is illustrated in Figure 1–11A for a simple one-syllable word, "bean" → /bin/. The syllable is constructed of multiple "tiers," with each tier holding different subsyllabic units. The highest subsyllabic tier in the syllable is the onset-rime tier. The rime is obligatory, which means that every syllable must have a rime (R) but the onset (O) is optional because some syllables do not have one (consider "beat" versus "eat"). The syllable /bin/ can be split into two parts, [b]$_O$[in]$_R$, with the initial consonant in the onset and the vowel and final consonant in the rime.

The next tier down shows that the rime can also be split into parts, an obligatory nucleus (N) with an optional coda (Co). Some words have no coda in the rime, for example "bee" → [b]$_O$[i]$_N$ compared with "beet" → [b]$_O$[i]$_N$[t]$_{Co}$. Some syllables have a consonant in the nucleus slot, in which case the consonant is called a syllabic consonant, such as in the second syllable of the word "bottle" → [baɖl̩], indicated by the small diacritic below the [l̩].

The next tier down is called the skeletal tier: it holds timing units that are marked C for nonsyllabic units (roughly equivalent to consonants) and V for syllabic units (including vowels and syllabic consonants). The timing units allocate time for the production of the segments to which they are associated but are nonetheless independent of those segments; this means that there can be more segments than timing units (e.g., in the case of affricates) and more timing units than segments (e.g., in the case of long vowels). Furthermore, the onsets and codas may have more than one consonant in them, in which case they are referred to as complex onsets and complex codas, as opposed to singleton onsets or singleton codas. Examples of these more complex options are shown in Figure 1–11, illustrating complex onsets and codas that contain more than one C unit as well as syllable nuclei with a long vowel (Figure 1–11B) or a diphthong (Figure 1–11C) necessitating more than one V unit in each case.

It is easily seen, when looking at Figure 1–11, that some words are intrinsically more complex than others, even when

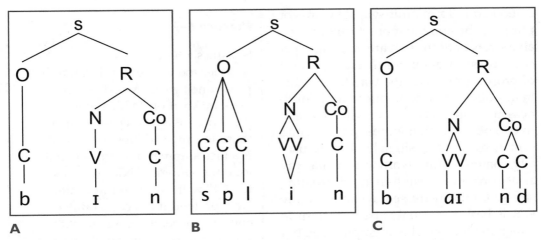

Figure I–II. *Diagram of syllabic and subsyllabic units for three words: (A) "bin" contains simple onset and coda and short vowel; (B) "spleen" contains a complex onset and a long vowel; (C) "bind" contains a complex coda and a diphthongal vowel. S = strong syllable, O = onset, R = rime, N = nucleus, Co = Coda, C = nonsyllabic timing unit, and V = syllabic timing unit. Used with permission from Susan Rvachew.*

they share the same number of syllables. A word with more optional elements should be more difficult for a child to learn to say. There is another consideration, however, and that is compliance with the **Sonority Sequencing Principle**. According to this principle, each phoneme from the nucleus toward the edge of the syllable is expected to be less sonorant that its predecessor. The sonorancy hierarchy, from most to least sonorant, is low vowels → high vowels → glides → liquids → nasals → voiced fricatives → voiceless fricatives → voiced stops → voiceless stops (Ball, Müller, & Rutter, 2010). The word "bean" → [bin] in Figure 1–11A is compliant with this principle because the [b] is the least sonorant, the following vowel is the most sonorant, and the nasal in the coda is less sonorant than the vowel that precedes it. The word "bind" → [baɪnd] in Figure 1–11C has a more complex structure but it too is compliant

with the sonority sequencing principle. On the other hand, the word "spleen" → [splin] in Figure 1–11B violates this principle: the /s/ stands out as being more sonorant than the /p/ and, thus, it does not "fit." Some linguists even propose that the /s/ does not even belong in the onset because the violation is so great (for further discussion of these issues, see Bernhardt & Stemberger, 1998). We will not address this aspect of linguistic theory here except to point out that this violation of the sonority sequencing principle may explain why these particular complex onsets (/s/-clusters) are often difficult for children with SSD to learn, as will be discussed further in Chapter 2.

1.4.4 Prosody

One important aspect of syllables is that they carry stress and when they are combined to form multisyllabic words or phrases, the combinations form predictable stress patterns that are language specific. These stress patterns are an aspect of prosody, meaning the way that talkers manipulate duration, pitch, and loudness to emphasize some syllables relative to others within words, phrases, and sentences. In English, syllables are usually combined into words in such a way as to produce a rhythm of alternating stressed and unstressed syllables. Many words have a **trochaic stress pattern** in which the first syllable is emphasized but the second carries less stress: "butter" → ['bʌɾɚ], "camping" → ['kæmpɪŋ], "nasal" → ['neɪzl̩]. Less frequently, English words have an **iambic stress pattern** in which the second syllable is more stressed than the first: "support" → [sə'pɔɚt], "return" → [ɹə'tɝn], "today" → [tə'deɪ]. **Spondees** have approximately equal stress on the two syllables: "backpack" → ['bæk'pæk], "half-time" → ['hæf'taɪm]. These different stress patterns can be combined, as in "banana" → [bə'nænə], butterfly → ['bʌɾɚ'flaɪ], and "backpacker" → ['bæk'pækɚ].

English has **lexical stress** such that the meaning of a word can be dependent on its stress pattern: consider "record" (noun) → ['ɹɛkɚd] in comparison to "record" (verb) → [ɹə'kɔɚd] (notice the change to lax vowels in the unstressed syllables). When words are combined into sentences, an **intonation** pattern will be overlain on the lexical stress pattern to signal attitudes and emotions, pragmatic functions, and boundaries between words, phrases, and utterances. It is important to describe these suprasegmental aspects of a child's speech at the word and phrase levels because interactions between preferred prosodic patterns and phonemes may account for mismatches between adult targets and child speech output.

Practice 1–9

Say the sentence "Nice weather today" out loud, carefully pronouncing each word as if it were in isolation. Which word in the sentence is a **trochee**? Which word is an **iamb**? Now pretend it is a nice summer day, and say out loud the sentence "Nice weather today!" with cheerful **intonation**. Next pretend it is a cold, rainy day and say the sentence again, with sarcastic intonation. Finally, pretend you are unaware of the forecast and asking your partner "Is it nice weather today?" What differences do you notice between each of these productions?

1.4.5 Syllabifying Words

Determining the syllable structure of single syllable words is relatively straightforward, as shown in Figure 1–11. Diagramming the syllable structure of multisyllabic words can be more difficult, especially when syllables are combined to form sequences of word internal consonants. Prosody and phonotactic rules play a large role in sorting out where the syllable boundaries are in more complex words. Figure 1–12 illustrates the syllabification of two words that contain word-internal consonant sequences. In Figure 1–12A, the word "elderly" contains no complex onsets or codas because the sequence /ld/ is not a legal onset in English, and therefore the /l/ is placed in the coda of the first syllable and the /d/ in the onset of the second. In Figure 1–12B, the word "extra" contains a four-consonant sequence /kstɹ/. The three consonants to

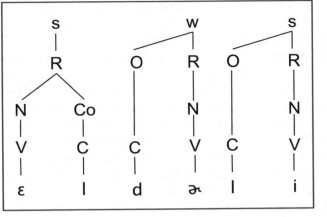
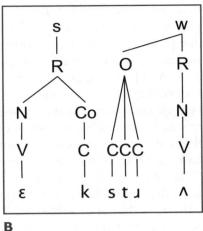

A　　　　　　　　　　　　　　　　　　　**B**

Figure I–I2. *Illustration of the syllabic and subsyllabic units for two words with word-internal consonant sequences: (**A**) "elderly" contains no complex onsets because the consonant sequence does not form a legal English onset; (**B**) "extra" contains a four-consonant sequence that is split to place the legal three-consonant sequence in the onset of the second syllable, leaving the /k/ in the coda of the first syllable. Used with permission from Susan Rvachew.*

the left of the second nucleus /stɹ/ form a legal word-initial cluster, and are therefore placed in the onset of the syllable and the /k/ is placed in the coda of the preceding syllable.

Practice 1–10

Make a diagram to show the syllable structure of the word "stopwatch." Follow these steps: (1) identify the syllable nuclei (the vowels) and connect them to the nucleus and rime symbols; (2) identify all consonants to the left of the nuclei that form a legal cluster and connect these to the onset of the appropriate syllable; (3) connect all remaining consonants to the coda of the appropriate syllable; (4) connect the onset and rime symbols to the appropriate syllable symbols.

In words with a trochaic stress pattern, consonants in the middle of the word between vowels can have an ambiguous status. Consider the words "butter" → ['bʌɾɚ] and "putting" → ['pʰʊɾɪŋ]. Notice that the /t/ is not pronounced [tʰ] as in "take" → [tʰeɪk] or "rattan" → [ɹə'tʰæn]. That is because the /t/ in the words "butter" and "putting" is simultaneously in the onset of the second syllable and the coda of the first syllable; therefore, we say that these consonants are **ambisyllabic**. Sometimes ambisyllabic consonants will be replaced by a glottal stop instead of the flap, as in "bottle" → [bɑʔl] or "button" → [bʌʔn̩]. Deaspiration of ambisyllabic consonants is also common, as in "happy" → ['hæpi], whereas /p/ would be aspirated if it were properly in the syllable onset, as in "support" → [sə'pʰɔɚt]. It is important to be able to identify the onset, coda, and ambisyllabic positions because children are very likely to have error patterns that are specific to particular syllable positions. For example, a child who cannot pronounce the /s/ phoneme might produce it like [tʰ] in the onset, [ts] in the coda, and [ʔ] in the ambisyllabic position. More often, however, children treat ambisyllabic consonants as if they were codas, that is, pronouncing the target consonant the same in these two positions (Bernhardt & Stemberger, 2002; Kehoe & Lleo, 2002; Marshall & Chiat, 2003; Rvachew & Andrews, 2002). An illustration of this pattern is shown in Table 1–4. This child produces the fricative sounds as fricatives in the ambisyllabic and coda positions but as stops in the onset position. This case exemplifies another characteristic of children's speech errors: often the child's errors are patterned in terms of **distinctive features** rather than being unique to specific phonemes.

1.4.6 Consonant Features in Nonlinear Phonology

Infants learning their native language hear various speakers produce a wide variety of phones in different contexts. Yet despite this high variability in the speech input, they learn the phonemes and phonotactic rules of their language. For example, a toddler learning English will learn that /p/ and /t/ form a minimal pair of consonants, since "pea" [pi] and "tea" [ti] have different meanings. These two words differ by a single phoneme, initial [p] and [t], and the difference between them is linguistically important in English. How are these phonemes different, and how are they similar? Looking at the IPA chart, we see that both consonants are plosives and voiceless, but their place of articulation differs ([p] is bilabial, and [t] is alveolar). Think also of different contexts in which

you are producing speech, such as talking to a classmate while walking quickly to your next class, talking to your roommates as you are chewing gum, and video chatting with a friend at the end of the day when you are tired and mumbling. How do your listeners understand what you are saying in view of the articulatory variation of your speech? In other words, how do learners of a language discover which articulatory and acoustic differences are allophones versus phonemes?

Different systems of characteristics that distinguish phonemes from one another have been proposed. A **distinctive feature** is an articulatory or acoustic parameter—its presence or absence defines a phonetic category. Speech sounds that share a distinctive feature can be grouped together into **natural classes** of sounds such as "stops/plosives," "front vowels," and "nasals." The system proposed by Chomsky and Halle (1968) is often the most familiar to speech-language pathologists. Since then, further investigation of children's acquisition of their phonological system and of cross-linguistic work have led to the development of more contemporary feature systems. In this textbook, we present the feature specifications described by Bernhardt and Stemberger (1998, 2000). Figure 1–13 depicts the feature hierarchy for consonants and Table 1–5 describes the place and manner features for the consonants. It is important to understand the feature organization of phonemes because children's speech error patterns can be explained by their knowledge of features. Furthermore, this feature explanation organizes many different errors into one pattern. The hierarchical organization of the features shown in Figure 1–13 is important because knowledge of features higher up in the hierarchy will impact use of all the features lower down

Table 1–4. *Unique Error Pattern for Fricatives in Onset versus Ambisyllabic and Coda Position*

Target	Word-Initial Onset		Word-Internal Onset		Ambisyllabic		Word-Internal Coda		Word-Final Coda	
/f/	fish	[pɪs]	uniform	[jubo]	muffin	[mʌfɪn]	halftime	[ʔæftaɪm]	giraffe	[dəwæf]
/θ/	thumb	[dʌm]	panther	[pædoɪ]	Cathy	[kæfi]	bathtub	[bæθtʌb]	mammoth	[maɪnəf]
/s/	sadly	[dɑdi]	casino	[katino]	glasses	[wæsəs]	police-chief	[wɪstʃɪf]	yes	[jes]
/ʃ/	shovel	[dʌʃəl]	machine	[mətin]	washing	[wæʃɪŋ]	fish-hook	[pɪsʔʊk]	rubbish	[wʌbɪs]

Source: Adapted from Rvachew, S., and Andrews, E. (2002). The influence of syllable position on children's production of consonants. *Clinical Linguistics and Phonetics, 16,* Table 5, p. 193. Used with permission of Taylor and Francis Ltd.

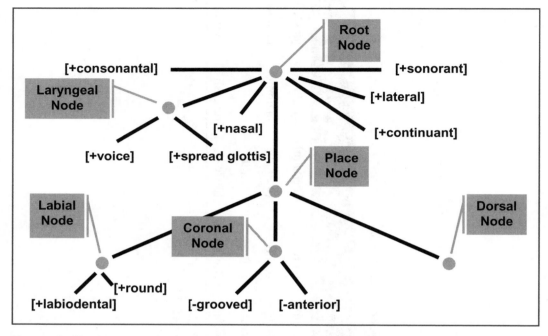

Figure 1–13. *Diagram of the feature hierarchy for consonants. Used with permission from Susan Rvachew.*

in the hierarchy. For example, if the young child has knowledge of the sonorant feature but not the consonant feature, the child might say "bee" → [wi] and "shoe" → [ju]. A complete understanding of **nonlinear phonology** is an advanced topic covered in more detail in Bernhardt and Stemberger (2000) and in Rvachew and Brosseau-Lapré (2018).

Another characteristic of the nonlinear feature hierarchy that is important for explaining children's speech development and speech errors is **underspecification**. This concept explains the difference between the description of the consonants provided in section 1.2.1 and the description shown in Table 1–5. Specifically, in Tables 1–1 and 1–2 the consonants are described according to all the place, manner, and voicing features that are relevant to their articulation. The more abstract picture provided in Table 1–5 provides an underspecified characterization of the consonants in that only the features that are required to differentiate one consonant from the others are associated with that consonant. For example, in Table 1–2 the /f/ and /v/ sounds are described as labiodental. However, in Table 1–5, the only **specified** phonological place feature for these phonemes is [Labial] because all the labial fricatives in English are labiodental; therefore, it is not necessary to specify [+labiodental] in order to differentiate the fricatives /f,v/ with [Labial] place from the fricatives /s,z/ with [Coronal] place: the [Labial] fricatives are assumed to be [+labiodental] in English. Some languages do have [Labial] /ɸ,β/ fricatives that contrast with the [Labial]:[+labiodental] pair /f,v/ in which case it would be necessary to specify the [+labiodental] feature.

Table 1–5. *Description of Features with Relevant Consonants*

Feature	Definition	Consonants[*]
Major Sound Class Features		
Consonantal [± cons]	Result from closing off the vocal tract, narrowing the vocal tract, or interrupting the airflow within the oral cavity	/m,n,ŋ/ /p,b,t,d,k,g/ /f,v,θ,ð,s,z,ʃ,ʒ,tʃ,dʒ/ /l,ɹ/
Sonorant [± son]	Result from an open or fairly open vocal tract	/w,j/ /l,ɹ/
Manner Features		
Nasal [± nasal]	Result from passage of air through the nasal cavity	/m,n,ŋ/
Continuant [± cont]	Produced without interrupting the airflow	/f,v,θ,ð,s,z,ʃ,ʒ,tʃ,dʒ/
Lateral [± lat]	Air flows around the sides of the tongue	/l/
Laryngeal Features		
Voice [± voice]	Produced with vibration of the vocal folds	/b,d,g/ /v,ð,z,ʒ,dʒ/
Spread glottis [± s.g.]	Produced with a wide opening of the vocal folds	/h/
Place Features		
Labial [Labial]	Speech sounds produced with the lips	/p,b,f,v/
Coronal [Coronal]	Produced with the tongue tip or the tongue blade raised	
Coronal [Coronal]:[-grooved]	Tongue is flat and tip between the teeth	/θ,ð/
Coronal [Coronal]:[-anterior]	Tongue blade retracted behind the alveolar ridge	/ʃ,ʒ,tʃ,dʒ/
Dorsal [Dorsal]	Produced with the back of the tongue (tongue dorsum)	/k,g,ŋ/

Note. *The consonants listed are specified for the feature as described. Other consonants may share this feature description by default. In particular, notice that Coronal is the default place feature corresponding to /n,j,t,d,s,z,l/; in other words, as these phonemes have no specified place they default to Coronal.

Some features are not specified because they are redundant. For example, [+voice] is a **default** feature for the sonorant and nasal phonemes and therefore [+voice] is not specified for these phonemes even though the vocal folds are obviously vibrating during the production of these sounds. In other words, if [+sonorant] or [+nasal] is specified, [+voice] is assumed and said to be a default feature for those phonemes. In English, the default place is usually [Coronal], which means that [Labial] and [Dorsal] must be specified; if no place is specified, the consonant place defaults to [Coronal]. For this reason, a developing child who has no knowledge of [Dorsal] place would produce words such as "key" → [ti], "go" → [do], and "tongue" → [tʌn]. One of the challenges of phonological development is to learn the language-specific system of feature specifications for the sounds of the language. The application of underspecification and nonlinear phonological rules to speech-language pathology assessment and treatment practice is covered in more detail in Bernhardt and Stemberger (2000) and in Rvachew and Brosseau-Lapré (2018).

1.4.7 Phonological Processes

One approach to the description of children's speech error patterns takes advantage of the way in which sounds naturally group according to features and syllable positions. **Phonological processes** are error patterns that (1) apply to natural classes of phonemes that are linked by a common feature or syllable position; (2) result in a simplification of the target phoneme; and (3) occur commonly in child and even adult speech. Table 1–6 contains a list of naturally occurring phonological processes that are commonly found in

child speech along with examples of these error patterns. Examples of errors that may be mistaken for these error patterns are also provided. This is only a partial list of phonological processes that may occur because Shriberg and Kwiatkowski (1980) excluded error patterns that are difficult to transcribe reliably.

> ### Practice 1–11
>
> Over the next 24 hours, make a list of simplification errors that you hear in your own speech when speaking quickly or casually. Label these speech productions using the list of **natural phonological processes** described in Table 1–6.

Final consonant deletion is manifested by complete omission of the coda. Omission of one member of a final cluster or substitution of a glottal stop for the final consonant would not be coded as this process. Omissions of liquid consonants in the coda position are more likely to be liquid simplification unless other types of consonants are also omitted word finally.

Substitution of alveolar consonants for velar consonants is usually **velar fronting**: in this case the [Dorsal] place feature has been omitted, leaving the default [Coronal] place feature, as in "key" /ki/ → [ti]. Phones that sound like [t͡ʃ] or [k͡ʃ] are better described as distortions and are therefore not phonological processes. Substitution of labials or other front consonants for velars are not properly coded as velar fronting, as they are not typical fronting errors and therefore not "natural." Most likely, these other front substitutions can be explained by some other rule or process such as assimilation.

Table 1–6. List of Phonological Processes with Examples and Counter Examples

Process	Good Exemplar	Dubious Exemplar	Not an Exemplar
Final consonant deletion	"dog" → [dɑ] "pants" → [pæ]	"far" → [fa] "boat" → [boʔ]	"toast" → [tos] "bottle" → [bado] "car" → [kɑo] "butter" → [bʌɾə]
Velar fronting	"sing" → [sɪn] "cob" → [tab] "go" → [do]	"dog" → [dad] "cone" → [t̪jon]	"key" → [kji] "coffee" → [pafi]
Stopping of fricatives or affricates	"sew" → [do] "shy" → [taɪ] "chew" → [tu]	"house" → [ʔaʊs]	"zoo" → [ju] "peach" → [pits] "push" → [pʊs] "see" → [tsi]
Palatal fronting	"sheet" → [sit] "chalk" → [tsɑk] "measure" → [mɛzɚ] "jump" → [zʌmp]	"shock" → [pɑk]	"show" → [tʃo] "jello" → [wɛwo] "she" → [θi] or [s̺i] or [ʃi]
Liquid simplification	"rat" → [wæt] "lake" → [jeɪk] "run" → [jʌn] "bar" → [bɑo] "little" → [wɪɾə]	"row" → [ɹ̠oʊ] "rabbit" → [ɹ̠æbɪt]	"bird" → [bʊd]
Unstressed syllable deletion	"about" → [baʊt] "telephone" → [tɛfon]	"probably" → [prabli]	"alligator" → [æʔɪgeə] "button" → [bʌʔn̩]
Cluster reduction	"spot" → [pat] "post" → [pos] or [pot] "bread" → [bɛd] "grow" → [woʊ] "steep" → [θip] "strike" → [twaɪk]	"card" → [kad]	"swim" → [θwɪm] "broke" → [bwok] "batman" → [bæmæn]
Assimilation	"dog" → [gag] "cups" → [pʌps] "knife" → [maɪf] "lamb" → [næm] "boat" → [bop] "band" → [bænd] "dress" → [bwɛs]	"black" → [bwæk]	"down doggie" → [gaʊŋ gagi]

Stopping describes the substitution of a stop for a fricative or an affricate, usually one similar in place of articulation to the target. Other errors may occur for fricative or affricate targets that do not involve stopping. Substitution of an affricate for a fricative (e.g., /s/ → [t͡s] or /z/ → [d͡z]) is called affrication rather than stopping. Note that affrication actually makes the target sound more complex and may not be a natural phonological process because these patterns are expected to simplify the target.

Palatal fronting is coded when a post-alveolar fricative or affricate is produced with alveolar place of articulation: these errors involve omitting the [-anterior] feature, leaving the default [Coronal] place feature. Other fronted substitutions would not typically occur and probably should not be coded as palatal fronting. Other errors for post-alveolar fricatives such as affrication or distortion do not count as palatal fronting either.

Liquid simplification includes liquid gliding (substitution of glides for liquids in the onset position) and vocalization/vowelization (substitution of vowels for liquids in the coda position). Distortions such as labialized or derhotacized variants of [ɹ] are not natural phonological processes but are included in the liquid simplification category in the Shriberg and Kwiatkowski (1980) system. Errors on rhotic vowels would not be coded as liquid simplifications because the target sounds in this case are vowels rather than liquid consonants.

Unstressed syllable deletion requires that the entire syllable be absent from the target word. When identifying these errors it is necessary to take local norms for the pronunciation of words into account (in fact, this is true for all phonological processes). The pronunciation of "probably" as [pɹɑbli] is so pervasive in some dialects that this could be an example where weak syllable deletion would not be a reasonable description of the child's production, especially in the case of a preliterate child.

Cluster reduction involves deleting one or more consonants from a sequence of consonants in a complex onset or complex coda. The consonant sequence must be contained within the onset or the coda of the same syllable for the sequence to be coded as a cluster. Therefore the production of "Batman" as [bæmæn] should be coded as final consonant deletion rather than cluster reduction because the omitted /t/ is in the coda of the first syllable, whereas the /m/ is in the onset of the second syllable. Word-final liquid+obstruent sequences form questionable clusters because the liquid might be considered to be part of the syllable nucleus. Therefore, "card" → [kɑd] could be described as omission of a rhotic vowel rather than cluster reduction. Similarly, syllabic nasals and liquids should not be coded as clusters and therefore "puddle" ([pʌdl̩]) → [pʌd] should be coded as weak syllable deletion rather than cluster reduction.

The identification of all phonological processes requires that the entire speech sample be taken into account because processes must apply to a natural class of phonemes. It is necessary to identify error patterns across the sample rather than isolated instances of sound changes such as those shown in Table 1–6. In the case of **assimilation** errors, the error pattern must occur in a specific context. For example, with regressive velar assimilation, the most commonly observed assimilation error, it is important to show that /d/ and /g/ are pronounced correctly in other words where there is no opportunity for assimilation to occur, therefore "dime" → [daɪm], "game" → [geɪm], but "duck"

→ [gʌk]. Similarly, "black" → [bwæk] is unlikely to be labial assimilation (as opposed to liquid simplification) unless /l/ was normally produced correctly, for example, "glass" → [glæs]. Other place and manner features are subject to regressive assimilation too and, although less common, progressive assimilation does occur. Assimilation can occur between coda and onset, between coda and vowel and between the two consonants in a complex onset or coda.

Box 1–4. Phonological Concepts: Key Points

- Phonology is the study of the sound system of languages.
- A phoneme is the smallest unit of speech that distinguishes the meaning of one word from another in a language.
- A minimal pair consists of two words that differ by only one phoneme and have different meanings.
- Phonotactics is the description of the permitted sequences of consonants and vowels in a language.
- A syllable is composed of an optional onset and an obligatory rime, which in turn contains a nucleus and an optional coda.
- A distinctive feature is an articulatory or acoustic parameter that defines a phonological category.
- Speech sounds that share a distinctive feature can be grouped into natural classes of sounds.
- Error patterns that apply to a natural class of sounds are called phonological processes.

Chapter 1 Study Questions

Compare and contrast the concepts listed in each row:

- Phonetics, phonology
- Acoustic phonetics, articulatory phonetics
- Articulation, articulatory-phonetic representation
- Perception, acoustic-phonetic representation
- Respiratory subsystem, phonatory subsystem, articulatory subsystem
- Vowels, consonants
- Co-articulation, assimilation
- Place of articulation, manner of articulation

- Fricatives, affricates
- Broad transcription, narrow transcription
- Frequency (acoustic) cue, amplitude (acoustic) cue
- Waveform display, spectrogram
- Voicing lead, short-lag voicing, long-lag voicing
- Identification test, discrimination test (of categorical perception)
- Phone, phoneme, allophone
- Onset, rime, coda
- Trochaic stress pattern, iambic stress pattern

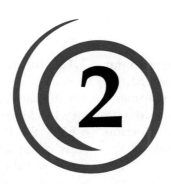

2

Phonological Development

Learning Objectives

- Describe the shift from language-general to language-specific phonetic perception.
- Explain the shift from phonetic to phonemic knowledge of the sound system of the native language.
- Describe the five stages of infant vocal development.
- Describe the expected phonetic and phonotactic repertoire for a 24-month-old child.
- Define customary production and mastery.

- Describe the criteria for identifying developmental, nondevelopmental, and atypical error types.
- List phonological error patterns that may be expected in the speech of 2-year-olds, 3-year-olds, and 4-year-olds.
- List some speech errors that are atypical at any age.
- Describe factors that may explain errors in the production of individual phonemes, weak syllables, and onset clusters.

The incremental but rapid acquisition of speech in infants, toddlers, and children is fascinating. Babies are born with the ability to vocalize (and cry!) but are unable to produce a variety of vowels and consonants or combine phonemes to produce words. Yet by the time children are 4 years of age, they usually produce meaningful speech in well-formed sentences that are understood by their communication part-

ners. By 9 years of age, adultlike speech accuracy has been achieved. Understanding this developmental trajectory is an important foundation for clinical practice. The speech-language pathologist (SLP) must be able to describe the important milestones in speech development between birth and late childhood and understand the underlying processes that contribute to normal speech development in order to assess or treat speech sound disorders (SSDs). Therefore, this chapter covers normal phonological development, starting in the speech perception domain and progressing to speech production milestones, in both cases following the trajectory from the prelinguistic through the preschool and early school-age periods. The focus is on a description of the most important developmental events that occur as the child progresses toward the achievement of an adultlike phonology. A deeper understanding of the biological mechanisms, cognitive learning processes, social-emotional factors, and environmental influences that contribute to normal phonological development is provided by Rvachew and Brosseau-Lapré (2018).

2.1 SPEECH PERCEPTION DEVELOPMENT

Critical events in the development of speech perception from birth to the early school years are presented in Table 2–1 and described in detail in the text.

2.1.1 Infants

The human fetus (assuming normal auditory function) hears speech in the womb during the last trimester of pregnancy. Newborns prefer to listen to their mother's voice over the voices of other female talkers (DeCasper & Fifer, 1980). Newborns only a few days old also prefer to listen to speakers of their native language compared with speakers of foreign languages that have a different prosodic pattern (e.g., Moon, Cooper, & Fifer, 1993; Nazzi, Bertoncini, & Mehler, 1998). Between birth and 6 months of age, infants can discriminate a range of phonetic contrasts, including: differences between vowels (Trehub, 1973); voicing contrasts among stop consonants (Hoonhorst et al., 2009); differences in place of articulation among stops and glides (Jusczyk & Thompson, 1978); differences in manner of articulation, such as stops versus glides (Hillebrand, Minifie, & Edwards, 1979) and stops versus nasals (Tsao, Liu, & Kuhl, 2006). Although infants can discriminate many different kinds of phonetic contrasts, it is not true that they can perceive every possible contrast from all of the world's languages.

Table 2–1. *Critical Events in the Development of Speech Perception*

Approximate Age Range	Event
0–6 months	Language-general phonetic perception
6–12 months	Shift to language-specific phonetic perception
1–2 years	Emergence of phonemic perception
2–5 years	Gradual acquisition of implicit phonological awareness skills
5–12 years	Learning of explicit phonological awareness skills

For example, Eilers and Minifie (1975) found that English-learning infants aged 4 to 6 months were unable to perceive the voicing contrast between [sa] and [za]. In general, the perception of contrasts involving fricatives seems to be challenging for infants and children (Nittrouer, 2001) although the perception of these difficult contrasts improves with experience. Nonetheless, infants demonstrate **language-general phonetic perception** until approximately 6 months of age and are able to discriminate a wide range of phonetic contrasts, both those that are present in the language(s) they are exposed to and those that are not phonemic in the language(s) in their ambient environment. This stage of language-general phonetic perception is said to be **universal** because the characteristics of speech perception for hearing infants are roughly similar for all infants during this period, regardless of their language experience (Kuhl, 2004). Notwithstanding the universality of language-general perception in early infancy, there are individual differences in perceptual performance even among infants learning the same language; while some contrasts are easier to perceive than others for all infants in general, some infants are more successful than others at perceiving even the easy contrasts. Differences in the ease with which speech is processed at birth may be heritable and may have implications for the emergence of speech, language, or reading disabilities later in life (Lohvansuu, Hämäläinen, Ervast, Lyytinen, & Leppänen, 2018; Lyytinen et al., 2004).

During the first year, infants gradually shift from language-general to **language-specific phonetic perception**. Progressively, starting at the age of 6 months, there is a decline in infants' sensitivity to non-native vowel contrasts they could discriminate at younger ages (e.g., Kuhl, Williams, Lacerda, Stevens, & Lindblom, 1992; Polka & Werker, 1994). The shift to language-specific perception for consonants occurs a bit later, as shown by Werker and colleagues, who tested infants' ability to perceive consonant contrasts produced in Hindi or Salish: infants learning English were no longer able to discriminate these consonant contrasts by 10 months of age, whereas infants exposed to one of these languages from birth maintained perception of the native-language contrast throughout the first year (e.g., Werker & Lalonde, 1988; Werker & Tees, 1983, 1984). In the early days of infant speech research, it was speculated that the transition from language-general to language-specific speech perception was caused by selective elimination of brain cells responsible for perceiving speech sounds; according to this hypothesis, sensory cells that do not receive sufficient environmental stimulation are eliminated. Although neural pruning and reshaping of neural pathways does occur during development in response to experience, this process does not explain early speech perception development. In fact, studies using sophisticated brain imaging techniques show that the brain remains alert to foreign-language differences in speech sound inputs, even after the infant stops responding to them in behavioral experiments (Cheour et al., 1998). Furthermore, the brain remembers heard speech patterns over long intervals. For example, some researchers have studied the perceptual abilities of adults who were adopted from foreign countries as infants. In general, these individuals do not find it easier to regain their birth language in a functional way but they do have an advantage on basic perceptual tasks, such as discriminating Chinese tone contrasts that they have not heard for over 10 years, as revealed by brain imaging technology (Pierce, Klein, Chen, Delcenserie, & Genesee, 2014).

That is not to say that brain responses to speech are not shaped by the environment; indeed, unique patterns of brain responses arise due to environmental inputs that are heard even before birth (May, Byers-Heinlein, Gervain, & Werker, 2011). The research shows that infants gradually learn language-specific strategies for perceiving speech sounds that are functionally significant in their ambient language(s). For example, even though English-learning infants are exposed to [t] in words such as "stop," they learn to perceive [t] as an allophone of /t/ or /d/ depending upon acoustic characteristics and phonetic context. Sensitivity to the English-specific voicing contrast between short lag and long lag voicing is enhanced during the first year of life, whereas perception of the contrast between voicing lead and short lag voicing declines. English infants learn to assimilate [ta] to the /da/ category in contrast to [tʰa], which is perceived as a member of the /ta/ category. French- and Spanish-learning infants learn to perceive these same stimuli in a different manner but in accordance with the voicing categories that occur in their native languages. In other words, the infant's perceptual performance takes into account the acoustic-phonetic details of the speech input as well as distributional characteristics that permit acquisition of phonetic category boundaries even before meaningful words are learned. One learning mechanism that accounts for these changes in perceptual sensitivity is **statistical learning**: memory traces of speech sounds are retained and grouped according to frequency of occurrence in a con-

text-sensitive fashion to form categories. Over time, speech input is perceived in relation to **bottom-up factors** (the acoustic information in the input) and **top-down factors** (the acoustic-phonetic categories that are being formed).

Infants are not exposed to individual phones and phonemes in the input. Rather, they are exposed to speech that is connected and has a language-specific prosodic structure. Prosody involves continuous changes in duration, pitch, and loudness, as described in Chapter 1. Prosodic information reaches the fetus before birth, so that the newborn is familiar with the rhythmic characteristics of the mother's language; in fact, the infant prefers to listen to this language over another with different rhythmic qualities. The infant's attention to the rhythmic qualities of the native language supports the development of word segmentation abilities. Segmenting words from the continuous stream of speech input is a difficult problem: words do not contain obvious boundaries between them, and adults rarely produce single words in isolation when speaking to babies (Gerken, 2009; Johnson, 2016).

Practice 2–1

Watch this short video clip of the news in Italian (https://www .youtube.com/watch?v=Ph0kiJdvz7w). Try to identify words as you listen to the continuous speech input. Was it difficult to identify some of the words? Which words were easier to identify, and why do you think you were able to identify them?

The infant's attention to the prosodic structure of the input language provides initial language-specific strategies to segment smaller units from the continuous speech input (Kehoe, 2013). Word boundaries are likely to happen at clause boundaries; prosodic cues to clause boundaries, such as pauses and characteristic intonation contours, help infants recognize language they have heard previously in their input. For example, an English-learning child might hear utterances such as "Look! That's a spider," "Look! That's a rabbit," and "Look! That's a doggie." When paying attention to the pauses at clause boundaries the infant can learn that words usually begin with stressed syllables ([lʊk], [spaɪ], [ɹæ], [dɑ]) and that two-syllable words have a trochaic stress pattern (['spaɪ,də-], ['ɹæ,bɪt], ['dɑ,gi]). Between the ages of 4 to 9 months, infants prefer to listen to language-specific word stress patterns, which aids in discovering a variety of word boundary cues. In particular, attention to prosody and stress patterns leads the child to discover information about phonotactic cues to word boundaries before 12 months of age: for example, in English many words begin with [sp] but words cannot begin with the sequences [ts] or [kt]. This is called the **prosodic bootstrapping hypothesis**. The relationship between learning about prosody and learning about phonetics is reciprocal, however: prosody aids in the processing of phonetic information, and the child's developing phonetic knowledge furthers the infant's ability to segment continuous speech into smaller prosodic units. During the first year, the infant has thus accomplished a shift from language-general to language-specific processing of phonetic and prosodic elements. The infant is now aware of phonetic contrasts, allophones, rhythmic patterns, and phonotactic characteristics of the language being learned.

2.1.2 Toddlers

During the first year of life, the infant's speech perception skills are considered to be phonetic, as the infant does not yet use this perceptual knowledge for meaningful communication. During the second year of life, toddlers make another qualitative shift in perceptual development as they transition from phonetic to phonemic knowledge of the sound system of the ambient language. Toddlers develop **phonemic perception** skills as they use their phonetic perceptual abilities to recognize meaningful words and associate those words with the appropriate referents. In the early stages of word learning, words are represented as "chunks" at the level of phrases and whole words; although infants can discriminate similar sounds such as [p] and [b], the ability to encode lexical representations such as "pear" and "bear" emerges gradually over the second year of life. During the first year of life, discrimination of [p] and [b] is accomplished by auditory mechanisms; during the second year, auditory representations are integrated with semantic representations and stabilize so that it is increasingly difficult to change these representations as the child ages (Kuhl et al., 2008; Zhang et al., 2009). It is for this reason that it is difficult to acquire a new language without an "accent" at an older age.

Early word learning skills have been extensively studied in laboratory tasks in which toddlers are repeatedly presented with nonsense words and taught to associate them with novel objects or pictures. The conditions under which toddlers can map novel words to objects can be determined in these studies because the stimuli and learning conditions are controlled by the experimenter. These studies show that most toddlers can learn to associate new words with novel objects at 14 months if the words are very different from each other (e.g., "lif" and "neem"). By the age of 20 months, many toddlers can map novel words to objects, even if the nonsense words are minimal pairs (such as [bɪ] and [dɪ]). There is individual variability observed during this age range, such that some toddlers age 14 months are able to map minimal pair nonsense words to novel objects, but some older toddlers cannot (Werker, Fennell, Corcoran, & Stager, 2002). The child's vocabulary size is in fact a better predictor of word learning ability than age during this period. As toddlers get older, they gain more experience with variable speech input in meaningful contexts. Their perceptual representations of words become increasingly detailed to allow for some differentiation of misarticulated words from their correctly produced targets. There appears to be a reciprocal relationship between speed of language processing and vocabulary acquisition in early childhood that has implications for language development over the long term (Marchman & Fernald, 2008). The shift from phonetic to phonemic perception of speech is gradual, and there is continuity in the development of speech perception skills from the first to the second year of life. This continuity is indicated by correlations between speech perception performance in the first year of life and later language development. For instance, perception of word stress patterns at 4 months correlates with language test performance at 5 years (Höhle, Pauen, Hesse, & Weissenborn, 2014).

Toddlers are able to use knowledge about native-language phone categories and rhythmic structures to extract words from the speech input and associate these spoken words with specific referents. However, the perceptual knowledge of toddlers is far from mature, as will be shown in the sections on speech perception development in preschoolers and school-age children.

2.1.3 Preschoolers

Preschoolers' knowledge of acoustic-phonetic characteristics of the phonemes in their native language improves with age and is significantly correlated with measures of language development such as vocabulary size (Claessen, Heath, Fletcher, Hogben, & Leitão, 2009). A mispronunciation detection task is often used to assess the phonological representation of words by preschoolers. Using this type of task, the child is presented with a picture of a target word, hears a pronunciation of the vocabulary item, and indicates nonverbally whether the word was produced correctly or incorrectly. These mispronunciations can involve omissions or transpositions of segments (e.g., "train" /tɹeɪn/ → [teɪn], "helicopter" /hɛlɪkɑptɚ/ → [hɛlɪtɑpkɚ]), whereas others represent substitution errors (e.g., "sandwich" /sænwɪtʃ/ → [sɪnwɪtʃ], "sun" /sʌn/ → [fʌn]). McNeill and Hesketh (2010) found that preschoolers, as a group, had the most difficulty detecting the substitution errors, especially those involving vowels (McNeill & Hesketh, 2010). Furthermore, the speech perception performance was correlated with vocabulary size in this sample.

During the preschool years, children gradually acquire implicit phonological awareness skills. **Phonological awareness** is the knowledge that spoken words are composed of smaller units such as syllables, onsets and rimes, and phonemes (Rvachew & Grawburg, 2006). Phonological awareness is a crucial prereading skill that sometimes develops more slowly than expected in children with speech and language impairments. Therefore, assessment of phonological awareness has become an important part of speech-language pathology practice. Phonological awareness tests are not measures of speech perception ability per se, but performance on these tasks is closely related to the child's speech perception abilities (Joanisse, Manis, Keating, & Seidenberg, 2000; Lyytinen et al., 2004; Rvachew & Grawburg, 2006).

Phonological awareness tasks vary along three dimensions that determine the difficulty level of the task. First, the task may require **implicit** knowledge or an **explicit** response. Implicit tasks require less conscious awareness, whereas explicit tasks require the child to manipulate linguistic units in a way that demonstrates high level **metalinguistic knowledge**. For example, a matching task in which the child groups pictures of "cane," "can," and "cup" together requires only implicit knowledge of word onsets. On the other hand, a "pig latin" game in which the onset must be consciously moved and transformed ("anecay," "ancay," "upcay") is difficult to play unless the child has advanced knowledge of the sound system of the language. Second, phonological awareness tasks may require the child to access linguistic units at any level of the phonological hierarchy, with larger or higher-level units typically being easier to access than smaller, lower level units. Segmenting a sentence into words or a word into syllables should be easier to accomplish than segmenting a syllable into its onset and rime or a rime into its constituent phonemes. Awareness of phonemes in syllables and words is called **phoneme awareness** and is especially important for the acquisition of reading. Finally, materials and instructions used to help the child complete the task can be varied to make it easier or more difficult. Younger children will benefit from the use

of pictures, repeated instruction, and non-verbal responses, whereas older children can demonstrate metalinguistic abilities in tasks that require verbal responses to questions with no other supports.

Age expectations for children's phonological awareness abilities are not perfectly understood because most research has not properly controlled the three factors described here. For this reason, it is sometimes difficult to know why younger children were not able to complete a task. However, it is generally agreed that preschool-aged children do have some implicit phonological awareness abilities beginning at approximately age 3 years. Some children have demonstrated implicit awareness of rhyming words at the age of 3 years on the "oddity" task, although the ability to do this task varies with social class and the child's vocabulary size (MacLean, Bryant, & Bradley, 1987). In this task, children are shown three pictures which are then named (e.g., fish, dish, book) and asked to point out the one that does not rhyme or does not belong. Implicit awareness of phonemes is not typically seen in children younger than 5 years of age (Lonigan, Burgess, Anthony, & Barker, 1998). This is the case even in the onset position of consonant-vowel-consonant (CVC) words (e.g., when asking the child which word does not belong among "bat," "bug," "rock," and "bin"). Phoneme awareness is also difficult in the coda position (e.g., when asking the child which words end with the same sound among "cat," "cap," and "hat"). The implicit awareness of individual phonemes remains unstable in kindergarten students.

The first three important milestones in early speech perception during the first year of life, second year of life, and the early preschool years are illustrated in Figure 2–1.

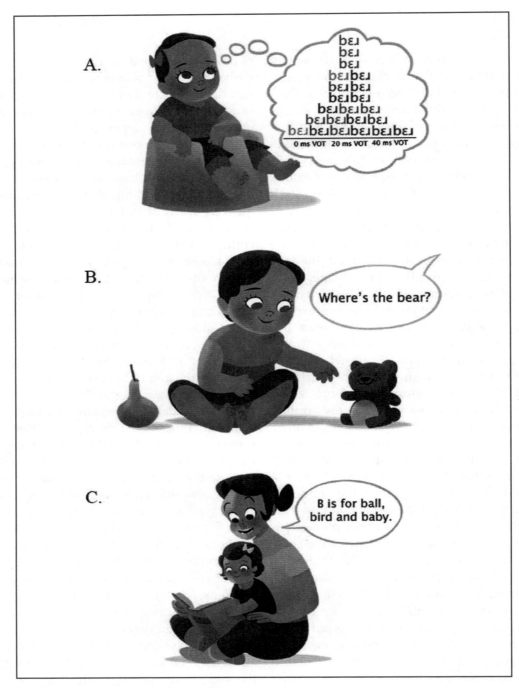

Figure 2–1. *Illustration of three important milestones in early speech perception.* **A.** *During the first year of life, the infant shifts from language-general to language-specific processing of phonetic categories.* **B.** *During the second year of life, the toddler learns to use phonetic categories to acquire and differentiate meaningful words, leading to the emergence of perceptual knowledge of phonemic contrasts.* **C.** *During the third year of life, the child demonstrates beginning implicit awareness of similarities among words based on shared onsets or rimes. Illustrations by Edith Lebel. Used with permission from Susan Rvachew.*

2.1.4 School-Age Children

Most 2-year-old children are able to identify clear exemplars of words that differ by a single phonetic feature, such as "pear" and "bear." However, when word identification skills are assessed using synthetic speech continua as opposed to clear, live-voice exemplars of words, speech perception abilities of children are shown to mature through very late childhood. In particular, vowel perception is not yet adultlike in children ages 9 to 12 years (Jacewicz & Fox, 2014). Speech perception of words presented in noise also develops gradually throughout childhood. When speech stimuli are presented against a steady-state noise background (as if there is noisy air conditioning overhead), 10-year-old children can perceive those stimuli approximately as well as adults; when the speech is presented against a background of speech (like listening in a noisy coffee shop), adultlike performance is not achieved until the age of 16 years (Erickson & Newman, 2017). Generally, it is important for the SLP to remember that children do not perceive speech as well as adults unless the **signal-to-noise ratio** is greater: this means that the speech signal needs to be much louder than the noise. For this reason, some of the therapy techniques discussed in Chapters 6 through 8 require amplification devices to be effective.

With regard to phonological awareness abilities, kindergarten-age children do not appear to have explicit awareness of phonemes as measured by elision tasks (Chiappe, Siegel, & Gottardo, 2002). Elision tasks require the child to break the word into individual phonemes and recognize the word that remains when a spe-cific phoneme is deleted. The child might be asked to delete a sound from anywhere in the word, such as "say *meat* without the /m/" or "say *meet* without the /t/," in which case the expected answers are "eat" and "me" respectively. By third grade, many children are able to perform elision tasks that involve omitting a phoneme from a complex onset, such as "say *plan* without the /l/" (McBride-Chang, 1995).

In summary, speech perception abilities continue to improve gradually and are not yet adultlike at the age of 12 years. As children continue to accumulate experience with language, they become increasingly skilled at encoding detailed acoustic-phonetic representations for words. Eventually, the school-age child is able to recognize words even when they are presented in a noisy environment or when they are ambiguous exemplars of the target item.

Practice 2–2

Find a partner in your class. Select four words from one of the following lists without telling your partner what words you chose. Next, produce the words while looking away from your partner. Your partner's task is to write the words he or she heard before changing roles with you. Were both of you able to identify the words produced by your partner in the noisy classroom environment? How do you think a child would perform compared with you, and why?

Word lists: (1) can, fan, man, pan, tan, van; (2) bat, cat, fat, hat, mat, rat, sat.

Box 2–1. Speech Perception Development: Key Points

- Infants shift from language-general to language-specific phonetic perception between 6 and 12 months of age.
- Toddlers develop phonemic perception skills as they use their phonetic perceptual abilities to recognize meaningful words.
- Preschoolers gradually acquire implicit phonological awareness of onsets and rimes.
- Good speech perception and a large vocabulary support phonological awareness.
- Explicit phoneme awareness is a crucial prereading skill that is learned after school entry.
- Adultlike ability to perceive speech-in-noise is not achieved until approximately 16 years of age.

2.2 EARLY SPEECH PRODUCTION DEVELOPMENT

Speech production is one of the most complex motor acts performed by humans. Producing speech requires the coordination of respiratory, laryngeal, and articulatory subsystems involving over 100 muscles (Kent, 2004). At birth the infant has very little control over these subsystems. After 6 or 7 months, the infant has gained enough control to begin producing speech-like syllables in vocalizations that are called **babble** (Oller, 2000). The first meaningful words follow a few months later. These early stages of speech development are described in this section.

2.2.1 Prelinguistic Vocal Development

Oller and colleagues (e.g., Oller, 1980, 2000; Oller, Eilers, Neal, & Schwartz, 1999) described infant vocal development in terms of sequential stages, each associated with a characteristic type of vocalization. These stages are summarized in Table 2–2 and described below. Although the progression of infant vocal development during the first 18 months is presented as passing through distinct stages, there is much overlap between them. A vocalization that is said to characterize one stage may occur at low frequencies during the preceding stages and continue at high frequencies during subsequent stages. Therefore the relationship between a stage and any vocalization type is one of relative frequency of occurrence and not one of absolute likelihood of occurrence. There is also variation among children in the rate of vocal development, and therefore the ages listed for each stage are approximate.

At birth, infants cry and produce other **reflexive sounds** such as coughing and burping; these sounds are related to the infant's physical state and seem to be produced automatically. In terms of speech development, the **phonation stage** is from birth to approximately 2 months of age, a period when the infant's vocal tract anatomy is starkly different from the adult vocal tract (Vorperian, Kent, Gentry, & Yandell, 1999). Briefly, infant anatomical features protect the airway by encouraging nasal airflow and restricting options for tongue movement (as described in more detail in Rvachew & Brosseau-Lapré, 2018). During this stage, the primary nonreflexive, nondistress vocalization is the quasi-resonant vowel. **Quasi-resonant vowels (QRVs)** typically consist of a short utterance produced with

Table 2–2. Five Stages of Infant Vocal Development

Approximate Age	Stage	Brief Description
0–2 months	Phonation	Primary nonreflexive vocalization is the quasi-resonant vowel (QRV).
1–4 months	Primitive articulation	Peak in the frequency of goos. Fully resonant vowels occasionally occur.
4–7 months	Expansion	Fully resonant vowels, squeals, raspberries, and marginal babbling.
7–10 months	Canonical babble	Well-formed canonical babbling (single syllables and reduplicated syllables).
10–18 months	Integrative	Canonical, reduplicated, and variegated babbling in combination with meaningful words.

Source: Adapted from Oller, Eilers, Neal, and Schwartz (1999) and Oller (2000).

the vocal tract in a more or less resting position. QRVs may be produced with normal phonation and duration, and often occur in rhythmic sequences. They are produced without deliberate shaping of the vocal tract so that they sound rather nasal in quality. Older children and adults also produce QRVs in their speech, when saying "um" and "hmm."

Practice 2–3

Produce clear vowels, such as "o," "ah," "eee." Observe the shape of your mouth as you produce these vowels. Then produce "filler sounds" such as "uh," "um," and "hmm" and note differences in how you produced these QRVs in contrast to the clear vowels.

The second stage is the **primitive articulation stage**, which occurs between the ages of 1 and 4 months. During this

stage, there is a peak in the frequency of goos, which are highly variable vocalizations that occur when phonation is interrupted by brief closures of the vocal tract. The closing gesture is produced in the back of the oral cavity and may be partial or complete. The articulatory gesture that closes the vocal tract is said to be **undifferentiated** because the infant does not voluntarily raise a specific part of the tongue to produce the closure; rather, a passive, possibly even accidental, positioning of the whole tongue, jaw, and pharynx results in partial or full closure of the tract, creating a sound that is perceived to be somewhat consonantal in nature. The closure is usually combined with a QRV, and often a series of goos are produced on a single exhalation.

The third stage is associated with significant reshaping of the vocal tract that permits more variable tongue movements from about 4 months of age. The new vocal behaviors that appear during this **expansion stage** are not directly caused by maturation of the vocal tract or the brain mechanisms that support speech. Rather the relationship between vocal tract structure and function is **reciprocal**, meaning there are influences in both directions. Social and linguistic inputs from adults stimulate the infant to produce vocalizations that are more speech-like, especially in the form of vowels (Bloom, 1988). Infants are also self-motivated to produce sounds that are novel or have salient characteristics (Twomey & Westermann, 2015). New articulatory movements themselves help to reshape the vocal tract as, for example, tongue pressure expands the size of the oral cavity and changes in muscle strength change the shape of the pharynx. During the **expansion stage** the infant systematically explores many parameters of speech, leading to a greater variety of vocalizations. The infant's vocal behavior during the expansion stage has also been called "vocal play," since the infant produces particular vocalizations repeatedly, giving the impression of deliberate experimentation and practice (Stark, Rose, & Benson, 1978). During this period, infants vary loudness: they whisper and yell. They play with laryngeal parameters to produce low-pitched creaky voiced utterances (growls) as well as high-pitched utterances often containing sudden pitch changes (squeals). Infants also produce a variety of vocal tract closures in the form of **raspberries**—loud trill-like sounds produced with the lips or the tongue, or the lips and tongue at the same time. The signature vocalization for this stage, however, is the appearance of **fully resonant vowels (FRVs)**, the most speech-like vocalization to emerge thus far, produced with an open vocal tract typically positioned for a central or mid-front vowel (such as schwa, /ə/). Some vocal-

izations produced in the expansion stage are perceived as **marginal babbling**, as they seem to be composed of consonant-vowel (CV) or vowel-consonant (VC) combinations even though they may not sound speech-like due to unusual loudness, resonance, or timing (Oller, 2000). Furthermore, marginal babbling is highly variable, with each marginal vocalization being different from the last.

The fourth stage, **canonical babbling**, is easily identified by parents and untrained observers. Canonical babbling occurs on average at the age of 7 months, and always by 11 months in normally developing infants (Eilers & Oller, 1994; Oller, Eilers, & Basinger, 2001). Normal hearing is essential to the emergence of canonical babbling during the first year of life. Canonical babbles are well-formed utterances that sound like speech due to a clear syllable margin, smoothly changing but rapid formant transitions combined with a fully resonant vowel produced with normal phonation and a relatively short duration. Single syllables such as "ba," "dee," and "gu" may be classified as canonical; reduplications such as "baba-bababa" are produced with increasingly regular timing as the infant gets older and is a defining feature of the canonical babbling stage. Infants are happy to vocalize when they are alone (even in the middle of the night!), as babbling is not communicative in function. Rather, the infant practices the production of certain syllables, using sensory feedback to achieve consistency. Brain imaging research suggests that neural pathways that link acoustic-phonetic representations, articulatory-phonetic representations, and motor plans are strengthened at this time (Imada et al., 2006). The canonical babbling stage does overlap with the emergence of intentional communication, but the infant will use nonverbal gestures or more primitive vocalizations such as yelling to demand attention (McCune, Vihman, Roug-Hellichus, Bordenave Delery, & Gogate, 1996).

The final stage is the **integrative stage**, which lasts roughly to the age of 18 months. During the integrative stage the child continues to develop control of the respiratory, laryngeal, and supralaryngeal articulatory systems to produce speech in single syllable babbles, **reduplicated babbles** ("dadadada"), and **variegated babbles** ("badagabama"). Although babbling itself is not communicative, there is a relationship between babbling and meaningful speech. First, children who produce several consonant sounds consistently in their babble at an early age tend to produce referential language at an earlier age as well (McCune & Vihman, 2001). Furthermore, the sounds that the child produces in babbling will be used to form the toddler's first words (Vihman, Macken, Miller, Simmons, & Miller, 1985). During the integrative stage, babbling and meaningful speech overlap. While babbling continues, the child is also producing an increasing number of meaningful words. Meaningful words may be combined with nonmeaningful syllables, the whole produced with a sentence-like pitch contour, creating **jargon**.

2.2.2 First Words

Children's first meaningful words appear around their first birthday. First words are identified on the basis of context as much as phonetic form (Vihman and McCune, 1994). For example, if a child says [bʊ] consistently when looking or pointing at a book, this would probably be considered

a word. However, if the child produces [bʊ] repeatedly when looking at a book, a stuffed toy, a ball, and a toy car, this is more likely to be babble. However, early word productions are extremely variable, so that this child might produce the word "book" as [bʊ], [bʊt], [put], [tʊ], [gʊ], and [dut], thus complicating identification of the child's first words. At a young age, the children's emergent phonological knowledge is word based—they attempt to produce words as chunks, without yet demonstrating knowledge that words are composed of smaller units, phonemes.

There is continuity between a child's babbling and first words, meaning phones and word shapes that the child produced often when babbling are likely to be present in the child's first words. Vihman and Croft (2007) proposed that toddlers select templates from the language input and adapt other words to their preferred templates. Templates are selected based on: (1) constraints imposed by the developing speech production mechanism; (2) the most salient or accessible features of the language input, especially word shape characteristics; and (3) individual factors related to the child's history of production practice and experience. It is important to note that the selection and avoidance of words applies to the child's expressive vocabulary only: while toddlers will select which words to produce based on their preferred templates, this does not influence their receptive vocabulary development, as they continue to learn the meaning of words of all shapes and containing all phonemes (Kay-Raining Bird & Chapman, 1998; Schwartz, Leonard, Loeb, & Swanson, 1987).

For young children at the first words stage, an **independent analysis** of their speech is ideal (Stoel-Gammon, 2001).

An independent analysis considers the child's use of speech sounds and word shapes independently of the adult target. In Chapter 1 we demonstrated the procedure for deriving a **phonetic repertoire** from the broad transcription of a child's speech; another independent analysis is the repertoire of the word or syllable shapes produced by a child, also called **phonotactic repertoire**. Independent analyses can be used with young children who produce both babbling and first words. In addition, meaningful words at this stage are difficult to associate with the adult target, as it is not always clear what the child intended to say. Furthermore, as described earlier in this chapter, infants represent words as "chunks" at the whole-word level and independent analyses do not assume adultlike underlying representations and are appropriate for describing a word-based phonology.

Kent and Bauer (1985) described the vocalizations of 1-year-old infants using phonetic and phonotactic repertoires based on broad transcription of the of the child's speech, recorded when they were 13 months old. The most frequent utterance observed was a single vowel; central and front vowels such as [ə, a, e, ɛ] were preferred over back and low vowels such as [ɑ, o], and [i] and [u] were rarely produced. When they produced CV syllables, the preferred consonant was the voiced bilabial stop [b]. Fricatives were most likely to occur in the syllable-final position and were more frequent than stops in this position. The frequency of occurrence of consonants in CV syllables is shown in Table 2–3 by manner of articulation, place of articulation, and voicing category. It is important to note that these data are specific to these English-learning infants. Generally, the speech sound repertoires of infants and toddlers are quite similar

Table 2–3. *Frequency of Occurrence of Word Shapes and of Consonant Features in CV Syllables by Place, Manner, and Voicing Category*

Phonological Unit	Frequency of Occurrence, %
Syllable Shapes	
V	60
CV	19
CVCV	8
VCV	7
Manner of Articulation	
Stops	74
Nasals	10
Fricatives	11
Glides	5
Place of Articulation	
Labial	62
Apical (Alveolar)	18
Palatal	3
Velar	10
Pharyngeal, Glottal	7
Voicing Category	
Voiced	85

Note. C = consonant, V = vowel.

Source: Adapted from Kent and Bauer (1985). Vocalizations of one-year-olds. *Journal of Child Language, 12,* pp. 491–526.

regardless of the language being learned; however, word shapes are influenced by environmental language input. Vihman (2006) described a greater frequency of multisyllabic, VCV, and CVC word templates appearing in the speech of toddlers learning languages other than English.

Practice 2–4

Derive the phonetic and the phonotactic repertoires from the broad transcription of these nine words produced by a 15-month-old girl: [mama], [dada], [babe], [no], [dʌ], [bæ], [bɛʔ], [tʌp], [bʌf]. Based on the description of the vocalizations of 1-year-olds by Kent and Bauer (1985), are you surprised these are the first words produced by this toddler? Why?

Although the child's speech capability at age 1 year is quite limited, the toddler at age 2 years is able to produce a good range of phones and word shapes when an independent analysis is applied to a free speech sample. Stoel-Gammon (1985) followed 34 infants between 9 and 24 months of age; the children were seen every three months twice for 30-minute recording sessions. During the sessions, the children were playing with toys and interacting with a caregiver. Based on the results of this study, Stoel-Gammon (1987) described the profile of phonetic and phonotactic repertoire, presented in Table 2–4 for the typical 24-month-old child.

Note that requirements 1 through 4 in Table 2–4 are based on the repertoire of phones and word shapes produced by the child, meaning the child's productions were analyzed independently of the adult target. For example, the expectation for one or two consonant clusters in word-initial position does not require that the child produce the clusters accurately. If the child produced "blue" → [bwu] and "swing" → [fwɪn], these productions that contain the substitution of /l/ → [w] would meet the requirement. The last requirement, however, is a rela-

Table 2–4. *Phonological Skills of the Typical 24-Month-Old*

Sampling Conditions	Expectations
1. Children were recorded two times.	1. CV, CVC, CVCV, and CVCVC *word shapes.*
2. Sessions were 30 minutes.	2. A few *consonant clusters* in word-initial position and maybe one or two in word-final position.
3. First 100 fully or partially intelligible words were included in the analysis.	3. Nine or 10 *initial consonants*, including exemplars from the classes of stops, nasals, fricatives, and glides.
4. No word was included more than twice.	4. Five or six *final consonants*, mostly stops but including a representative of the nasal, fricative, and liquid classes.
5. Second tokens were included only if the second token of a word differed from the first.	5. *Seventy percent consonants correct,* when matching to consonants in the adult target word.

Source: Adapted from Stoel-Gammon (1987). Phonological skills of two-year olds. *Language, Speech, and Hearing Services in Schools, 18,* pp. 327–328. Used with permission of the American Speech-Language-Hearing Association.

tional analysis, meaning the productions of the child are analyzed in relation to the adult target. In this case, the expectation is that 70% of the consonants produced by the child would be correctly produced.

Shriberg and Kwiatkowski (1982) initially described the measure of **percentage of consonants correct (PCC)**, calculated by dividing the number of consonants produced correctly by the total number of consonants in the sample (correct and incorrect). The number is then multiplied by 100 to obtain a percentage. The rules for collecting a speech sample and scoring the phones as correct or incorrect vary depending upon the age of the child, the type of transcription applied to the sample, and the goals of the SLP. For

example, there are different rules and normative data to take distortion errors into account or to ignore these errors (Shriberg & Kwiatkowski, 1982). When ignoring distortion errors, PCC increases quite gradually, to approximately 80% at age 4 and only reaching 98% at age 12 years. The calculation rules will not be covered in detail in this book as the calculation of PCC from free speech samples occurs more frequently in research contexts than in clinical practice. However, more information and demonstrations can be found in Rvachew and Brosseau-Lapré (2018).

Another issue with the calculation of PCC from the free speech sample produced by a toddler is that it focuses attention on the accuracy of individual phonemes produced by the child. However, in the early stages of speech development, the primary phonological unit is the word. As children expand the size of their lexicon, there is a need to produce different but similar words in distinctive ways in order to maintain **lexical contrast**. In other words, a child who says [gəgə] for "cookie" and "egg" might be motivated to change "cookie" to [kəkə] or [gəgi:]. Ingram (2002) introduced **whole word measures** of speech accuracy to describe the complexity and the consistency of the word productions attempted by the child, as well as their proximity to the adult target. Consider, for example, the speech sample reproduced in Demonstration 1–1. This child produced the pet names "Coco" and "Dito" in several different ways and thus inconsistency in the sample was high. If the child settled on [koxo] and [dɪdo] as consistent ways to say these names, his speech intelligibility would improve. Another way to index improvement in this child's speech accuracy over time would be to simply count the number of words that are produced

---

Practice 2–5

Consider the following speech sample produced by a 24-month-old boy, recorded while the child played with a toy farm and interacted with his mother for 30 minutes. Use Stoel-Gammon's profile of the typical 24-month-old to determine whether this boy's speech abilities meet expectations, or are delayed for his age.

"baby" /beɪbɪ/ → [bebi]; "cat" /kæt/ → [tæt]; "chicken" /tʃɪkən/ → [tɪtən]; "cow" /kaʊ/ → [tao]; "dirty" /dɝti/ → [dədi]; "dog" /dɑg/ → [dɑ]; "duck" /dʌk/ → [dʌt]; "farm" /fɑɹm/ → [paʊm]; "go" /go/ → [do]; "horsie" /hɔɹsi/ → [ɔʊti]; "mommy" /mɑmi/ → [mɑmi]; "outside" /aʊtsaɪd/ → [aʊtaɪd]; "pig" /pig/ → [pig]; "sleep" /slip/ → [twip]; "tractor" /tɹæktɚ/ → [twætɚ]; "wagon" /wægən/ → [wædən].

completely correctly: in this sample it might be said that "Dito" was said correctly and therefore whole word correctness was only 7% for the entire sample. Increases in this statistic would indicate improvements in speech accuracy over time. However, improvements might also be noticed if the child's productions became closer to their targets even while not becoming accurate. For example, the word "TV" was produced as [βi] and [ti]; if the child started to say [tiβi], this inaccurate production would have closer proximity to the word he is attempting to produce. The instructions for calculating these whole word measures can be found in other sources (e.g., Ingram, 2002; Rvachew & Brosseau-Lapré, 2018).

2.3 PHONOLOGICAL DEVELOPMENT

The toddler's initial word productions, differentiated in terms of whole word templates, place a limit on language development. Older children want to produce more words and express more complex messages in longer sentences. In order to produce these longer sentences, the older child must learn to access lexical items quickly. Efficient lexical access requires an efficient filing system: specifically, it helps to represent words in terms of their smaller sublexical parts. Furthermore, intelligible production of these longer utterances requires better phonological planning skills: children must access and order individual phonemes in increasingly complex sequences. As the child makes the transition from word-based to phoneme-based lexical representations, it is possible to describe the child's phonological knowledge using a **relational analysis**. This means that the child's use of sounds in words is considered in relation to the adult target. The phonemes that the child uses when speaking can each be scored as correct or incorrect. Consistency in the production of each phoneme of interest can be determined for one child or a group of children, at one time or over a period of time. The SLP needs to know the ages at which children typically acquire different speech sounds in order to know whether a particular child is developing as expected in comparison to his or her age peers. This kind

---

Box 2–2. Early Speech Production Development: Key Points

- The five stages of infant vocal development are: phonation, primitive articulation, expansion, canonical babbling, and integrative.
- Canonical babbling occurs on average at 7 months of age, and always by 11 months in normally developing infants.
- During the integrative stage, when first words and babbling co-occur, the most commonly produced utterances are a single vowel, although CV syllables also appear quite often.
- By the age of 24 months, the toddler should produce a range of word shapes, including two-syllable words with coda consonants.
- The 2-year-old toddler should produce consonants from all manner classes in the phonetic repertoire even if they are not produced correctly on a consistent basis.

of information is referred to as normative data or **norms**. Norms for the acquisition of speech sounds (phonemes) will be presented in the next section.

2.3.1 Phoneme Acquisition Norms

Sander (1972) makes the point that phoneme acquisition does not happen all at once: it occurs over a period of time for most children. If you are describing phoneme acquisition for an individual child that you are assessing, the child's accuracy for any given phoneme will be anywhere between no accuracy and perfect accuracy. If you follow the child over time, repeating your assessments at regular intervals, you may observe the child's accuracy change for some phonemes, with gradual improvements observed along this continuum from no accuracy toward perfect accuracy. Sander (1972) identified two points along this continuum as being important for the purposes of clinical description: (1) **customary production**—the child produces the phoneme correctly more often than not, or at least 51% correct; and (2) **mastery**—the child produces the phoneme with almost or perfect accuracy, that is, at least 90% correct. Some examples of these concepts are shown in Table 2–5.

Normative studies describe phoneme acquisition for groups of children. Sander (1972) reviewed a number of normative studies based on single word naming tests that sampled all the consonants in English. Then he identified the ages at which 50% of children had achieved customary production (median age of acquisition) and the ages at which 90% of

had achieved customary production for these consonants (normal limit for acquisition). For example, 50% of children had achieved customary production for /k/ at or before the age of 2 years; 90% of children achieved customary production for /k/ at or before the age of 4 years. For some sounds, the median age of acquisition and the normal limit were even further apart. In particular, 50% of children achieved customary production for /s/ at or before the age of 3 years; but the age at which 90% of children had achieved customary production was 8 years. It is important to be aware of how much variability there is in the acquisition of speech sounds, even among children who do not have any developmental delays. A parent or preschool teacher may be concerned about a child who cannot pronounce /k/ or /s/ correctly. This is a reasonable concern because many children in the preschool classroom will be able to pronounce these sounds correctly much of the time. However, many other children in the same classroom will continue to struggle with these sounds for another year or more. Additional information will be required to determine if there is reason for concern.

Given the extreme variability in the ages at which children acquire speech sounds, it is common to pay close attention to the normal limit for acquisition in clinical practice. In other words, the SLP will not be very concerned about a child's phonological development unless the child is older than the age at which 90% of children have acquired the sound in question. Consider again the examples shown in the left-hand side of Table 2–5. If the child was 3 years old the SLP would "wait and see" if the child's /k/ produc-

Table 2–5. *Examples of Customary Production and Mastery of /k/ in Single Words and Connected Speech*

Customary Production (at least 51% ✓)	Mastery (at least 90% ✓)
Single Word Naming Examples	
"cup" /kʌp/ → [tʌp]	"cup" /kʌp/ → [kʌp]
"car" /kɑɹ/ → [tao]	"car" /kɑɹ/ → [kao]
"duck" /dʌk/ → [dʌk]	"duck" /dʌk/ → [dʌk]
"quack" /kwæk/ → [kwæk]	"quack" /kwæk/ → [kwæk]
"monkey" /mʌŋki/ → [mʌŋki]	"monkey" /mʌŋki/ → [mʌŋki]
4✓/6 = 66%✓	6✓/6 =100%✓
Connected Speech Examples	
I see a donkey eating a carrot. I don't like carrots. I like corn, and zucchini. I don't like cabbage or pickles. Sometimes my mom makes cabbage with pickles. I can't eat that!	I see a donkey eating a carrot. I don't like carrots. I like corn, and zucchini. I don't like cabbage or pickles. Sometimes my mom makes cabbage with pickles. I can't eat that!
[aɪ si ʌ dɔŋki itɪn ʌ kɛɹət] [aɪ don waɪt kɛɹəts] [ai waɪt kɔɚn en zutini] [aɪ don waɪt kæbɪdʒ ɔɚ pɪklz] [sʌmtaɪmz maɪ mɔm meɪts kæbɪdʒ wɪf pɪklz] [aɪ tænt it dæt]	[aɪ si ʌ dɔŋki itɪn ʌ kɛɹət] [aɪ don waɪk kɛɹəts] [ai waɪk kɔɚn en zukini] [aɪ don waɪk kæbɪdʒ ɔɚ pɪklz] [sʌmtaɪmz maɪ mɔm meɪts kæbɪdʒ wɪf pɪklz] [aɪ kænt it dæt]
8✓/14 = 57%✓	13✓/14 = 93%✓

tions would become increasingly more accurate with time. However, if the child was 5 years old, the SLP would be concerned because the child is older than the normal limit for acquisition of /k/.

The Iowa-Nebraska Articulation Norms Project (Smit, Hand, Freilinger, Bernthal, & Bird, 1990) identified the age at which boys and girls should have acquired consonants and consonant clusters in English. In this study a large sample of children aged 3 to 9 years named pictures that elicited consonants and con-

sonant clusters in the word-initial and word-final positions, usually two productions per consonant per word position (for a total of four attempts per consonant). The number of correct productions for each consonant was aggregated across all the children and all words at each age level. The age of acquisition was identified as the earliest age at which consonant accuracy was at least 90% and therefore these data pertain to the age of mastery. These normative data are reproduced in Table 2–6.

Table 2–6. *Recommended Ages (Years;Months) of Acquisition by Phoneme or Cluster, Based on 90% Level of Acceptable Articulation*

Phoneme	Females	Males	Phoneme	Females	Males
/m/	3;0	3;0	/ʃ/	6;0	7;0
/n/	3;6	3;0	/tʃ/	6;0	7;0
/-ŋ/	7;0–9;0	7;0–9;0	/dʒ/	6;0	7;0
/h-/	3;0	3;0	/l/ /l-/	5;0	6;0
/w-/	3;0	3;0	/-l/	6;0	7;0
/j-/	4;0	5;0	/ɹ/ /ɹ-/	8;0	8;0
/p/	3;0	3;0	/-ɚ/	8;0	8;0
/b/	3;0	3;0	/tw kw/	4;0	5;6
/t/	4;0	3;6	/sp st sk/	7;0–9;0	7;0–9;0
/d/	3;0	3;6	/sm sn/	7;0–9;0	7;0–9;0
/k/	3;6	3;6	/sw/	7;0–9;0	7;0–9;0
/g/	3;6	4;0	/sl/	7;0–9;0	7;0–9;0
/f/ /f-/	3;6	3;6	/pl bl kl gl fl/	5;6	6;0
/-f/	5;6	5;6	/pɹ bɹ tɹ dɹ kɹ gɹ fɹ/	8;0	8;0
/v/	5;6	5;6	/θɹ/	9;0	9;0
/θ/	6;0	8;0	/skw/	7;0–9;0	7;0–9;0
/ð-/	4;6	7;0	/spl/	7;0–9;0	7;0–9;0
/s/	7;0–9;0	7;0–9;0	/spɹ stɹ skɹ/	7;0–9;0	7;0–9;0
/z/	7;0–9;0	7;0–9;0			

Source: Adapted from Smit et al. (1990). The Iowa Articulation Norms Project and its Nebraska replication. *Journal of Speech and Hearing Disorders, 55,* Table 7, p. 795. Used with permission of the American Speech-Language-Hearing Association.

Practice 2–6

Consider each pair of phonemes and indicate which one is earlier developing, using the norms in Table 2–6 for girls: (1) /m/ versus /n/; (2) /j/ versus /k/; (3) /l-/ versus /θ/; (4) /ɹ-/ versus /dʒ/.

Consider each pair of phonemes and indicate which one is earlier developing, using the norms in Table 2–6 for boys: (1) /j/ versus /w/; (2) /v/ versus /j/; (3) /ð/ versus /ɹ/; (4) /g/ versus /θ/.

The norms that are shown in Table 2–6 can be used to determine if a child's errors are developmental or nondevelopmental. A **developmental** error is a speech error that the child is expected to "grow out of." Therefore developmental versus nondevelopmental error types are largely differentiated on the basis of the child's age, in relation to the normal limit for acquisition of the error sound. If the child is younger than the expected age of acquisition, the error is developmental because there is still some time for the child to acquire the phoneme. A **nondevelopmental** error is a speech error that will probably not correct unless the child receives speech therapy. If the child is older than the expected age of acquisition, there is no reason to believe that the child will acquire the phoneme without help because research shows no improving trend after this age point. Developmental and nondevelopmental errors may be substitutions, omissions, or distortions as long as the error is one that occurs commonly in the speech of young children. Unusual persistence of a commonly occurring error might suggest that the child will not grow out of the error without the assistance of an SLP. For example, a 4-year-old child might substitute [t] for /s/; this type of error should not be heard in a child's speech past the age of 3 years and is therefore cause for concern even though the normal limit for acquisition of /s/ is not until age 8 years. More typically a child will progress from the [t] substitution to dental distortion of the /s/ sound and eventually to increasingly correct production.

When the error is very unusual, occurring in the speech of fewer than 5% of children at any age, the error is **atypical**. Atypical errors should be treated regardless of the child's age because research shows that these errors will persist without intervention. Nondevelopmental errors should be treated because the child is past the expected age of acquisition. Developmental errors are not usually treated if there are no nondevelopmental or atypical errors in the child's speech. However, if the child's speech problem is significant enough overall to require treatment, as discussed further in Chapter 5, developmental errors may be selected for treatment along with the other errors in the child's speech. Examples of developmental, nondevelopmental, and atypical errors are shown in Table 2–7.

The order in which phonemes are learned, as presented in Table 2–6, is sometimes assumed to reflect relative **articulatory complexity**. In this case, the order of acquisition might inform treatment planning: some SLPs choose to treat phonemes in order according to the order of acquisition with the assumption that early acquired sounds are easier to learn than later acquired sounds. The production of stop phonemes such as /p, t/ require less fine force control than fricatives, in which it is necessary to create just the right amount of vocal tract closure to create turbulence in the air flow. Some phonemes have difficult articulatory configurations, such as the narrow groove in /s/ or the three places of constriction in /ɹ/. **Input frequency** also plays a role, however: if the child hears a sound frequently in the input language, that sound is likely to emerge earlier in the child's speech (Stokes & Surendran, 2005). The phoneme /s/ is a very frequently occurring phoneme in English, which explains why it has an early age of customary production; the late age of mastery may be due to its articulatory complexity. Some phonemes occur frequently and are easy to produce but are acquired late nonetheless: consider /ð/, which is acquired between

Table 2–7. *Examples of Developmental, Nondevelopmental, and Atypical Speech Sound Errors*

Example of Error	Error Type	Justification
Girl, aged 3;9		
"ham" /hæm/ → [hæm̃]	Atypical	Less than 5% of children aged 3 to 8 years denasalize nasals.
"coat" /kot/ → [tot]	Nondevelopmental	More than 5% of children front velars between age 2 and 3 years but /k/ should be mastered by 90% of girls before age 3;6.
"leaf" /leaf/ → [wif]	Developmental	Normal limit for acquisition of /l/ in girls is 5 years.
Boy, aged 6;6		
"sun" /sʌn/ → [ʂʌn]	Atypical	Lateral lisp is always atypical; less than 5% of children aged 3 to 8 produce this error and there is no improving trend with age.
"ban" /væn/ → [bæn]	Nondevelopmental	Although common at age 2 years, this error is rare past the age of 5 years.
"jam" /dʒæm/ → [dzæm]	Developmental	The age of acquisition for /dʒ/ in boys is 7 years.
Boy, aged 4;6		
"deer" /diɚ/ → [giɚ]	Atypical	Backing of coronal consonants is always atypical; less than 5% of children aged 3 to 8 years produce this error.
"leaf" /lif/ → [lis]	Nondevelopmental	Substitution of s/f is common at younger ages but /f/ should be mastered at 3;6.
"sun" /sʌn/ → [ʂʌ]	Developmental	The age of acquisition for /s/ in boys is 7 to 9 years and dental distortion is a common error at all ages.

4;6 and 7 years even though it occurs very often in English. One hypothesis for its late occurrence is low **functional load**, meaning that the phoneme does not form many minimal pairs in English. When a phoneme has low functional load, there is no loss in meaning if the child mispronounces the sound and the child may fail to learn the phonological contrast. Imagine, for example, if the child says "I need the coat" /aɪ nid ðə kot/ → [aɪ nid də tot]; the mother may misunderstand and give the child the "tote" that is in the closet alongside the "coat" but she will have no trouble understanding the word "the." In this scenario, there is more information provided to learn the /t/-/k/ contrast. The phoneme /v/ is another phoneme that has low functional load, possibly explaining its late emergence in English even though it is acquired early in other languages in which it has high input frequency and functional load. The impact of all these variables means that it is difficult to predict whether any given phoneme will be easy or difficult for a child to learn because the error may be due to input factors (the child's experience with or perception of the input), phonological factors (the child's organization of representations abstracted from the input), and/or output factors (the child's ability to produce the articulatory gestures). Furthermore, it is usually more efficient to consider patterns of phoneme error when planning treatment for a child with many speech errors.

2.3.2 Phonological Process Norms

One indication that a toddler is transitioning from a word-based to a phoneme-based phonology is the appearance of predictable phonological processes in the child's speech, that is, speech error patterns of the type described in Table 1–6. These error patterns suggest that the child is abandoning lexical contrast as phoneme level knowledge emerges in the lexicon. Consider as a hypothetical example a toddler who has a preference for a CVCV word template with reduplication. The child produces velar consonants with great inconsistency: "egg" /ɛg/ → [gəgə], "tiger" /taɪgɚ/ → [taɪtaɪ], "piggie" /pɪgi/ → [pibi], "chicken" /tʃɪkɪn/ → [xɪxɪ], "rocket" /ɹɒkɪt/ →[wʌtʌ], and "cracker" /kɹækɚ/ → [kɹækə]. A year later, after much reorganization of his phonology, these productions change to: "egg" /ɛg/ → [ɛd], "tiger" /taɪgɚ/ → [taɪdɚ], "piggie" /pɪgi/ → [pɪdi], "chicken" /tʃɪkɪn/ → [tsɪtɪn], "rocket" /ɹɒkɪt/ →[wɔtɪt], and "cracker" /kɹækɚ/ → [twætə]. Many changes have occurred: the shape of each word is now matched and the production of specific consonants is now predictable. The velar consonants are now consistently fronted, which means that the word "cracker," which was produced more or less correctly in the past, is now produced incorrectly to fit with the patterns of velar fronting and liquid gliding. These simplification errors rise rapidly during this transition period and then disappear as the child's knowledge of phoneme contrasts increases during the preschool period. For this reason, phonological process errors are most frequent during the ages 2 and 3 years and decline through the age of 5 years.

In order to determine if a child is producing a phonological process error, it is best to elicit at least five exemplars of each speech sound in word-initial and word-final positions and use strict criteria for identifying the presence of each process. Three different kinds of phonological error patterns might be observed in the child's speech: (1) **syllable structure processes** change the shape of the target words, usually by deleting segments or entire syllables; (2) **harmony processes** simplify the word by making the segments in the word more similar to each other; and (3) **substitution processes** neutralize phonological contrasts by substituting one phoneme for another.

> **Practice 2–7**
>
> Review the phonological processes listed in Table 1–6 of Chapter 1 and classify each process by type (either a syllable structure process, a harmony process, or a substitution process).

The criteria that are applied to identify phonological processes are meant to ensure that the errors observed in the child's speech actually form a phonological error pattern. Therefore, errors that apply to one specific speech sound will be excluded and errors that are not phonological in nature will also be excluded. These criteria are summarized in Table 2–8. First, a phonological process error must simplify the target sound or word shape. The error must be phonological in nature, typically leading to neutralization of a phonological contrast. This means that distortion errors are excluded from the category of phonological processes. The error must occur across a natural class of phonemes. For example,

if the pattern appears to be stopping of fricatives, several fricative phonemes must be subject to stopping. If stopping is only observed for the phoneme /ð/, the pattern is not stopping. This is a common miscoding of phonological processes; /ð/ → [d] occurs frequently but usually the other phoneme in this class is produced /θ/ → [f]. The fact that these two interdental fricatives are not subject to the same pattern shows that neither error is a phonological process. Rather each is an isolated articulation error that applies to a specific phoneme. In contrast if all the sibilant fricatives /s,ʃ,z,ʒ/ are produced as stops, then it is proper to conclude that the child is stopping these fricatives. Within a natural class of phonemes the

Table 2–8. *Criteria for Identifying Phonological Processes (Phonological Error Patterns) in a Speech Sample*

Include	Exclude
The error must simplify the target phoneme or word shape, e.g., "sunshine" /sʌnʃaɪn/ → [sʌnsaɪn]	Complex errors, as in phonemic paraphasias, e.g., "sunshine" /sʌnʃaɪn/ → [ʃʌnseɪn] e.g., "sunshine" /sʌnʃaɪn/ → [sʌnʃaʊwɚ]
The error must be phonemic, e.g., "sunshine" /sʌnʃaɪn/ → [tʌntaɪn]	Distortion (phonetic) errors are excluded, e.g., "sunshine" /sʌnʃaɪn/ → [s̺ʌnʃaɪn]
The error applies to a natural class of phonemes that share similar features, e.g., "sunshine" /sʌnʃaɪn/ → [tʌntaɪn]	Isolated phoneme errors are excluded, e.g., /ð/ → [d] and /θ/ → [f] or /ɹ/ → [ɻ] and /l/ → [n]
The error must be predictable even if not consistent, e.g., "sunshine" /sʌnʃaɪn/ → [tʌntaɪn], "suntan" /sʌntæn/ →[tʌntæn], "sunny" /sʌni/ → [sʌni]	Errors that are unpredictable and inconsistent, e.g., "sunshine" /sʌnʃaɪn/ → [tʌnsaɪn], "suntan" /sʌntæn/ →[jʌntæn], "sunny" /sʌni/ → [ʃʌni]
The error must occur with sufficient frequency, e.g., in at least 20% of the obligatory contexts	The error occurs only occasionally or only when producing certain words.

error should be predictable even if it is not consistent. There may be an alternation between correct productions of the target and the error pattern but there should not be random, unpredictable errors. Finally, the error patterns should occur with at least 20% frequency across the obligatory contexts that are affected by the rule. For example, if it appears that the child is stopping in the onset position, then all of the sibilant fricatives in the word-initial position should be examined for the occurrence of stopping; if stopping occurs on more than 20% of these targets, then it can be concluded that the child is using the stopping process.

The child's use of phonological processes can be compared with age expectations. With respect to phonological processes the researcher investigates the age at which children use the process frequently (this is the **expected age** for use of the process) and the age at which children typically stop using the process (this is the **age of suppression** or the age at which use of the process is suppressed). There are several studies that have documented phonological process use by young children (Cahill Haelsig & Madison, 1986; Dodd, Holm, Hua, & Crosbie, 2003; Hodson & Paden, 1981; Lowe, Knutson, & Monson, 1985; McIntosh & Dodd, 2008; Porter & Hodson, 2001; Preisser, Hodson, & Paden, 1988). Unfortunately the amount and type of speech data collected varies widely and the coding systems used in these studies can be rather idiosyncratic. These kinds of discrepancies across studies in methods are known to impact the outcomes of normative studies (Edwards & Beckman, 2008). Characteristics of the word stimuli have a significant impact on children's production accuracy. In other words, a child might produce a phoneme such as /ʃ/ correctly in a simple word

("bush" /bʊʃ/ → [bʊʃ]) but have difficulty when the phoneme appears in a complex context ("shrew" /ʃɹu/ → [swu]) or in a word that has more syllables ("toothbrush" /tuθbɹʌʃ/ → [tufbwʌts]). Elicitation, scoring, and transcription procedures also have an important impact on outcomes. Even though there is not perfect agreement across studies for the ages at which certain processes can be expected in young children's speech, a rough guide can be created by looking for areas of consensus.

Table 2–9 lists phonological error patterns according to the ages at which they commonly occur. The phonological patterns may be expected at the age indicated and at all younger ages but they should be suppressed at all older ages. If a child is

Table 2–9. Expected Age Ranges for Occurrence of Phonological Error Patterns

Age Range	Error Patterns
1 to 2 years	Assimilation patterns Voicing and devoicing patterns Final consonant deletion Fronting (velars, palatals) Stopping
2 to 3 years	Glottal replacement Cluster reduction Weak syllable deletion
3 to 5 years	Liquid simplification Deaffrication
Atypical at any age	Denasalization Affrication Gliding of fricatives Backing alveolars to velar place

producing the error pattern with greater than 20% frequency and is older than the "expected age" as indicated in this table, there would be cause for concern about the child's speech development. Harmony patterns include labial and alveolar assimilation as well as prevocalic voicing and postvocalic devoicing. These are most likely to occur before the age of 2 years and decline rapidly thereafter. Fronting errors may involve both velar stops and palatal fricatives; the age of suppression is reported to be as early as 24 months in some studies and as late as 36 months in others. It seems clear that fronting should not be a pervasive pattern in the child's speech past the age of 24 to 30 months, with the exception of n/ŋ substitutions in words such as "running" /ɹʌnɪŋ/ → [ɹʌnɪn]. Similarly, stopping should be suppressed before the third birthday with the exception of isolated speech errors such as "this" /ðɪs/ → [dɪs]. Between the ages of 3 and 4 years cluster reduction, glottal replacement, and weak syllable deletion should show a marked reduction in frequency, although these errors may reappear at later ages when the child is attempting complex words. In other words, at age 36 months the child may produce "clown" /klaʊn/ → [kwaʊn] and "banana" /bənænʌ/ → [bənænʌ], indicating suppression of cluster reduction and weak syllable deletion. Nonetheless, words such as "spaghetti" /spəgɛɾi/ → [pʊsgɛɾi] and "vegetables" /vɛdʒtəblz/ → [vɛʒboz] might be difficult for several more years. The liquid simplification errors of liquid gliding in syllable onsets and vowelization of liquids in the nucleus or coda position are common between 3 and 5 years. Thereafter some children will produce correct productions of /ɹ/, while others will produce a derhotacized distortion before acquiring this late developing phoneme. The frequency of occurrence of deaffrication errors (as in "church" /tʃɝtʃ/ → [ʃɝʃ]) is unclear in the literature: the normal limit for acquisition of /tʃ/ and /dʒ/ is not until age 6 or 7 years; the typical phonological process is difficult to establish because children produce a variety of errors for these phonemes, including stopping, fronting, and deaffrication, but none of the error types occur with greater than 20% frequency in all studies. Finally, some error patterns are seen on clinical caseloads but are very rare in the general population of English-speaking children, specifically gliding of fricatives, affrication, denasalization, and backing. These error patterns are clear indicators of an SSD when they occur with greater than 20% frequency in the child's speech.

Describing children's speech errors in terms of phonological patterns has significant clinical implications. First, the phonological process norms provide an important perspective on the child's level of phonological development. If a 5-year-old child misarticulates the /s,ʃ,z,ʒ,tʃ,dʒ/ sounds, the SLP could conclude that the child is producing developmental errors that are not particularly concerning because the normal limit for acquisition of these phonemes is between 6 and 9 years of age. However, if the child is stopping all of these phonemes, the phonological process norms indicate that this pattern should be suppressed before the age of 3 years, and it becomes clear that this is in fact a very significant speech delay.

Describing children's errors in terms of phonological processes also has implications for treatment planning. As will be discussed in more detail in Chapter 5, all the phonemes that are affected by the phonological process can be targeted in speech therapy with the goal of helping the child to suppress the process of stopping these sibilants. This approach is more efficient than treating each phoneme as an isolated speech error.

There are some pitfalls to the phonological process approach that should be considered when applying this approach to assessment or treatment planning. The underlying theory assumes that the children have adultlike phonological representations for the phonemes that they are learning. Speech errors arise from an innate mechanism that simplifies the phonemes according to universal rules, anticipating inevitable constraints on speech motor control in early development. As the child matures, the processes are gradually suppressed, following a predictable schedule. These assumptions are not supported by research evidence, as reviewed in Rvachew and Brosseau-Lapré (2018). Most importantly, it is clear that many children with SSD do not have adultlike underlying phonological representations; therefore it is necessary to assess underlying perceptual and phonological knowledge directly and to conduct deeper analyses of the children's phonological systems in many cases before selecting treatment goals and an approach to treatment. Furthermore, it is necessary to be aware that children's speech error patterns are often less consistent than one would expect from the phonological process perspective. For example, Smit (1993) noted that prevocalic voicing applied to stop consonants but not fricatives. Stopping occurred with greater frequency for /f v ð z/ than for /θ s ʃ/. Stopping and fronting were much more common in word-initial than word-final position. Final consonant deletion was much less likely for targets /k g tʃ dʒ/ in comparison to other obstruents.

In addition to these differences in process production across word posi-

tions, a great deal of variability in the types of errors that are produced within a word position can occur, even by the same child. Furthermore, and especially on clinical caseloads, many children produce error patterns that are difficult to discern because they are idiosyncratic and yet fully predictable. For example, Rvachew and Andrews (2002) present a detailed case study in which the child substituted glides for voiced sounds but only in the ambisyllabic position. At first glance the child's speech error patterns were inconsistent but ultimately her errors were found to be predictable in every case. When children have SSD it is necessary to consider that they may not have adultlike underlying representations and that they may have error patterns that are more complex than the discrete set of natural phonological processes presented in Table 1–6.

2.3.3 Acquisition of Prosodic Units

A phonological process description of child speech considers error patterns that affect phonemes (substitution processes) and error patterns that affect word structure (harmony and syllable structure processes). Taking syllable structure into account was a significant advance over the traditional analysis by SODA (substitutions, omissions, distortions, additions), which considered only phoneme accuracy. However, the description of the child's syllable structure errors is somewhat constrained by the limited number of patterns that are considered in most clinical analyses. Although weak syllable deletion, final consonant deletion, and cluster reduction are the most frequently occurring patterns in English, many other kinds of syllable structure errors may be observed, especially on clinical caseloads. Some of these rare syllable structure errors make phonological sense when viewed from the perspective of nonlinear phonology. A full understanding of the underlying nature of these error patterns requires a detailed nonlinear analysis, as described in Bernhardt and Stemberger (2000), Velleman (2002), and Rvachew and Brosseau-Lapré (2018). Although nonlinear analysis will not be covered here, some of the more common error types that occur during the acquisition of weak syllables and consonant clusters will be presented so that they can be recognized when encountered in children's speech.

Several studies have documented in detail the difficulties that young children have when attempting to produce multi-syllabic words (Echols, 1993; Klein, 1981; Snow, 1998). These studies confirm some universal patterns for simplifying difficult words. In English, deleting weak syllables in an iambic context is especially common. However, it is not the only strategy used by young children. A variety of patterns involving **syllable deletion** and **syllable weakening** are shown in Table 2–10. The examples are drawn from various samples recorded for research purposes from 18- and 24-month-old children with normally developing speech or from older children with SSDs (MacLeod, Laukys, & Rvachew, 2011; Rvachew & Andrews, 2002). It can be seen that weak syllables are sometimes deleted in the trochaic context (strong-weak) as well as in the iambic context (weak-strong). More surprisingly, strong syllables are sometimes deleted as well. Another pattern that reduces the number of syllables in the word is **coalescence**, in which one syllable combines the phonetic characteristics of two. Some syllable weakening strategies serve

to maintain the number of syllables in the word: at the same time, reduplication and assimilation reduce the phonetic challenge by repeating syllables or sounds. Neutralization also simplifies the word, in this case by substituting glides for consonants in weak syllables. Finally, some children employ a "filler syllable" that can be substituted for weak syllables as a kind of place holder for the actual phonetic content. Presumably filler syllables reduce the phonological planning challenge when the child is aware of the syllable but not quite sure of the sounds that are in it. The example shown in Table 2–10 is taken from a longer sample in which the child substituted a variant of [ɪn] for every weak syllable in iambic and trochaic contexts.

Snow (1998) and Echols (1993) have proposed that these strategies for simplifying multisyllabic words are used because the child has poor perceptual knowledge of the acoustic-phonetic information in syllables that are weakened or deleted. This hypothesis is justified by the finding that syllables with **low perceptual prominence** are most vulnerable to weakening or deletion. The syllables within an utterance that have the lowest perceptual prominence are those that have the least duration, amplitude, and pitch change. Furthermore, there is some experimental evidence that children store salient stress patterns of words along with incomplete phoneme information when learning new words. The stored representations for the most prominent parts of speech input will be more complete and the representations for the least prominent input will be less complete. Therefore, if the mother says, "Eat your apple honey," the stressed syllables may have the most complete representations because they are produced louder with prominent pitch changes:

Table 2–10. *Error Patterns Involving Syllable Deletion or Syllable Weakening*

Error Pattern	Examples
Syllable Deletion	
Weak syllable deletion (iamb)	"spaghetti" /spəˈgɛɾi/ →[dɛɾi]
	"umbrella" /əmˈbɹɛlʌ/ → [bɹɛlʌ]
	"banana" /bəˈnænʌ/ → [nænæ]
Weak syllable deletion (trochee)	"water" /ˈwɑtɚ/ → [waɪ]
	"button" /ˈbʌtən/ → [bæ]
	"butterfly" /ˈbʌtɚˈflaɪ/ → [bʌfaɪ]
Strong syllable deletion	"ladybug" /ˈleɪdiˈbʌg/ → [idɑħ]
	"elevator" /ˈɛləˈvetɚ/ → [vetɚ]
Coalescence	"flowers" /ˈflaʊɚz/ → [fæs]
	"balloons" /bəˈlunz/ → [bɹunz]
Syllable Weakening	
Reduplication	"table" /ˈteɪbəl/ → [bʌbʌ]
	"umbrella" /əmˈbɹɛlʌ/ → [bələlʌ]
Assimilation	"doggie" /ˈdɑgi/ → [gɑgi]
Neutralization	"potato" /pəˈteɪtoʊ/ → [bədejo]
	"tomato" /təˈmeɪtoʊ/ → [wəmejo]
Filler syllable	"cabin" /ˈkæbɪn/ → [tænɪn]
	"Kellog" /ˈkɛlɔg/ → [tɛnɪn]
	"wagon" /ˈwægən/ → [wanɪn]
	"pocket" /ˈpɑkət/ → [pɑtɪn]

"EAT your APple HONey." The second syllables in the words "apple" and "honey" are also unstressed, but they have some extra prominence because word-final and sentence-final syllables are lengthened: "EAT your APple HONey." The word "your" in this sentence will be produced with a short unstressed vowel, [jɚ], and will be the most difficult one for the child to learn as it has the lowest perceptual prominence. Descriptive and experimental studies (Gerken, 1996; Richtsmeier, Goffman, & Hogan, 2009; Snow, 1998) show that language learning is determined by a combination of input factors (How frequent and salient is the input?), perceptual factors (How easy is it for the child to process particular parts of the input?), linguistic factors (How complex is the underlying linguistic structure?), and production factors (How difficult is it to articulate the structure?).

Practice 2–8

Consider the sentence "She watches the baby." Write this sentence down but use ALL CAPS for the stressed syllables and underline syllables at the end of words and at the end of the sentence. Which syllables are most likely to be deleted or produced incorrectly by a young child? Repeat this process with the word "alligator."

(4) age of acquisition for a cluster is often the same as the age of acquisition for the phonemes that make up the cluster.

Practice 2–9

Make a list of words, each with a unique cluster in the word-initial position. Make another list of words with clusters in the word final position. How many different clusters do you find in these positions for the English language?

Difficulties with perceptual knowledge may also account for errors in the production of consonant sequences, in combination with articulatory and phonological factors (Kirk & Demuth, 2005; Rvachew, Leroux, & Brosseau-Lapré, 2014; Yavas & McLeod, 2010). Certainly the English language presents a particular challenge to young children with the great variety and complexity of clusters that occur in onsets and codas in word-initial, word-final, and within-word positions. At least 17 different error patterns have been observed for word-initial clusters alone and the developmental path toward mastery of clusters is long and winding (McLeod, Van Doorn, & Reed, 2001). Very few generalizations about the development of clusters may be made because there is much variability between children. Furthermore, children may each change the way they produce different clusters from one incorrect form to another before they settle on the correct form. However, it is safe to say that (1) complex codas tend to be acquired before complex onsets (Kirk & Demuth, 2005); (2) two-element clusters are usually acquired before three-element clusters; (3) the typical pathway is from cluster reduction through cluster simplification and then completely correct production;

Phonologists have proposed explanations for children's variable cluster productions that assume developmental change in knowledge of underlying phonological structure as well as accumulating knowledge of the phonetic input. Different types of cluster realization for syllable initial clusters (also known as **complex onsets**) will be discussed here. As shown in Table 2–11, the earliest realization of these forms involves reduction to a single phoneme. Typically the least sonorant phoneme in the cluster is retained. At the earliest stage of cluster reduction, some children appear to have no underlying knowledge of the structure that is called **branching onset** in nonlinear phonology: this is the structure that permits two consonants in the onset of the syllable. In this case the child puts one of the consonants in the onset—specifically the least sonorant member of the pair. The child ignores the other consonant and in fact may have no perceptual awareness of it. Several examples of this pattern are shown in Table 2–11 and one is illustrated in Part A of Figure 2–2. The end result is a syllable that conforms to the **Sonority Sequencing Principle** discussed in Chapter 1: the least sonorant sounds should be

Table 2–11. Various Cluster Realization Types in Syllable Initial Position

Cluster Type	Specific Forms	Example Word
Reduce Cluster to Least Sonorant Consonant		
Stop + liquid	/pɹ/, /bɹ/, /tɹ/, /dɹ/, /kɹ/, /gɹ/, /pl/, /bl/, /kl/, /gl/	"bleed" /blid/ → [bid]
Fricative + glide/liquid	/sw/, /θɹ/, /fɹ/, /vɹ/, /ʃɹ/, /sl/, /fl/	"sweep" /swip/ → [sip]
Fricative + nasal	/sn/, /sm/	"snow" /snoʊ/ → [soʊ]
/s/ + stop	/st/, /sp/, /sk/	"stop" /stɑp/ → [tɑp]
Reduce Cluster to More Sonorant Consonant		
Fricative + nasal	/sn/, /sm/	"smoke" /smok/ → [mok]
Reduce Cluster with Coalescence		
Fricative + glide/liquid	/sw/, /fɹ/, /ʃɹ/, /sl/, /fl/	"sweep" /swip/ → [fip]
Cluster Simplification		
Stop + liquid	/pɹ/, /bɹ/, /tɹ/, /dɹ/, /kɹ/, /gɹ/, /pl/, /bl/, /kl/, /gl/	"grow" /gɹoʊ/ → [dwoʊ]
Fricative + glide/liquid	/sw/, /fɹ/, /ʃɹ/, /sl/, /fl/	"fly" /flaɪ/ → [fwaɪ]
Fricative + nasal	/sn/, /sm/	"sneeze" /sniz/ → [s̩niz̩]
/s/ + stop	/st/, /sp/, /sk/	"speɪs" /speɪs/ → [s̩peɪs̩]
Epenthesis		
Stop + liquid	/pɹ/, /bɹ/, /tɹ/, /dɹ/, /kɹ/, /gɹ/, /pl/, /bl/, /kl/, /gl/	"play" /pleɪ/ → [pəleɪ]
Fricative + glide/liquid	/sw/, /fɹ/, /ʃɹ/, /sl/, /fl/	"fry" /fɹaɪ/ → [fəɹaɪ]
Fricative + nasal	/sn/, /sm/	"snake" /sneɪk/ → [səneɪk]

at the edges of the syllable and the most sonorant sounds should be at its center.

Gradually, however, the child acquires greater knowledge of the two consonants in the onset and reorganizes phonological knowledge of the underlying structure. At this stage the child's speech output will be unchanged for most clusters. In other words, clusters will be produced with a single consonant, typically the least sonorant member of the pair, as indicated in Table 2–11. Part B of Figure 2–2 indicates that the underlying structure of the complex onset has changed, however, to represent the branching onset: both consonants are represented underlying but one has been **delinked** so that it does not appear in the output. In some clusters the difference in sonorancy between the two consonants in the cluster is so small that it is hard to work out which one should remain in the surface form. Specifically,

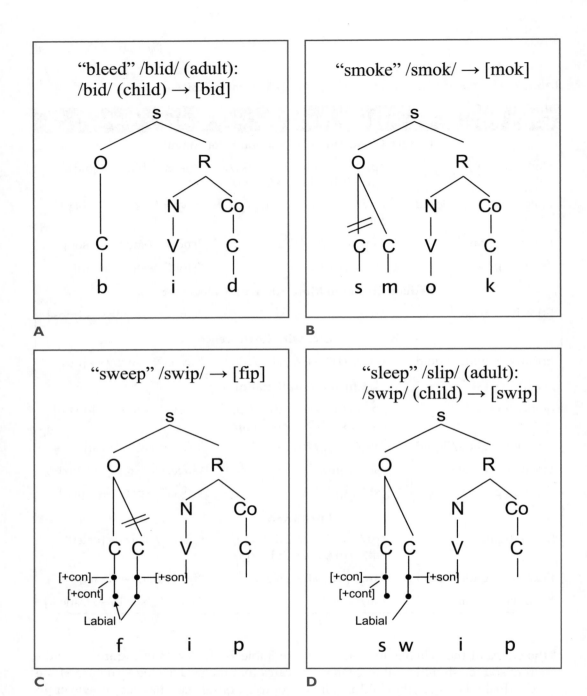

Figure 2–2. *Illustration of underlying representations for four words with incorrect cluster realization in the surface form.* **A.** *No knowledge of branching onset leads to representation of the least sonorant consonant in the onset and cluster reduction.* **B.** *Although the branching onset is represented underlying, the first segment is delinked, resulting in cluster reduction in the surface form. Either the /s/ or the /m/ may be delinked because they are close in sonority.* **C.** *The [Labial] place feature spreads from the second segment, which is delinked, to the first segment, resulting in coalescence.* **D.** *The branching onset structure is represented underlyingly and two segments are produced in the surface form but /l/ is simplified to [w].*

fricatives and nasals are both relatively sonorant in comparison to stop consonants. In the case of /s/ + nasal clusters, the child may alternate between /s/ onset ([sok]) and nasal onset ([mok]) productions. The other cluster types will continue to be produced as before because the least sonorant consonant is easier to identify.

A pattern that confirms the presence of the branching onset in the underlying representation is **coalescence**. In Part C of Figure 2–2 the onset is represented with two segments: a fricative ([+consonantal] [+continuant]) that is unmarked for place, meaning that it defaults to [Coronal], that is /s/; and the glide [+sonorant] that is specified as [Labial] place. The coalescence is shown as the spreading of the feature [Labial] from the second segment [w] to the place node of the first segment [s] which turns it into /f/. The second segment is delinked, which creates "sweep" /swip/ → [fip]. Coalescence can occur without delinking of the second segment and therefore the child might also produce "sweep" /swip/ → [fwip]. In either case, a segment was produced that combines features from the two phonemes that are supposed to be in the cluster; therefore, the production indicates that the underlying representation contains both segments, /s/ and /w/. Spreading errors provide important clues to the child's underlying representations because features will only spread to unmarked nodes. Additional examples of interesting spreading patterns are shown by Bernhard and colleagues (Bernhardt & Stemberger, 1998, 2000; Bernhardt & Stoel-Gammon, 1994) as well as by Rvachew and Brosseau-Lapré (2018).

Once the branching onset structure has been acquired in the underlying phonology, cluster reduction patterns may give way to cluster simplification. This pattern involves producing both consonants, but at least one will be produced with a nonstandard articulation. Particularly common between 2 and 3 years of age is the production of glide clusters in place of liquid clusters, as shown in Table 2–11 and Part D of Figure 2–2. In these productions the branching onset structure is present but the second segment is represented as a glide rather than a liquid. Later, the child may acquire knowledge of the liquid features ([+consonantal] [+sonorant]) but produce distortions in place of the liquid sounds in the clusters, as in "pretty" /pɹɪɾi/ → [pwɪɾi] at age 30 months but "pretty" /pɹɪɾi/ → [pɹɪɾi] at age 42 months.

Another strategy for simplifying the production of clusters in the onset is **epenthesis**—as shown in Table 2–11, a neutral vowel is inserted between the two segments so that the word sounds as if it has an extra syllable. It is possible that the child is creating a new syllable structure to avoid the branching onset in the underlying representation. Alternatively, the underlying representation may be adultlike but epenthesis results from slow articulation that eases production of consonant sequences that are difficult to coarticulate.

One final point about cluster realization patterns is that acquisition of /s/ + stop clusters may take a different path than that observed for the other /s/ clusters. Some phonologists suggest that the underlying structure of /s/ + stop clusters is unique because these clusters violate the Sonority Sequencing Principle: in a word such as "stop," the first segment /s/ is less sonorant than the second segment /t/. Therefore it is proposed that the /s/ is not part of the onset; in fact it is not even part of the syllable but is an "appendix." On the other hand in a word such as "sweep," the second segment /w/ is more sonorant than /s/ and the middle segment /i/ is the most sonorant of all and therefore the word is perfectly consistent with the Sonority Sequencing Principle. All the clusters that begin with a stop or a fricative followed by a glide, liquid, or nasal are consistent with this principle. Therefore it is not surprising that the most frequent complex onsets observed in the phonetic repertoires of toddler speech were /w/ clusters followed closely by nasal clusters in the longitudinal study reported by McLeod, Van Doorn, and Reed (2001). Furthermore, the /l/ clusters were the earliest clusters to be produced correctly by the 2-year-olds followed by McLeod et al. (2001). Acquisition of the /s/ + stop clusters was variable, however, with some children producing these clusters early and others later in their third year. In fact, these studies of cluster development reveal the most important truths about phonological development: children achieve adultlike speech ability in their own way; further, a mix of perceptual, articulatory, and phonological factors accounts for variability in this developmental course between children. In order to determine if any one child requires special assistance to achieve adultlike speech within the expected time frame, careful assessment of the child's skills in all these domains is required.

Box 2–3. Phonological Development: Key Points

- Customary production means the child is producing the phoneme correctly more often than not.
- Mastery means the child is producing the phoneme correctly at least 90% of the time.
- The age of acquisition is the age at which 90% of children have mastered the phoneme or are producing it at the level of customary production (depending upon the norms).
- The consonants in English are mastered by the age of 9 years in typical development.
- It is common for children to misarticulate a natural class of sounds with the same error pattern. These error patterns are referred to as phonological processes.
- Many phonological processes are suppressed before age 3 years and all should be suppressed before age 5 years with small exceptions for complex words.
- The course of phonological acquisition for each child is determined by input factors (input frequency and saliency), phonological factors (knowledge of underlying representations), and output factors (articulatory complexity).

Chapter 2 Study Questions

In each paragraph, fill in the blanks with the number of the appropriate words or phrases shown in the list at the bottom.

Question 1: Speech Perception Development

The first stage of speech perception development is said to be _____ because the characteristics of speech perception for hearing infants are roughly similar for all infants during this period. Between the ages of 6 and 12 months, the infant transitions from the _____ to the _____ stage of perceptual development. One famous study found that English-learning infants stopped responding to a Hindi consonant contrast after this transition. One mechanism that causes this change in perceptual responding is _____. Changes in perception in the first year are not just about speech sounds. The infant is also attending to phonotactics and stress patterns in words. The infant's learning about one aspect of speech supports learning about other aspects of speech, a mechanism called _____. At the end of the first year, the infant is aware of phonetic contrasts, allophones, rhythmic patterns, and phonotactic characteristics of the language being learned. The next transition, in the second year of life, is the shift to _____ as toddlers use their phonetic perceptual abilities to recognize meaningful words and associate those words with the appropriate referents. Early speech perception development is correlated with later language skills, especially growth in vocabulary, which in turn supports the emergence of _____. However, _____ may not emerge without reading instruction in school.

1	language-specific phonetic perception
2	phonemic perception
3	language-general phonetic perception
4	explicit phonological awareness skills
5	prosodic bootstrapping
6	universal
7	statistical learning
8	implicit phonological awareness skills

Question 2: Early Speech Production Development

The phonation stage is from birth to approximately 2 months of age and is characterized by the infant's production of _____. There is a peak in the frequency of goos during the _____. During the _____ the infant systematically explores many parameters of speech, leading to a greater variety of vocalizations. The most speechlike vocalization produced during this stage is the _____. The fourth stage, _____ occurs on average at the age of _____, and always by _____ in normally developing infants. The final stage is the _____, which lasts roughly to the age of _____.

1	expansion stage
2	18 months
3	7 months
4	canonical babbling
5	11 months
6	fully resonant vowel
7	integrative stage
8	primitive articulation stage
9	quasi-resonant vowels

Question 3: First Words

The most common utterance type observed in the speech of 1-year-olds was the _____. Also common were _____, produced with approximately 20% frequency. By 2 years of age, toddlers have expanded their syllable shape repertoire to include _____ and _____. In terms of consonants, toddlers should produce 9–10 _____, including exemplars from the classes of _____. They should also produce 5–6 _____, mostly _____ but including a representative of the _____ classes.

1	closed syllables
2	final consonants
3	glide clusters
4	CV syllables
5	initial consonants
6	stops, nasals, fricatives, and glides
7	stops
8	nasal, fricative, and liquid
9	single vowel

Question 4: Phoneme Acquisition Norms

Two important points along the continuum from no accuracy to perfect accuracy for a speech sound are: (1) _____—the child produces the phoneme correctly more often than not, or at least 51% correct; and (2) _____—the child produces the phoneme with almost or perfect accuracy, that is, at least 90% correct. The age at which 90% of all children have acquired a phoneme is called the _____ or the _____. Often but not always, _____ acquire phonemes earlier than _____. In general, _____ tend to be acquired before _____. If the child is younger than the expected age of acquisition, the error is _____ because there is still some time for the child to acquire the phoneme. A _____ error is a speech error that will probably not correct unless the child receives speech therapy because the child is older than the expected age of acquisition. When the error is very unusual, occurring in the speech of fewer than 5% of children, the error is _____.

1	stops and glides
2	boys
3	nondevelopmental
4	normal limit for acquisition
5	age of acquisition
6	liquids and fricatives
7	customary production
8	developmental
9	mastery
10	atypical
11	girls

Question 5: Phoneme Acquisition and Phonological Process Norms

Pretend that you have assessed the speech of a boy aged 4 years and 0 months. You notice that he produces the errors "key" /ki/ → [ti], "pocket" /pɑkɪt/ → [pɑtɪt], and "pack" /pæk/ → [pæt]. This error pattern is called _____ and is _____. Although all the other fricatives are produced correctly, you notice that he says "this" /ðɪs/ → /dɪs/ and "tooth" /tuθ/ → [tuf]; these errors are called _____ errors and are _____. A group of errors affecting /l/ and /ɹ/, including "rat" /ɹæt/ → [wæt], "carry" /kɛɹi/ → [kɛɹi], "ball" /bɑl/ → [bɑo], "car" /kɑɹ/ → [kɑo], and "puddle" /pʌdl/ → [pʌdo], represents _____ and is _____.

1	expected
2	liquid simplification
3	fronting
4	not expected
5	developmental
6	isolated phoneme errors

Question 6: Acquisition of Prosodic Units

Pretend that you have assessed the speech of a girl aged 18 months and have noticed a variety of prosodic errors in her speech. Her production of weak syllables represents a number of different types of error, including weak syllable deletion (e.g., _____), strong syllable deletion (e.g., _____), coalescence (e.g., _____), reduplication (e.g., _____), and neutralization (e.g., _____). Her production of word-initial clusters represents a number of different realizations, including cluster reduction (e.g., _____), coalescence (e.g., _____), cluster simplification (e.g., _____), and epenthesis (e.g., _____).

1	"sleep" /slip/ → /fip/
2	"tomato" /təmeɾo/ → [meɾo]
3	"zucchini" /zukini/ → [zkini]
4	"basket" /bæskɪt/ → [bæbæ]
5	"dinosaur" /daɪnosɔɚ/ → [daɪjɪtɔə]
6	"apple" /æpl̩/ → [po]
7	"fried" /fraɪd/ → [fwaɪd]
8	smile /smaɪl/ → [səmaɪo]
9	please /pliz/ → [pis]

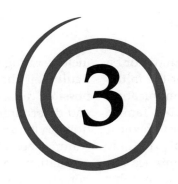

Assessment

Learning Objectives

- Describe the main purposes of an assessment.
- Compare standardized, informal, norm-referenced, criterion, static, and dynamic types of measurement tools.
- Identify the background information collected through the case history.
- List the typical components of a speech assessment.
- Describe advantages and disadvantages of single-word measures of speech accuracy.
- Define cultural competence.

Chapter 2 described the course of normal phonological development, which involves the integration of complex knowledge at multiple levels of representation. As the child is gradually acquiring intelligible and accurate speech, he or she becomes increasingly independent at interacting socially with others, learning new skills, and participating in activities with family members and in the community. However, when a child is not acquiring speech at the same rate and in a similar way as other children of the same age, the speech-language pathologist (SLP) will likely be asked to assess the child's communication skills.

Parents will often contact an SLP to express concerns about their child's speech following a change in the environmental context. For instance, a transition from home to daycare or to a new child care center, a new sibling, or upcoming school entry may provide opportunities to notice differences in their child's speech relative to other children of the same age. Transitional events may challenge their child's capacity to function or participate in their home or in the community, likely increasing anxiety and frustration by the child or parent in the face of those challenges. When parents identify a problem with their child's speech, their description will usually have a comparative aspect: the child is not speaking as clearly as expected. In some cases, referral for a speech-language assessment may not be initiated by the parents; rather the initial concern about the child's communication skills may be raised by another family member, the child's teacher, or a medical professional, leading to a referral to the SLP.

Assessing the child's communication abilities is one of the most important roles of the SLP, since a comprehensive evaluation is the foundation for the design of the speech-language intervention. "Our treatment programs follow directly from the assessment and diagnosis of the disorder and therefore, can only be as effective as the assessment is thorough and the diagnosis is accurate" (Gierut, 1986, p. 1). In this chapter, the main purposes of an assessment are covered before different types of measurement tools are described. Subsequently, planning the assessment session is discussed and the components of an assessment are described with obligatory components receiving the most attention. Finally, we provide an overview of the SLP's cultural competence and considerations for dialect speakers, children speaking English as a second language, and multilingual children.

3.1 PURPOSES OF EVALUATION

The main goal of the initial speech assessment is diagnosis, that is, describing the child's speech behaviors in order to decide whether the child has a speech problem and, if present, to identify the nature of that speech problem. Therefore, the first step in the diagnostic process is to determine whether the child's speech performance is below age expectations. Additional goals of the speech assessment

include rating the severity level of the difficulties if they are present, identifying possible causes of the speech difficulties, and determining a direction for intervention (Tyler & Tolbert, 2002). Table 3–1 summarizes the purposes of the speech evaluation and provides example questions related to each purpose.

3.1.1 Screening Assessment

Speech-language pathologists collect data through screening measures or more in-depth assessment procedures. The purpose of a speech screening is to identify children who require further testing because, upon brief assessment, they appear to be at risk for speech difficulties. In other words, screening measures help determine whether speech difficulties can be ruled out or if more in-depth testing is required to identify the presence of a speech sound disorder (SSD). Screening assessments may be conducted by SLPs in some clinics in order to provide a timely and cost-efficient service upon initial referral. Screening assessments can also be conducted by paraprofessionals, such as communication disorders assistants, and by other professionals who are not SLPs, such as community health nurses, teachers, or physicians. Screening programs to identify children in the general population who are at risk for speech and language difficulties should be designed and supervised by SLPs, however, and therefore it is necessary to be familiar with common screening tools and screening methodology.

Important characteristics of screening assessments are ease of administration and accuracy of identification. In other words, the test should identify those children who are most likely to have an SSD,

Table 3–1. *Purposes of the Speech Evaluation*

Purpose	Example Questions
Identification	Is further testing required by the SLP?
	Is further testing required by other professionals?
	Is the child's speech developing typically?
	Does the child have speech difficulties relative to age peers?
Severity Rating	What is the severity of the SSD?
Diagnosis	What factors may be causing the child's SSD?
	What is the type of SSD?
	Are there concomitant impairments?
Treatment Planning	Does the child need treatment?
	If necessary, who should treat the child?
	What are the treatment goals?
	What is an effective treatment approach?
	Should the child be discharged?

using a procedure that is quick and easy to administer. The accuracy of a screening measure is expressed in terms of sensitivity and specificity. The sensitivity of the measure is the ability to accurately identify children who are confirmed to have SSD upon more in-depth testing; the specificity is the ability to identify children who actually have normally developing speech. Sensitivity and specificity values range from 0 to 1.0, with values over .90 being optimal (Plante & Vance, 1994). In other words, a screening test that identifies children with SSD with 90% accuracy and identifies children with typical speech with 90% accuracy would be an ideal speech screener. This level of sensitivity and specificity is rare in screening tests, however; usually, a screening test that is very sensitive will have somewhat lower specificity, in that too many children with typical speech will be flagged

for further assessment. The SLP and other members of the health care team will need to consider the costs and benefits of different screening procedures when designing the screening program.

3.1.2 Diagnostic Assessments

If the child performs below expectations on the screening, the SLP will complete a comprehensive diagnostic speech assessment, which consists of a series of tests, measures, and activities described in sections 3.3 and 3.4 of this chapter. Not all children who are referred for a speech assessment will be assessed with the same measures: factors such as the child's age and reason for referral will influence which measures and activities the SLP will decide to include in the child's assessment. In addition, depending on the clinical setting, available time, and reason for referral, the SLP may perform a full diagnostic assessment without first completing a screening. An in-depth assessment of the child's communication skills is necessary to rate the severity level of the speech difficulties if they are present, reach a diagnosis, and determine a direction for intervention. Assessment is an ongoing process: some components of the assessment may be completed in a second evaluation session, or during the initial therapy sessions. In some cases, a diagnosis cannot be reached without gathering information from other professionals, and therefore referrals for additional assessments may be required. Finally, the results of the assessment can be used to monitor progress because the child's performance during intervention can be compared with baseline measures obtained during the initial assessment sessions.

Box 3–1. Purposes of Evaluations: Key Points

- Screening measures are used to identify children who are most likely to have speech difficulties and therefore require a full evaluation to confirm the presence of a speech disorder.
- The primary purpose of an evaluation is to confirm whether a speech or other communication disorder is present and to rate the severity level of those difficulties if present.
- The full evaluation may also allow the SLP to reach a diagnosis or refer the child for additional assessments that may be required for diagnosis.
- The evaluation also provides a direction for intervention.

3.2 TYPES OF MEASUREMENT TOOLS

When conducting a diagnostic assessment, three main types of measurement tools can be used for assessment purposes: standardized measures versus informal measures; norm-referenced measures versus criterion-referenced measures; and static versus dynamic measures. These types of measurement tools are described below.

3.2.1 Standardized versus Informal Measurement Tools

Standardized measures of speech are an essential part of the assessment process for children suspected of presenting with an SSD. **Standardized tests** use the same test materials and are administered and scored in a consistent manner. In other words, standardized tests have specific procedures to follow to elicit speech, and a manual that describes how to record and score the child's answers. Most speech assessment tests that are available for purchase are standardized. The child is typically presented with a series of colored pictures in the same order and the SLP asks the same question each time she presents a picture to the child. After each response, the SLP records the child's answer on a scoring sheet provided with the test using standardized rules for coding correct and incorrect responses. Standardized tests can be either norm-referenced or criterion-referenced, as will be discussed in more detail in subsection 3.2.2.

Most standardized speech measures have been designed to provide a description of the child's speech production accuracy with respect to the phonological characteristics of the language and usually in relation to the performance of other children of the same age. This description can be used to support the diagnostic process, but the test results do not by themselves determine whether the child has SSD.

Sometimes the SLP needs to observe speech abilities that are not targeted by standardized tests or in contexts that are more natural than permitted by the standardized test procedures. For example, the SLP may be interested in the child's ability to produce word-internal codas accurately, a structure not often included in the words on standardized tests. Alternatively the SLP may wish to observe the child's speech accuracy when playing with peers on the playground. In situations like this, SLPs often devise informal measurement tools that do not have detailed and standardized descriptions of how to administer, score, and/or analyze the child's speech. Skahan, Watson, and Loft (2007) investigated the procedures used by SLPs when assessing children referred with suspected speech problems. Many SLPs reported using informal measurement tools in combination with standardized tests, especially to assess children speaking languages for which standardized tests are not available. However, SLPs also reported developing informal measures to assess monolingual English-speaking children, to supplement the data provided by standardized tests. In particular, clinicians may probe the production of longer and more complex words than those typically included on a standardized test of articulation.

3.2.2 Norm-Referenced versus Criterion-Referenced Measurement Tools

The purpose of a norm-referenced test is to compare the performance of an individ- ual with the performance of a reference sample of individuals drawn from the larger population (Flipsen & Ogiela, 2015; McCauley & Swisher, 1984). This reference sample is called a normative sample because when it is large, the scores produced by the sample will be distributed on the normal curve. A normal distribution of scores shows the average range of scores as well as scores that are above or below the average range. Scores that are below the average range are below the normal limits—usually defined as the scores in the bottom 16% of scores obtained from the reference sample.

Norm-referenced tests are typically standardized, and the manual will contain detailed information about the normative sample, such as the individuals' age, sex, language background, geographical location, and socioeconomic status (SES). When choosing a norm-referenced test, it is important to be sure that the individuals in the normative sample are similar to the child that is being assessed. If the normative sample is composed of children aged 5 to 7 years, the test cannot be used to assess a child aged 9 years. Similarly, if the normative sample for a test was middle class children from Australia, the test should not be used to assess a child from a low SES home in the United States. If the normative sample for the test was children who speak Mainstream American English, the test will not be a valid measure of the speech produced by children whose primary dialect is African American English. Therefore, it is important that the SLP read the manual carefully when choosing tests to assess any given child. After a test has been selected, information in the manual is also important for interpreting the child's test performance. The test designer may have deliberately included children with speech and language delays in the normative sample, or such children may have been deliberately excluded: this decision will have an impact on the likelihood that any given child will score below normal limits on the test. Sometimes, test data are provided separately for samples of children who did and did not present with a communication disorder, which helps to interpret the child's test performance for diagnostic purposes (Spaulding, Plante, & Farinella, 2006).

The examiner manual contains tables with the raw scores obtained by the normative sample, usually broken down by age and sometimes also by gender. The individual's raw score can be compared with the normative sample, and the clinician can derive a standard score and a percentile rank for the individual, as illustrated in Figure 3–1. A **standard** score represents the child's performance as a distance from the mean of the normative sample, in standard deviation units: most commonly these scores have a mean of 100 and a standard deviation of 15, so that a standard score of 85 is equivalent to 1 standard deviation below the mean of the corresponding reference group. A child who obtains a standard score of 80 has very clearly scored below normal limits and would be considered to have a delay or disorder in most circumstances. A **percentile rank** indicates the percentage of children in the normative sample who scored the same or worse: therefore, if you assess a child who obtains a percentile rank of 16, approximately 84% of same-aged children obtained a better score, whereas the remainder obtained a similar or worse score. A child who scores

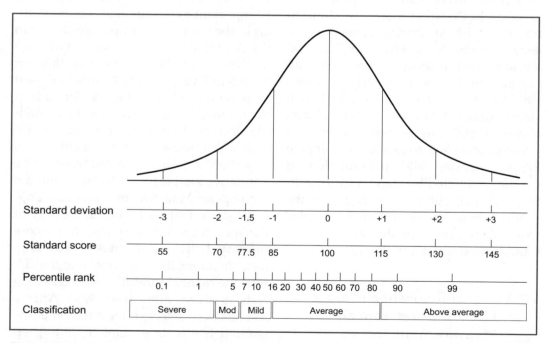

Figure 3–1. *Normal curve with percentile and standard score equivalents in relation to severity intervals. Used with permission from Françoise Brosseau-Lapré.*

at the 10th percentile on the test has very clearly scored below normal limits and would be considered to have a delay or disorder in most circumstances. Percentile ranks derived from the test allow the clinician to assign a severity ranking of the child's speech difficulties, and are very convenient for showing parents how their child is performing in comparison to peers. Finally, percentile ranks are sometimes required to qualify for services or third-party payments (Tyler & Tolbert, 2002).

Criterion-referenced assessments measure the child's strengths and weaknesses with regard to a particular skill but do not compare the child's performance to results obtained by other children. Rather, the comparison is to a criterion level of performance that may be required for some specific purpose. For example, a treatment program may require that the children who receive the treatment present with a minimum of three consistent speech errors while being able to speak in sentences at least three words long. Criterion-referenced measures are often used to compare the child's performance at different points in time. Therefore, in the example just given, a criterion-referenced measure could be used to determine the child's suitability to enter the speech therapy program as well as the child's continued eligibility to remain in the program at three-month intervals. Criterion-referenced assessments can be standardized or informal, and are often dynamic, as described below.

3.2.3 Static versus Dynamic Measurement Tools

Most standardized, norm-referenced tests are **static assessments**. Static assessments require the individual to complete a specific task, such as naming a picture, without receiving feedback about performance accuracy and without cues or assistance from the person administering the test. The individual's performance is measured under the same conditions as the other individuals from the normative sample. It is essential that the SLP resist the urge to deviate from the test instructions in order to provide additional assistance to the child when administering a static standardized test.

Dynamic assessments aim to elicit the child's optimal performance by giving different amounts of assistance and identifying the strategies that are most helpful for the child, such as providing a verbal model, using tactile cues to help the child produce the target sound, and/or segmenting the target response into smaller units (Olswang & Bain, 1991). Dynamic measures can be standardized or informal, and are criterion-referenced, meaning the performance of the child can be compared over time, but not with those of other children, since the specific cues and strategies used to elicit the best performance will vary for each child depending on the child's capacity to complete the task.

Practice 3–1

Search online for child speech and language measures commonly used by SLPs. Determine whether they are standardized, informal, norm-referenced, criterion-referenced, dynamic, or static. Indicate what information helped you classify them in these categories.

Box 3–2. Types of Measurement Tools: Key Points

- A standardized test is administered and scored in a consistent manner.
- Informal assessments do not have standardized instructions for administration or scoring.
- Norm-referenced measures compare an individual's performance with those of a similar group of test takers.
- Criterion-referenced measures determine whether the child meets or exceeds a criterion level of performance on a particular skill required for a given purpose.
- Static assessments measure performance under the exact same conditions for all individuals.
- Dynamic measures aim to elicit the very best performance and identify the specific strategies and cues that are helpful for each individual.

3.3 PLANNING THE ASSESSMENT

A critical aspect of the assessment process is the balance of thoroughness versus time constraints. An in-depth and multifaceted assessment of the child is necessary to reach a diagnosis and design an intervention. The SLP should gather sufficient information regarding multiple aspects of the child's speech skills; however, collecting information that is not valuable in the diagnostic or treatment planning process would be a waste of time for the clinician, the child, and the parents. To create an efficient assessment plan, the SLP identifies the minimum information required for diagnostic purposes and the most effective means to collect those data. Consider two children referred to an SLP for suspected speech difficulties: one child is 18 months old and does not yet produce words; the other is 8 years old, produces full sentences but is not easily understood by his teachers and classmates, and struggles with reading. Although both children were referred to the same SLP for a speech-language assessment, their profiles are very different. Therefore, the SLP must plan to gather different information using measurement tools that are individually suited to the ages and overall communicative abilities of these two clients. The assessment plan we recommend is illustrated in Figure 3–2; although a common structure can be used for all clients, it allows for flexibility in the choice of assessment components and specific measurement tools for each child. The assessment as planned may require only one session or as many as three, depending upon the complexity of the case.

In this section, important sources of information for planning the assessment are described, specifically the referral and the case history form. These documents, usually received prior to the child's first visit to the SLP, provide essential information for selecting and ordering measurement tools within the assessment process. Procedures for administering various measurement tools are described in subsequent sections.

3.3.1 Referral

The assessment process begins with a **referral**, the process of sending the child to the SLP. The referral is usually writ-

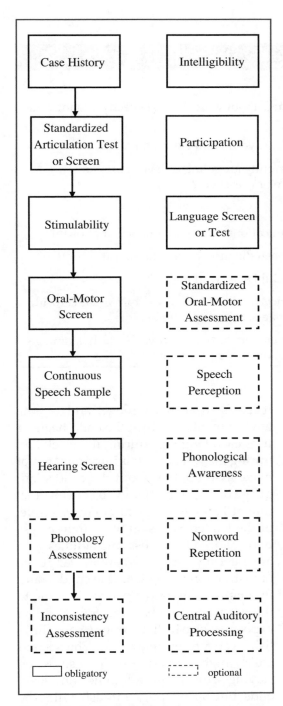

Case History	Intelligibility
Standardized Articulation Test or Screen	Participation
Stimulability	Language Screen or Test
Oral-Motor Screen	Standardized Oral-Motor Assessment
Continuous Speech Sample	Speech Perception
Hearing Screen	Phonological Awareness
Phonology Assessment	Nonword Repetition
Inconsistency Assessment	Central Auditory Processing

☐ obligatory   ⌐ ⌐ optional

Figure 3–2. *Recommended assessment plan requiring 75 to 120 minutes over one to three sessions. Used with permission from Susan Rvachew.*

ten (in the form of a referral letter or on a referral form completed by a pediatrician, family physician, audiologist, or other health professional). The referral may also be verbal (such as a phone call from the parent, or a conversation with the school teacher). SLP should know who referred the child for the evaluation, who initiated the referral process, and for what reason. It is important to know whether the parents are worried about their child's speech and language abilities, as their attitudes will influence how the SLP conducts the assessment, explains the results of the assessment, provides counseling, and plans follow-up interventions if required. Once a referral has been received, the SLP will plan the collection of data to assess the child. The first step in collecting data is usually the case history.

3.3.2 Case History

Many clinical settings use a standard case history form and ask parents to complete the document before the speech-language assessment; otherwise, the information is collected during the initial assessment visit. If the case history form is completed before the initial visit, the information provided by the parents may guide the choice of assessment components and measurement tools (see Figure 3–2). As we will discuss further in Chapter 4, the case history information may aid in diagnosis, referral decisions, and treatment planning. Most case history forms gather contextual information in two broad categories, environmental factors and personal factors, as listed in Table 3–2.

Pertinent **environmental factors** include the attitudes of the child's parents and family, especially their level of concern about the child's speech. These

Table 3–2. *Case History: Sample Questions*

Contextual Factors	Sample Questions
Environmental Factors	
Attitudes and Support	Are you concerned about your child's speech and language development?
Languages	What language(s) is your child exposed to?
Education History	Is your child currently attending or has he previously attended daycare or preschool?
Personal Factors	
Birth History	Were there complications during pregnancy or at birth?
Medical History	Has your child been diagnosed with a medical condition?
Developmental History	When did your child start walking?
Social Development	Do you have concerns about how your child interacts with friends, school mates, or family members?
Family History	Do any family members have a history of speech, language, reading, spelling, or learning disability?

attitudes may also include their feelings about the possibility that there is a speech problem, their opinion about possible causes and the best way to support the child if there is a problem. Information about the network of supportive relationships within the family and between the family and the community can also be important for assessment and treatment planning (McLeod & McCormack, 2007). Support provided by parents, siblings, and educators will impact the child's participation in activities at home, daycare, educational settings, and leisure activities.

Another relevant factor is the child's **language exposure**. This factor includes: (1) the number of different languages the child has been exposed to; (2) the age at which the child first began to learn each of the languages the child has been exposed to; (3) the amount of exposure the child receives to each language; and (4) the environments in which the child hears or uses each language during the week and during the weekend. It is important to not make assumptions about the child's language background but to objectively document language exposure. For example, in the United States an SLP might assess two children from Hispanic families who are entering a school where the language of instruction is English. One child's family might speak only Spanish at home to the extent that he has had only Spanish exposure since birth excepting some English exposure on television. The second child might experience Spanish when staying with the grandmother on weekends but speak only English with the parents during the rest of the week and attend an English-speaking preschool. These differences in language exposure will impact the choice and interpretation of measurement tools as well as post-assessment recommendations.

With regard to the child's **educational history**, parents would be asked about preschool and school attendance and any special services provided to the child since birth. Written or verbal information about the child's experience or performance in these other settings can only be obtained with the parents' written consent.

Personal factors covered on the case history form usually include the birth and medical history; developmental history, including social development; and family history (Bleile, 2002). Case history forms routinely ask parents about the child's **birth history**, such as whether there were complications during pregnancy or at birth, and whether the child was born at term or prematurely. With regard to the **medical history**, parents are asked about hospitalizations, medications, allergies, surgeries, and diagnoses the child may have received. Special attention should be paid to the child's hearing. Parents should be asked whether the child has had ear infections, and if so, at what age, what frequency, and what treatment was provided. Procedures to follow if the child's hearing has not been assessed are discussed later in this chapter. The **developmental history** may indicate the need to obtain more information regarding other aspects of development from other professionals (Hodson, Scherz, & Strattman, 2002). Parents are usually asked at what age their child achieved general motor and language milestones such as sitting for the first time, walking without support, onset of babbling, and first words. It is useful to know whether there have been recent changes in the child's rate of progress. Other personal factors such as the child's age, sex, disposition, and coping styles may also be considered during the assessment and when planning the intervention.

A family history of communication difficulties may be both an environmental and a personal factor. First, if other family members have communication difficulties, there will be impacts on the child's linguistic and social environment. For example, we can consider the hypothetical case of a young child whose mother works two jobs because the father has limited verbal abilities and is unemployed. This child may not be read to regularly, thus receiving poorer quality language inputs than is ideal unless accommodations are put in place to support the family. The nature of the father's communication problem will be relevant to the diagnosis: if the father has lost his speaking capacity subsequent to a traumatic brain injury, the diagnostic implications may be restricted to concerns about linguistic inputs; if the father and grandfather have developmental language and reading impairments, there is a possibility that the child has inherited similar or related impairments. Family history of communicative impairments are also relevant to the **prognosis**, i.e., a prediction about the course of the child's speech difficulties, because certain inherited communication difficulties are known to be especially persistent and some respond to treatment more easily than others, issues that will be discussed further in Chapter 4. It is recommended to collect a family history of speech, language, reading, spelling, and/or learning disability for three generations (Lewis & Freebairn, 1993): the child, siblings, and cousins are the first generation; the child's parents, uncles, and aunts are the second generation; and the grandparents are the third generation. The family history may be obtained through the case history questionnaire or by interviewing the parents or a combination of the two approaches.

Practice 3–2

Working in small groups, design a case history form that is appropriate for ONE of the following speech therapy clinic environments: a community health care clinic; a tertiary care hospital; a network of preschools; an elementary school board. Cover a broad range of environmental and personal factors on the form.

Box 3–3. Planning the Assessment: Key Points

- The assessment process usually begins with a referral, the process of sending the child to see the SLP.
- Information gathered from the case history may guide the choice of assessment components if it is completed before the initial visit; this information is also useful for diagnosis, referral decisions, and treatment planning.
- Contextual factors considered in the case history include environmental factors and personal factors.
- Environmental factors include the child's supporting network, language background, and educational experiences.
- Personal factors include birth, medical, developmental, and family history.

3.4 COMPONENTS OF THE SPEECH ASSESSMENT

In this section, we present an overview of the components that might be included in a speech assessment. Although the purposes of the speech assessment are multifaceted, the goal of the initial assessment is primarily to determine if there is an SSD or not. The SLP also decides during this initial assessment whether additional testing is required by the SLP, or by other professionals, in order to reach a diagnosis. Therefore, the procedures we list as **obligatory** during the first visit include measures of speech accuracy and screening tests for aspects of related function. Obligatory components must be assessed in one form or another regardless of the reason for the referral. For example, it is common for teachers to request an assessment of a child's speech accuracy for specific sounds ("please see this child whose 'r' sounds are unusual"). However, the SLP must go beyond listening to the child's speech articulation and establish that the child's hearing acuity, motor speech, and language skills are acceptable, using either formal or informal procedures. On the other hand, some assessment components are optional, and may be assessed only if there is a specific reason for concern.

The number of components that are tested on the first visit is limited by the time available and the ability of the child to remain focused and cooperative. If the child's results appear to be within normal limits, the assessment process may stop at the end of the initial visit: in other words, the child will be **discharged** from the service. Alternatively, the child may perform below age expectations, in which case multiple outcomes are possible. First, additional assessments may be required to reach a **diagnosis** (a conclusion about the nature of the SSD, if present, as discussed in detail in Chapter 4). In this situation, a second assessment session may be scheduled to gather more information about the child's speech-language functioning, or the child might be referred to other specialists to gather information that will aid diagnosis and support treatment planning. After a diagnosis has been reached, the child might be referred immediately for a speech-language intervention, scheduled for a re-assessment at a later date in order to monitor progress without treatment, or discharged. A discharge decision means that the child no longer requires services from the agency that conducted the diagnostic assessment, either because the child has no speech-language service needs or because the child's needs would be better met by another service provider. These various pathways are illustrated in Figure 3–3.

3.4.1 Norm-Referenced Single-Word Articulation/Phonology Test

The administration of a norm-referenced, single-word articulation/phonology test is an essential part of the assessment process and is the most commonly used assessment measure for children with suspected SSD (according to surveys in Australia: McLeod & Baker, 2014, and the United States: Skahan et al., 2007). Typically, the SLP will elicit spontaneous productions of single words by asking the child to name pictures, although objects are used in some tests. There are several **advantages** to using standardized, norm-referenced single-word articulation/phonology tests. First, the child's performance can be compared with that of a normative group in a time-efficient and standardized manner. Second, the target words included on the test were selected to include a **representative sample** of consonants

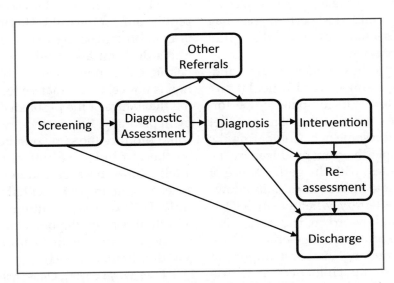

Figure 3–3. *Multiple possible pathways from screening through discharge. Used with permission from Susan Rvachew.*

and sometimes vowels: this means that all or at least frequently occurring phonemes in the language are targeted in the words elicited by the test procedure. A well-designed test will also target those phonemes in syllable or word positions that are commonly occurring in the test language. Another advantage is that the target words are known, which facilitates transcribing the child's responses phonetically and comparing what the child said with what the child attempted to say (Hodson et al., 2002).

Several **criticisms** of single-word tests have been reported. For instance, most of the test items are nouns, as they are easier to represent by drawings or pictures (Bernhardt & Holdgrafer, 2001). In addition, a continuous speech sample may be a better context to assess coarticulation and the impact of varied phonetic contexts on the child's accuracy. Furthermore, many tests require scoring the child's response as either correct or incorrect, which is not very informative. Finally, if the target words elicited by the test are not selected carefully, the child's test performance may not be representative of the child's typical speaking accuracy.

Although these criticisms are valid, the goal of a single-word articulation/phonology test is to compare the performance of the child with that of many other children of the same age. Comparing the number of speech errors produced by the child on the test with the performance of an appropriate reference sample allows the SLP to identify whether an SSD is present. Single-word articulation/phonology tests provide a time-efficient procedure for making that first important decision: does the child present with a speech impairment that warrants further investigation? Other decisions, such

as diagnosing the type of SSD, selecting treatment goals, or monitoring treatment progress, will require the collection and integration of additional assessment information (McCauley & Swisher, 1984). The norm-referenced single-word articulation/phonology tests that are most used in English clinical practice are presented in Table 3–3.

Single-word tests of articulation and phonology generally have the same format and require the child to name pictures. The main difference between single-word articulation tests and single-word phonology tests is in the analysis of the results. Commercially available, norm-referenced single-word tests include record forms to indicate and score the child's responses. Most single-word tests of articulation use **two-way scoring**, which means the child's production of each target sound is classified as correct or incorrect. Subsequently, the number of incorrect articulations of target sounds is summed to yield the total number of errors, and this **raw score** is used to obtain a standard score and percentile rank for the child. This information is an important source of evidence for the SLP's decision about whether the child has an SSD or not; however, this information is not very informative for determining the nature of the problem or for treatment planning. For instance, two children could produce the same number of errors on the test but have different levels of intelligibility because different types of speech errors impact intelligibility differently. For example, omitting consonants will diminish intelligibility more significantly than producing distortion errors (Gordon-Brannan, 1994)

Five-way scoring classifies the child's productions as belonging to one of five categories: (1) accurate production: the

Table 3–3. *Standardized Single-Word Tests of Articulation and Phonology Published Since 1990*

Name of Test	Author(s) & Year	Publisher	Age Range (norms)	Number of Words	Consonant Positions
Articulation Tests					
Arizona Articulation Proficiency Scale, 3rd ed. (ARIZONA-3)	Fudala, 2000	Western Psychological Services	1;5–18;0	42	IF
Goldman-Fristoe Test of Articulation, 3rd ed. (GFTA-3)	Goldman & Fristoe, 2015	Pearson	2;0–21;11	60	IMF
LinguiSystems Articulation Test	Bowers & Huisingh, 2010	Lingui-Systems	3;0–21;11	52	IMF
Photo-Articulation Test, 3rd ed. (PAT-3)	Lippke, Dickey, Selmar, & Soder, 1997	Pro-Ed	3;0–8;11	77	IMF
Structured Photographic Articulation Test, 2nd ed. (SPAT–II)	Dawson & Tattersall, 2001	Janelle Publications	3;0–9;0	45	IMF
Phonology Tests					
Bankson-Bernthal Test of Phonology (BBTOP)	Bankson & Bernthal, 1990	Special Press	3;0–9;0	80	IF
Hodson Assessment of Phonological Patterns (HAPP-3)	Hodson, 2004	Pro-Ed	3;0–8;0	50	n/a
Khan-Lewis Phonological Analysis, 3rd ed. (KLPA-3)	Khan & Lewis, 2002	Pearson	2;0–21;11	60	n/a
Articulation & Phonology Tests					
Clinical Assessment of Articulation and Phonology (CAAP)	Secord & Donahue, 2002	Super Duper Publications	2;6–8;11	44	IF

continues

Table 3–3. *continued*

Name of Test	Author(s) & Year	Publisher	Age Range (norms)	Number of Words	Consonant Positions
Diagnostic Evaluation of Articulation and Phonology (DEAP)	Dodd, Zhu, Crosbie, Holm, & Ozanne, 2006	Psychological Corporation	3;0–6;11	30	IF
Smit-Hand Articulation and Phonology Evaluation (SHAPE)	Smit & Hand, 1997	Western Psychological Services	3;0–9;0	81	IF

Note. The ARIZONA-3, DEAP, GFTA-3, and HAPP-3 also measure the accuracy of vowels.

child's production is the same as or acceptably close to the adult production, /sʌn/ → [sʌn]; (2) substitution: the target sound is replaced by another sound, /sʌn/ → [tʌn]; (3) omission: the target sound is deleted, /sʌn/ → [ʌn], sometimes transcribed as /sʌn/ → [Øʌn]; (4) distortion: the target sound is produced in an unusual manner that does not represent another phoneme, /sʌn/ → [s̪ʌn]; and (5) addition: a sound is added to the target, /sʌn/ → [stʌn]. The five-way scoring system is often referred to as accurate productions and SODA errors (for **s**ubstitution, **o**mission, **d**istortion, and **a**ddition). The examiner manuals of single-word articulation tests commonly recommend using the five-way scoring to derive more information about the child's speech production abilities than two-way scoring. At the same time, two-way scoring is often ideal for obtaining a raw score and comparing the child's performance to the normative sample. An example of two-way versus five-way scoring is shown in Demonstration 3–1. The items shown in the demonstration are

from the Diagnostic Evaluation of Articulation and Phonology (DEAP) diagnostic screen (Dodd et al., 2006), as produced by a girl aged 4;4. Five-way scoring is preferred for this screen because the nature of the child's errors determines which kind of test will follow (i.e., an articulation test if there are many distortion errors, a phonology test if the errors suggest the production of phonological error patterns).

Single-word tests of phonology typically analyze the child's productions according to phonological processes. While the clinician could administer a single-word articulation test, transcribe the full word productions of the child, and scan the sample to identify phonological processes, the record forms of tests of phonology were developed to assist the clinician in rapidly identifying the types and frequency of phonological processes used by the child during administration of the test. Regardless of the type of norm-referenced single-word test the clinician administers, we recommend that the child's picture-naming response be transcribed fully

Demonstration 3–1

Two-Way and Five-Way Scoring of DEAP Diagnostic Screen Responses

The second response to each screening test item is scored, above the expected consonant: correct ✓, incorrect ○ (with circle above rather than around the phonetic symbol for visual clarity), substitution /, omission -, distortion D, addition ^. Two-way scoring (left) reveals a percentage consonant correct of 75. Five-way scoring (right) shows that most of the errors are substitutions, additions, or omissions (with no distortion errors), indicating the need for a deeper phonological assessment.

Item	Two-Way Scoring							Five-Way Scoring						
wɑʧ	✓	✓						✓	✓					
watch	w	ɑ	ʧ					w	ɑ	ʧ				
fɪʃɪŋk	✓	✓		○				✓	✓		^k			
fishing	f	ɪ	ʃ	ɪ	ŋ			f	ɪ	ʃ	ɪ	ŋ		
gəlʌvz	○	✓		✓	✓			^ə	✓		✓	✓		
gloves	g	l	ʌ	v	z			g	l	ʌ	v	z		
spaɪtə˞	✓	✓			○			✓	✓			t/		
spider	s	p	aɪ	d	ə˞			s	p	aɪ	d	ə˞		
sæŋkju	○		✓	✓	✓			s/		✓	✓	✓		
thank you	θ	æ	ŋ	k	j	u		θ	æ	ŋ	k	j	u	
sɪsə˞s	✓		○		○			✓		s/		s/		
scissors	s	ɪ	z	ə˞	z			s	ɪ	z	ə˞	z		
hɛkɑtə˞	✓		○		✓		○ ✓	✓		-		✓		- ✓
helicopter	h	ɛ	l	ɪ	k	ɑ	p t ə˞	h	ɛ	l	ɪ	k	ɑ	p t ə˞
bɹɪʤ	✓	✓		✓				✓	✓		✓			
bridge	b	ɹ	ɪ	ʤ				b	ɹ	ɪ	ʤ			
ʌnbɹɛlʌ		○	✓	✓		✓			n/	✓	✓		✓	
umbrella	ʌ	m	b	ɹ	ɛ	l	ʌ	ʌ	m	b	ɹ	ɛ	l	ʌ
ɛlfʌnt		✓		✓		✓ ✓			✓		✓		✓ ✓	
elephant	ɛ	l	ə	f	ʌ	n	t	ɛ	l	ə	f	ʌ	n	t

using conventional International Phonetic Alphabet (IPA) notation.

Practice 3–3

Consider the word "rabbit," in which the first phoneme is the target, /ɹæbɪt/ as indicated by bolding. Imagine children have produced this word with the following misarticulations: [wæbɪt], [ɹʷæbɪt], [ɹæbɪ], [ɹʌbɪt], [dɹæbɪt], [ɟæbɪt], and [ɹʷæblɪt]. Classify the productions of the target phoneme according to the two-way scoring and five-way scoring systems.

3.4.2 Stimulability Testing

Stimulability is the child's ability to correctly imitate a phoneme when given a model by the clinician (Miccio, 2002; Rvachew, 2005). The results of the stimulability assessment provide valuable information regarding prognosis, as stimulable sounds may be mastered more readily than unstimulable phonemes (e.g., Miccio, Elbert, & Forrest, 1999; Tyler, 1996). After administering the single-word test of articulation/phonology, the SLP will have a list of the phonemes (usually consonants) that the child misarticulated. Determining whether the child is stimulable for these phonemes is simple: the clinician asks the child to "watch me and listen" and then presents a model of the target phoneme for imitation (Lof, 1996). Some standardized articulation tests provide specific stimulus materials for stimulability testing. For example, the Goldman-Fristoe Test of Articulation (Third edition; Goldman & Fristoe, 2015) provides a syllable, word, and sentence for each consonant singleton and cluster

that is targeted by the test. The DEAP articulation assessment recommends that each misarticulated consonant be elicited in a syllable (provided by the test) three times, and then if the child remains unsuccessful, three more times in isolation, as a measure of stimulability (Dodd, Zhu, Crosbie, Holm, & Ozanne, 2006). On this test, stimulability is tested only if the consonant is never produced correctly during articulation testing—in other words, completely absent from the phonetic repertoire.

Stimulability may also be assessed in different linguistic environments. Tyler and Tolbert (2002) recommend a stimulability task that varies with the child's articulation competence for each phoneme: (1) if the sound is absent from the inventory, assess stimulability in isolation, and if correct, then in CV and VC syllables; (2) if the sound is incorrectly produced in a particular word position, assess stimulability in that position in syllables and words; and (3) if the sound is produced accurately but inconsistently in words, assess stimulability of the sound at the word and sentence level. The Glaspey Dynamic Assessment of Phonology (GDAP; Glaspey & MacLeod, 2010; Glaspey & Stoel-Gammon, 2007) is a standardized dynamic assessment of stimulability. If the child can produce the target correctly, the linguistic environment is systematically made more complex. If the child mispronounces the target, cues are gradually added in a cumulative fashion.

3.4.3 Oral Mechanism Examination

The examination of the oral-peripheral mechanism is a mandatory part of the assessment. Results of this examination are essential to identify or rule out possible etiologies, that is to say, possible causes or causal factors underlying the SSD. The purpose of the oral mechanism examination is to determine if the structure and the function of the articulators are adequate for age-appropriate speech production. If the SLP suspects abnormalities in the oral-peripheral mechanism, the child would be referred to another health professional, such as a family physician, a pediatrician, a dentist, or an otorhinolaryngologist (ENT).

During the oral-peripheral mechanism examination, the SLP observes specifically: (1) the structural adequacy of the face, lips, dentition, tongue, palatal, and pharyngeal areas, and (2) the functional integrity of the articulators in simple and coordinated nonspeech and speech movements. Oral structure refers to the size, shape, and symmetry of the articulators, whereas function refers to range, speed, precision, and coordination of the movements of the articulators.

There are few standardized, norm-referenced tests of the oral-peripheral mechanism. The Verbal Motor Production Assessment for Children (VMPAC; Hayden & Square, 1999) was developed for use with children ages 3;0 to 12;0 and is currently the only tool that provides adequate descriptive information regarding its normative sample (McCauley & Strand, 2008). An Oral Motor Screen is included in the DEAP (Dodd, Zhu, Crosbie, Holm, & Ozanne, 2006) which is normed for children ages 3;0 through 8;11; the Oral Speech Mechanism Screening Examination, Third Edition (OSMSE-3; St. Louis & Ruscello, 2000) is another screening tool that has normative data for individuals ages 5;0 to 78;0. Many SLPs use a standardized protocol that is not norm-referenced as an initial screening tool. A sample form that can be used to administer a quick screening of the structure and function of the oral-peripheral mechanism is provided in Table 3–4. The observation and scoring procedure will be described briefly for each mechanism below, in order as listed on the form.

Facial characteristics should be observed at rest to assess the child's overall expression and appearance; size, shape, and symmetry of the head; and facial structures (Johnson-Root, 2015). The width of the face should be approximately the size of "five eyes": in other words, five vertical sections that are about the same width, specifically the sections between the outside and inside corners of each eye, the section between the inside corners of each eye, and the two sections between the outside corners of the eyes to their closest ear. While no human face consists of identical sides, the two sides of the face should be similar, in other words more or less symmetrical. Therefore, the clinician should note the presence or absence of facial drooping or sagging while the face is at rest or during movement. Drooping on one side of the face may indicate nerve damage. For example, individuals who have had strokes or cardiovascular accidents will often have unilateral facial drooping resulting in a visible asymmetry in the appearance of the face. In contrast, some children with very low muscle tone will appear to have bilateral drooping, that is, symmetrical sagging on both sides of the face. Horizontally, the face can be broadly divided into thirds: the top of the head at the hairline to the eyebrows, the eyebrows to just under the nose, and under the nose to the bottom of the chin; it is expected that these three portions will be approximately the same length. While no human is expected to conform to the perfect ratios of symmetry of the face, significant deviations from expected vertical

Table 3–4. *Sample Form for Screening the Oral-Peripheral Mechanism*

Face	Pass	Describe Deviation from Normal
Head size and shape		
Symmetry of the face		
Face: absence of drooping		
Lips		
Contact of the lips at rest		
Smile on demand		
Protrude lips on demand		
Teeth		
Gaps, missing or supernumerary teeth		
Occlusion (indicate type if malocclusion)		
Tongue		
Appearance		
Size in relation to oral cavity		
Protrude tongue on demand		
Move tongue upward on demand		
Move tongue downward on demand		
Move tongue left to right on demand		
Palatal and Pharyngeal Areas		
Appearance of the palate		
Absence of nasal emission		
Appearance of uvula		
Adequate velar movement during production of /a/		
Coordinated Nonspeech Movements		
Alternate lip rounding and retraction		
Alternate lip spreading and tongue protrusion		
Maximum Performance Tasks		
Repetition rate: [papapa]		
Repetition rate: [pataka]		

and horizontal proportions may indicate the presence of a genetic syndrome or neurological problem. It is not the role of the SLP to diagnose these syndromes but to make appropriate referrals when there are significant concerns or questions.

At rest, the lips should be closed with the left and right edges even. Lips that droop or remain partially open can be indicative of decreased muscle tone, muscle weakness, or paralysis. To assess lip function, the SLP observes retraction of the lips by asking the child to smile or produce the sound [i] while noting the range of motion, symmetry of the movement, and quality of the movement (did the lips move smoothly? Did the movement appear broken or irregular?). Protrusion of the lips is usually observed by asking the child to imitate a rounded lip posture or the sound [u]. Again, the symmetry of the movement, range of motion, and observations regarding the overall muscle tone of the lips would be noted.

Examination of dentition involves checking for three types of dental abnormalities: poor alignment of the teeth, malocclusions, and irregularities of the bite. These dental irregularities will be defined

in turn even though dental deviations may or may not have an impact on articulation skills, since children can adapt surprisingly well for their own oral structure despite changes as they mature. While missing teeth and malocclusions are associated with greater risk of poor articulation skills, they do not necessarily prevent the accurate production of speech (Bankson & Bernthal, 2004). Nonetheless, some problems with dentition can be significant causal factors for SSD, and orthodontic or surgical interventions are helpful treatments in some cases (Ruscello, Tekieli, & Van Sickels, 1985). Therefore it is important to know how to observe the dentition carefully.

With respect to procedure, use (1) a model for imitation, (2) verbal instructions, and (3) a tongue blade to help the child achieve the appropriate posture, which is teeth comfortably closed but lips open, providing a view of the front and back teeth. Note tooth decay, gaps, missing teeth, and supernumerary (extra) teeth protruding from the dental arch or from the palate. Dental abnormalities appear as significant deviations from the ideal as shown in Figure 3–4. When the

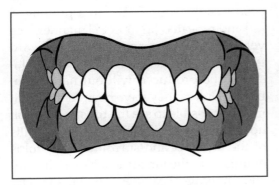 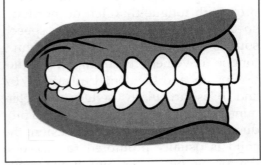

A **B**

Figure 3–4. *Normal occlusion and bite.* **A.** *Frontal occlusion.* **B.** *Lateral occlusion. Used with permission from Ellen Graham-Platt.*

teeth are aligned correctly in the dental arch, each tooth will fit smoothly side-by-side; when there is crowding, some teeth may appear to be turned to the side, creating **misalignment**. The state of molar **occlusion** is revealed by the relationship between the upper and lower **molars** (grinding teeth at the back of the mouth): the lower first molar should be slightly ahead of the upper first molar on each side. When the **bite** is normal, the top central **incisors** (sharp cutting teeth at the front of the mouth) will extend by about one-fourth of an inch over the bottom central incisors.

The **tongue** should first be observed at rest for general appearance and absence of lesions or growths. In terms of size, it should fit well within the oral cavity. Next, it is standard to prompt the child to raise the tongue tip to the alveolar ridge, behind the upper incisors. This movement permits observation of the **lingual frenum** (also called frenulum), a narrow fold of mucous membrane connecting the base of the tongue to the floor of the mouth. Tongue-tie, or **ankyloglossia**, occurs when the lingual frenum is short or when it is attached near the tip of the tongue. When a child with tongue-tie tries to protrude the tongue, it forms a heart-shaped edge of a "W" shape. Children with tongue-tie often do not have speech difficulties, since many speech sounds can be produced with minimal tongue movement. Focusing on production of /l/ and the dental fricatives /θ/ and /ð/ is particularly useful to help determine if ankyloglossia impacts speech production. In terms of tongue function, the child is usually prompted to protrude the tongue out of the mouth and move the tongue upward, downward, and then side to side. The tongue blade can be used

to provide a target for tongue tip placement in order to prompt these movements, or a model for imitation can be provided. The movements should be smooth without false starts or struggle. School-aged children should be able to move the tongue without moving the head or the jaw.

A flashlight will be required to properly observe the **palate and pharyngeal** areas, after asking the child to open the mouth with head slightly back. The palate forms the roof of the mouth. The soft palate, or velum, acts as a valve to build up pressure in the oral cavity required to produce many consonants. Regarding structure, note symmetry and the lack of abnormalities such as scars or changes in coloration. The hard and soft palate should be pink and white; a red palate points to inflammation, and a blue tint close to the midline of the palate may indicate a **submucous cleft**, meaning a gap in the underlying bone or muscle that forms the palate. The primary concern when inspecting the palatal and pharyngeal areas is whether the structures function properly to achieve velopharyngeal closure. Noticing the size, shape, and symmetry of the velum and its movement can be observed while the child produces the sound "ah" in a prolonged [a:] and repeated [aʔ aʔ aʔ aʔ] manner. The velum should rise symmetrically toward the back of the mouth, and the sound [a] should be produced without nasal resonance. Unless they have been removed, it may be possible to see the tonsils—lymph nodes embedded in the lateral (side) walls of the pharynx and surrounded by folds of muscle at the juncture between the oral and pharyngeal cavities called the **faucial pillars**; the presence of redness or swelling in these structures may indicate the presence of infection and therefore should be noted.

Practice 3–4

Find a mirror in a room that has good lighting. Open your mouth and move the tongue, looking in the mirror to identify your frenum. Inspect your hard and soft palate and the movement of your velum when repeating the sound [a] in a succession of short bursts.

Coordinated speech movements involve sequences of the simple movements of the lips and tongue that have been observed so far in the examination. Some children are able to produce oral movements individually but have great difficulty sequencing two or more movements. For example, a child might be able to smile when asked and protrude the tongue on command; the same child might nonetheless struggle if asked to alternate between spreading the lips and protruding the tongue. **Oral apraxia** refers to the poor ability to coordinate sequences of nonspeech oral movements of the articulators. A child with oral apraxia may or may not have **verbal dyspraxia**—difficulty coordinating speech sounds—and for this reason one last series of tasks is required on the oral-peripheral examination.

Maximum Performance Tasks are used to assess speech motor function and are especially useful to help diagnose the presence of motor speech disorders (as discussed further in Chapter 4). There are two broad categories of Maximum Performance Tasks: measures of **Maximum Phonation Duration**, in which the child prolongs a sound for as long as possible,

and measures of **Maximum Repetition Rate**, in which the child rapidly repeats either a single syllable or a sequence of syllables as quickly as possible. The oral-motor screening tool presented in Table 3–4 focuses on the repetition of syllables because it is difficult to obtain a reliable measure of maximum phonation time from a young child. Furthermore, only a limited number of syllable types are probed because it is a quick screener. If the child is having difficulty with these tasks, more extensive and standardized measures of speech motor control can be administered. The measurement of the maximum repetition rates, sometimes referred to as **diadochokinetic rates**, requires that the SLP obtain the child's best possible performance. This means that the SLP should allow the child several attempts and use any cues necessary to obtain the fastest rate that the child is capable of producing. A common difficulty that young children experience is coordinating the sequence of events—inhale, speak rapidly upon exhalation, inhale again. Often children will inhale, exhale, and then begin to speak, which makes it impossible to produce many syllables before the next inhalation. However, the goal is to produce many syllables rapidly on one exhalation. Drawings and gestures can help the child understand the requirements, as illustrated in Figure 3–5: in this example, the SLP would demonstrate to the child how to take a deep breath while sliding her finger up the drawing of the hill; produce one syllable each time her finger touches a bump on the slide; and take another breath once she has produced all the syllables and reached the bottom of the slide. After each attempt, the number of repetitions, time intervals required to produce the repetitions, accuracy of the

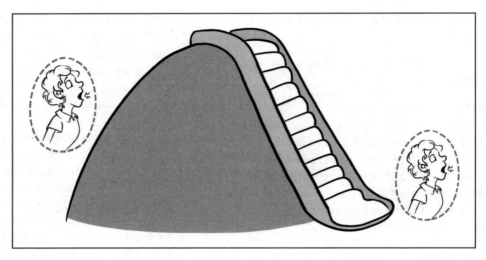

Figure 3–5. *Graphic cues to help child achieve maximum repetition rate. Used with permission from Ellen Graham-Platt.*

productions, and consistency of the productions are the outcome measures. The measures taken on the child's best attempt are recorded. It is most accurate to use a waveform editor to determine the child's repetition rate precisely, as demonstrated by Rvachew and Brosseau-Lapré (2018, see Demonstrations 5–3A and 5–3B). However, SLPs often make an informal judgment of adequate performance if the child repeats at least nine syllables in approximately three seconds, i.e., [papapapapapapapapa] in the monosyllable task or [patakapatakapataka] in the trisyllable task. If the child is younger or unable to pronounce the [k] sound, repetition of [pata] is acceptable as a multisyllable repetition task. Precise normative data are available for these tasks, but when using these data for diagnostic purposes it is necessary to administer the tasks exactly according to instructions and score the child's performance in accordance with the procedures used to gather the normative data. These procedures vary widely and influence the range of scores that are expected for children of different ages (Fletcher, 1972; Robbins & Klee, 1987; St. Louis & Ruscello, 2000; Williams & Stackhouse, 2000).

3.4.4 Continuous Speech Sample

The continuous speech sample is also a crucial part of the assessment process, but a minority of SLPs consistently elicit a spontaneous speech sample when assessing children suspected of presenting with an SSD (Skahan et al., 2007). Many clinicians see the amount of time required to elicit the speech sample and to transcribe it using the IPA as a significant barrier. However, time devoted to a thorough assessment process is time well invested; without an accurate diagnosis and description of the child's phonological system there is a chance of wasting time on an ineffective treatment approach or inappropriate therapy goals. Furthermore, the advantages and disadvantages of the single-word articulation test and the conversational speech sample complement each other. Therefore, the child's phonological knowledge should be assessed using a combination of the single-word articulation/phonology test and the continuous speech sample.

There are several **advantages** to collecting a continuous sample of speech to assess the child's production of speech sounds. First, this procedure has great **ecological validity**—eliciting the speech sample is more naturalistic, as the verbal interaction with the clinician will be similar to how the child interacts with other speakers in daily life, and therefore the child's speech production may be more representative of speech in daily life compared with picture naming. Second, the speech sample may reveal speech errors that occur in sentences, but not single words, provided that the SLP can elicit more complex utterances from the child during continuous speech sampling compared with picture naming. Several studies have shown that children produce different amounts of speech errors in connected speech versus single-word samples, with most studies finding that children produce more speech errors in connected speech (e.g., Healy & Madison, 1987). Third, all word types (such as nouns, verbs, adjectives, adverbs, pronouns, and prepositions) can be present in the speech sample. Finally, connected speech samples allow the assessment of the child's intelligibility, prosody, voice, resonance, and fluency as well as pragmatics and expressive language skills (Bernhardt & Holdgrafer, 2001; Miccio, 2002; Tyler & Tolbert, 2002).

Despite these benefits of continuous speech sampling, there are four potential threats to the validity of this measurement tool, as identified by Shriberg and Kwiatkowski (1985). First, the child may not say much at all. Second, if the child's intelligibility is limited and it is very hard to understand the child, it will be difficult to write down what the child attempted to say. Third, the speech sample may not be representative if the sentences produced by the child do not contain all the consonants and vowels of English, and/or word shapes such as longer words and consonant clusters. Finally, the child may react to the materials used to collect the speech sample and use unusual speaking registers, such as imitating characters' voices when playing with toys. Carefully planning an elicitation strategy is therefore necessary to maximize the information obtained from collecting a speech sample within 10 to 15 minutes.

Although there is no clear consensus on the optimum size of the conversational speech sample (e.g., Bernhardt & Holdgrafer, 2001; Morrison & Shriberg, 1992), Grunwell (1987) recommended a minimum of 100 different words for the length of the speech sample, with a sample of 200 to 250 words being preferable. Given the typical speaking rate of children in conversation (Pindzola, Jenkins, & Lokken, 1989), a speech sample of 100 to 200 words should be elicited in 10 to 15 minutes. If for some reason the child is unable to produce a large sample of words while conversing with the SLP over a 10-minute period, the experience of trying to elicit a continuous speech sample from the child will be informative in any case. Observation of the child coupled with those of the parent may reveal whether limitations in speech intelligibility, language skills, fluency, pragmatic skills, or temperament contributed to the size of the speech sample that was recorded.

The preferred method is for SLPs to elicit spontaneous conversation, although other methods are possible, such as free play, retelling stories, and sentence imitation tasks. Some studies observed similar levels of speech accuracy when children with typical speech engaged in spontaneous conversation versus imitation of sentences (e.g., Kenney, Prather, Mooney, & Jeruzal, 1984). However, when Goldstein, Fabiano, and Iglesias (2004) investigated the speech sound accuracy of young Spanish-speaking children with speech impairments in both sampling contexts, they found that child-specific factors played a role in their speech accuracy in spontaneous and imitative responses. Children who have previously received speech therapy and school-age children particularly may perform better when imitating sentences as opposed to producing sentences spontaneously. Therefore, sentence imitation should be used only if the child is not sufficiently talkative during a spontaneous speech task. When eliciting the spontaneous speech sample, the examiner should be careful not to talk more than the child. Table 3–5 presents a

Table 3–5. *Activities and Strategies for Obtaining a Continuous Speech Sample*

Activities	Strategies
Ask open-ended questions about a familiar topic of conversation (the child's pets, favorite movie, television show or activity).	Use fill-in-the-blank completion prompts. Model turn-taking routines. Avoid yes-no questions.
Use toys and allow the child to play freely while you comment on the child's actions from time to time.	Ask a choice question by providing two answers, one of which is clearly the correct answer.
Use a wordless picture book, flannel pieces, or stickers to elicit a story from the child.	Try commenting on the child's actions rather than repeatedly asking questions.
Set up an activity that involves verbal routines such as requesting items and indicating where they go.	Remain silent for several seconds or more if necessary while waiting for the child to respond.
When playing with the child, omit some pieces or mix up pieces from different games.	Follow the child's lead when replying to the child's response.
Ask the child to describe how to make cookies, build a snowman, etc.	Try to ensure balance in the conversation, with examiner and child talk being approximately equal.
Be prepared to use more than one activity and flexibly change elicitation strategies when required to keep the child talking.	Do not comment on or correct the accuracy of the child's speech.

summary of recommendations to obtain an adequate speech sample within 10 to 15 minutes.

Excellent quality recordings can now be obtained with low-cost digital recording devices, including cell phones, tablets, and portable computers. One challenge is positioning the microphone appropriately and ensuring that protective device covers or the child's fingers are not covering the microphone. The recording environment is also often noisy. Always test the sound quality of the recording device before use, and adjust the recording level of the device to the child's speaking level. Transcribing as much as possible the spontaneous speech sample while it is elicited will decrease the time required for transcription later. During the conversation, recast the child's utterances naturally: for example, if the child says, "the baby sleep," the SLP can answer "yes, the baby sleeps in his crib." Recasting is a conversational form of repeating what the child says, which is helpful for later transcribing what the child said and acknowledges the child's role in the conversation, thus increasing the child's speech output while collecting the sample.

Practice 3–5

Plan to elicit a spontaneous speech sample from a child age 4 years 6 months who had difficulties producing the sounds /k, g, s, z, ʃ, ʒ, ɹ, l/ during the single-word articulation test. Describe the materials and activities you would use to collect the speech sample. Choose the strategies that would be most useful to elicit a sample of 100 to 200 words within 10 to 15 minutes.

3.4.5 Hearing Screening

A hearing screening as per the ASHA Guidelines for Childhood Hearing Screening (American Speech-Language-Hearing Association, 1997) must be completed unless the child's hearing has recently been assessed or the child is scheduled to have an audiology assessment very shortly after the SLP assessment. As with the oral peripheral examination, it is essential to screen the child's hearing. Screening procedures typically involve visual inspection of the ear, tympanometry to assess the function of the middle ear and pure tone audiometry to assess detection of sounds at different frequencies. Depending on procedures specific to the SLP's clinical setting, children who fail the hearing screen will be referred to the family doctor, referring physician, ENT, or audiologist.

3.4.6 Inconsistency and Variability Assessment

Consistency of the child's error patterns has implications for diagnosis and treatment planning. Informal observation of consistency is possible by scanning the error types produced on the articulation/phonological assessment. If necessary, more formal measures of consistency can be conducted. Two types of consistency are of interest. **Within-phoneme inconsistency** is actually very common, if not the norm, when children produce phonological patterns (Iuzzini & Forrest, 2010; Rvachew & Andrews, 2002). This type of inconsistency is revealed as a predictable pattern of error types for a particular class of phonemes across different syllable positions, for example: "fan" /fæn/ → [pæn], "soap" /sop/ → [top] but "cuff"

/kʌf/ → [kʌf], "bus" /bʌs/ → [bʌs]. In this example, the child is stopping fricatives in the onset position but producing them correctly in the coda position, a frequently occurring error pattern. Similarly, it is common for children to front velars in the onset but not the coda, as discussed in Chapter 2. Sometimes the child might misarticulate the phoneme in all syllable positions, but the patterns are nonetheless predictable on the basis of syllable position, for example: "soap" /sop/ → [top], "shoe" /ʃu/ → [tu], "bus" /bʌs/ → [bʌtʃ], "wash" /waʃ/ →[watʃ], "messy" /mɛsi/ → [mɛji], "mushy" /mʌʃi/ → [mʌji]. Another form of within-phoneme inconsistency is the production of various types of distortions for the same phoneme across syllable positions: for example, /s/ → [s̪], [s̠], and [s̪] in an unpredictable fashion, as in "soap" /sop/ → [s̪op], [s̠op], and /bʌs/ → [bʌs̠], [bʌs̪].

Some children produce high rates of **within-word inconsistency**, which typically indicates a unique and severe type of SSD requiring intense treatment (Dodd, 2014). In this case, the same word is produced inconsistently over repeated attempts, and the errors often involve metatheses or productions that bear little relation to the adult target, such as /sop/ → [ops], [fot], [sæd], [swop]. These errors are more likely to occur when the target words are long or complex and therefore valid measurement of within-word inconsistency requires a special test procedure.

The Diagnostic Evaluation of Articulation and Phonology (Dodd et al., 2006) provides a subtest called the Word Inconsistency Assessment, which is a picture naming task that elicits 25 words, 8 being single-syllable words but the remainder being more complex, including items such as "umbrella," "helicopter," "chocolate cake," and "vacuum cleaner." The

25 words are elicited three times during the same visit, separated by other tasks or activities. Each set of three-word productions are scored for consistency rather than accuracy: for example, "shark" /ʃaək/ → [saək], [saək], [saək] is scored as consistent but "shark" /ʃaək/ → [tʃaək], [kaək], [skaək] is scored as inconsistent. According to Dodd and colleagues, children who produce 40% or more of the words in an inconsistent manner are considered to present with **Inconsistent Phonological Disorder** (Holm, Crosbie, & Dodd, 2013). The treatment implications of within-phoneme and within-word variability are discussed further in Chapters 6 and 8.

3.4.7 Intelligibility

Intelligibility refers to the degree to which the speaker is understood. Intelligibility is often confused with a related but different concept, **accuracy**, which refers to the correctness of the articulation of the target word. Children age 4 years are intelligible to unfamiliar listeners (McLeod, Crowe, & Shahaeian, 2015) but they do not necessarily produce all speech sounds accurately (Smit, Hand, Frellinger, Bernthal, & Bird, 1990). Other variables besides speech accuracy contribute to intelligibility so that a speaker who produces phonetically accurate speech could be unintelligible because the speech is not loud enough to be heard, or the language content is irrelevant to the topic of conversation, or the language form is grammatically incorrect, as illustrated in Figure 3–6.

For children with SSD, being intelligible is generally their long-term intervention goal. The child's intelligibility level helps to determine whether there is an SSD, whether the child should receive

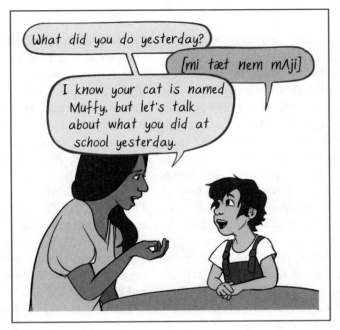

A

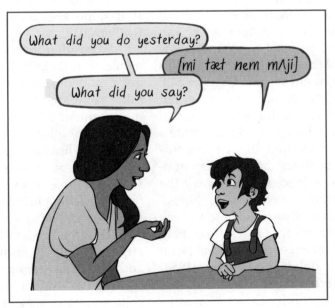

B

Figure 3–6. *Intelligibility is determined by many factors related to the talker, the talker's speech, and the listener. Notice that the child's speech accuracy is the same in both panels. What factors might help the adult listener understand the child's meaning in panel A? Used with permission from Ellen Graham-Platt.*

speech therapy, and whether the speech intervention is successful (e.g., Hustad, 2012). Intelligibility must be measured directly, and not inferred from the results of the single-word articulation test, which assesses speech production accuracy. For example, children with severe SSD may produce fewer omission errors but more substitution errors following intervention: this change in error patterns would improve intelligibility while not changing the raw score obtained on a measure of single-word accuracy. As another example, some children who score within the average range on a single-word articulation test are not as intelligible as they should be for their age. Although speech accuracy and intelligibility are related, they are distinct concepts and must be measured with different tools.

To measure speech intelligibility, rating scales may be used to estimate how much the speaker is understood. The child's intelligibility might be rated by the SLP from the continuous speech sample, but the validity of this rating will be limited because the child may not demonstrate a typical level of intelligibility during this brief interaction in an unfamiliar environment. A simple procedure is to ask the parent: *"How clear is your child's speech? That is, how much of your child's speech can a stranger understand?"* (1) less than half, (2) about half, (3) three-quarters, and (4) all or almost all. Coplan and Gleason (1988) found that children aged 22 months were 50% intelligible, children aged 37 months were 75% intelligible and children aged 47 months were 100% intelligible. These findings can be used as a rough indicator of whether a child's intelligibility is within or below expectations.

The Intelligibility in Context Scale (ICS; McLeod, Harrison, & McCormack, 2012) was developed for parents to report on how well their child is understood by the parents, immediate family, extended family, friends, acquaintances, teachers, and strangers. This 7-item scale is available in more than 60 languages. The scale has recently been validated for use with young children speaking a variety of languages (e.g., McLeod, Crowe, & Shahaeian, 2015; Ng, To, & McLeod, 2014; Washington, McDonald, McLeod, Crowe, & Devonish, 2017). Rating scales are an easy and ecologically valid way to screen the child's intelligibility, but they lack precision due to the subjective nature of this concept: two listeners might choose different ratings even when they find the same speaker to be equally intelligible; one listener might find a given speaker easy to understand while another listener finds that same speaker quite unintelligible (Miller, 2013).

Word-identification can be used to generate intelligibility percentages that are a more objective measure of intelligibility compared with rating scales (Gordon-Brannan, 1994). The procedures usually require the child to produce a list of words, and listeners write down the words they heard, or select an answer among a set of possible answers. The Children's Speech Intelligibility Measure (CSIM; Wilcox & Morris, 1999) was developed for use with children age 3 to 10 years, and takes approximately 20 minutes to administer and score. The examiner randomly selects 50 stimulus words to be produced by the child spontaneously or by imitation. One or two unfamiliar adults listens to the recordings of these production attempts; to respond, the listeners write down the words perceived, or select among 12 possible answers. The Beginner's Intelligibility Test (BIT; Osberger, Robbins, Todd, & Riley, 1994) assesses intelligibility at the sentence level. It consists of lists of 10 short sentences containing simple words that are one or two syllables in length; the child imitates or reads the sentences that are audio-recorded. Ideally, three unfamiliar listeners write down the child's productions, and the percentage of target words correctly identified, averaged across the listeners, is calculated.

Practice 3–6

Watch this short video of a 4-year-old boy with a severe SSD. Write down the number of words that were intelligible to you, and the number of words that you did not understand. Did this child produce most words accurately? In the conversational context of the video, was he more intelligible than you expected? Do you think you would understand him if you did not first hear the questions he was asked? youtube.com/watch?v=rlciHHC0uT4

3.4.8 Participation

Poor speech intelligibility is known to make it difficult for children to participate fully in activities of daily life (McLeod & Threats, 2008). During the case history, the child's parents may have described these difficulties explicitly. Parents may also be worried about potential upcoming challenges: if the child is soon to attend school for the first time, problems communicating in this new environment might be anticipated. The child's intelligibility level is related to **participation restrictions**, as not being easily understood by friends, teachers, or strangers will impact how well the child can participate in activities such as attending a play group, answer-ing a teacher's questions during story-time, and asking a child to have a turn on the swings at the playground. However, the child's personal factors, contextual factors, and speech impairment interact in an intricate manner to impact the child's participation in daily life activities (McLeod & Threats, 2008). For example, a child with very limited intelligibility may be skilled at using gestures to get her message across and be understood by her friends. On the other hand, another child with a mild SSD may be shy and refuse to participate in activities if his parents are not present to speak on his behalf. Therefore, participation is not only related to speech accuracy and speech intelligibility but arises from the interaction of the child in his or her environment.

Very few speech-language pathology outcome measures are available for the assessment of participation by preschool children. The Focus on the Outcomes of Communication Under Six (FOCUS; Thomas-Stonell, Robertson, Walker, Oddson, Washington, & Rosenbaum, 2012) measure was specifically developed to document change in functional communication skills for preschool children. Specifically, the FOCUS captures performance in life activities and the level of assistance required to successfully participate in the activity rather than measuring the communication impairment. Internal consistency, test-retest reliability, content, and construct validity have been established, and sensitivity to change over short intervals of intervention has been demonstrated with large samples of preschool-age children receiving speech and language interventions (Thomas-Stonell, Oddson, Robertson, & Rosenbaum, 2010). The FOCUS-34 is now available for free in English and other languages, and consists of 34 items that have been shown to have equal validity and sensitivity to the original FOCUS. The FOCUS includes many items related to domains of activities and participation, such as "My child is included in play activities by other children," "My child makes friends easily," and "My child participates in group activities." Clinicians currently using the FOCUS have reported collecting more information about the child's participation abilities in the community and selecting more treatment goals related to increasing participation levels and decreasing participation restrictions (Thomas-Stonell et al., 2010).

Practice 3–7

Think of three more situations in which a child with severe speech difficulties may experience restrictions in communicative participation.

3.4.9 Language Screen or Test

Language impairments frequently co-occur with SSD in preschool-aged children (e.g., Baker & Cantwell, 1982; Shriberg, Tomblin, & McSweeny, 1999) and therefore, at the very least a language screening should be administered. The speech sample obtained previously during the assessment session can also be used to analyze the child's expressive language skills. All aspects of the child's use of spoken language to communicate a message are indicative of expressive language ability: vocabulary includes selecting a variety of words that accurately represent the concepts to be expressed; morphology involves manipulating the form of words to communicate person, number, and tense; syntax pertains to the arrangement of words to create grammatically correct sentences; and pragmatics requires adjustments to the social situation and the needs of the listener. Tyler and Tolbert (2002), for instance, calculate mean length of utterance (MLU) in morphemes, based on 50 representative utterances to compare the child's expressive language performance to normative data from Miller and Chapman (1981). This means that the words in each utterance in the sample are divided up into their minimal meaningful units. For example, if the child said "I banged the trucks," there are four words but six morphemes, as in "I bang/ed the truck/s." Children's utterances contain more morphemes on average as they get older. Tyler and Tolbert (2002) recommended this detailed description of the child's morphology because bound morphemes are characteristically incorrect in the speech of children with developmental language impairments. Therefore, it is important to learn the specialized skills that are required for this type of analysis even though the procedure is beyond the scope of this book. However, in the case of children with unintelligible speech, it can be difficult to know whether the child lacks knowledge of the language structures or if the child is unable to pronounce the morphemes. For example, if the child does not articulate consonant clusters correctly the past tense morpheme will be difficult to produce. For this reason it might be more accurate to count the child's mean length of utterance in words when the child's speech is difficult to understand. Parker and Brorson (2005) found that the mean length of utterance in words (MLUw) is perfectly correlated with the mean length of utterance in morphemes (MLUm). This suggests that MLUw is a valid measure of language development for children with SSD even though MLUm is more commonly used in speech-language assessments. A useful normative reference is provided by Rice et al. (2010), who report MLUw and MLUm for children aged 2;6 through 8;11, including groups with typical language and groups with language impairment.

Preferably, a comprehensive language assessment will be completed, especially if the child fails the language screen or concerns with language comprehension or expression are noted in conversation. It is especially important to have a standardized measure of **receptive language skills** because otherwise difficulties with the comprehension of vocabulary, morphology, and syntax can be missed and children with these deficits often do not receive the services they need (Tomblin, Records, & Zhang, 1996; Zhang & Tomblin, 2000). Several comprehensive language assessments are available commercially for use with preschool or school-aged children, such as the Clinical Evaluation of Language Fundamentals–Preschool, Second Edition (CELF-P2; Semel, Wiig, & Secord, 2004); Clinical Evaluation of Language Fundamentals–Fifth Edition (CELF-5; Semel, Wiig, & Secord, 2013); and the Test of Integrated Language and Literacy Skills (TILLS; Nelson, Plante, Helm-Estabrooks, & Hotz, 2016). It may also be helpful to have a measure of the child's narrative abilities, an important precursor to the use of language for academic purposes (Schneider, 2004; Schneider, Hayward, & Vis Dubé, 2007).

If the child has a speech or language impairment, it is important to determine whether these difficulties are specific to the speech and language domains, in which case the impairments are deemed to be **primary**. Alternatively, the speech and language difficulties might be **secondary** to some other medical diagnosis or condition, including global developmental delay. Further assessments, such as evaluating the verbal and nonverbal cognitive skills of the child, may be required. SLPs are not qualified to administer tests to obtain an intelligence quotient (IQ), and valid measurement of IQ in children with speech and/or language difficulties may be complicated (Francis, Fletcher, Shaywitz, Shaywitz, & Rourke, 1996). However, the SLP can judge whether it is necessary to refer the child for assessment by a psychologist or a multidisciplinary developmental clinic to help in differential diagnosis and treatment planning. The SLP may ask the parents to complete a comprehensive questionnaire that screens multiple areas of development to help decide whether further referrals are necessary.

3.4.10 Phonological Processing

Phonological development, as described in Chapter 2, is clearly dependent at all stages upon phonological processing skills. Phonological processing itself is dependent upon the knowledge the child has accumulated about the sound system of the language. In other words, the processing of speech to gain new knowledge, and the knowledge that the child has previously learned, impact each other in a reciprocal fashion. First, as speech input accumulates, the child builds and stores representations of words in the **lexicon**. Over time, the child's phonological representations in long-term memory become increasingly detailed; consequently the **lexicon** expands and reorganizes itself to link words with similar phonological features (Metsala & Walley, 1998). Early in development the linkages may reflect fairly gross characteristics of words, so that "shine," "duck," "man," and "deep" may be linked because the words have only one syllable; subsequently, a link between "duck" and "deep" may emerge, recognizing the shared onset, /d/. This reorganization of the lexicon allows the child to process words at finer levels of phonological structure as vocabulary size increases.

Phonological processing skills refer to the child's ability to construct, store, access, and manipulate phonological representations (Claessen, Heath, Fletcher, Hogben, & Leitão, 2009). In this section, tools to measure three aspects of phonological processing are described, specifically speech perception, phonological awareness, and phonological memory. The assessment of auditory processing is also briefly discussed, even though this is distinct from phonological processing, since basic auditory processing abilities support the development of phonological processing skills.

The test of speech perception should determine whether the child's underlying acoustic-phonetic representations are adultlike (Claessen et al., 2009). There are few well-designed standardized tools to assess speech perception in young children. Often, SLPs use informal procedures to assess the child's ability to discriminate between phonemes in isolation, syllables, or words. The simplest type of discrimination task involves asking the child whether two sounds (or syllables, or words) sound the same or they sound different. This type of task is problematic for young children, since they are not always familiar with this vocabulary and may not understand the task; even when they do, it is difficult for children to decide "how different" two items need to be before a response of "different" is appropriate. For example, some children may answer that a green apple and a red apple are the

same, since they are both apples. There are other, more complicated measures of speech discrimination that are more valid (Locke, 1980a), but the more serious problem is that a measure of speech discrimination does not reveal the nature of the child's underlying representation for the target speech sound or phoneme contrast. In order to assess speech perception in a way that is relevant to a child's SSD, it is best to use a mispronunciation task (Bountress, Sever, & Williams, 1989; Vance et al., 2009). A mispronunciation identification task requires the child to perform a unique motor response if a correct pronunciation of the target word is heard, and an alternate motor response if a mispronunciation is heard. For example, if the task assesses the underlying representation of the word "rat," the child could be required to touch the picture of "rat" if the word was produced correctly as [ɹæt], and touch the picture of "X" if the child heard a mispronunciation such as [wæt], [ɹæt], or [jæt]. Notice that the child is not asked to verbally indicate that [ɹæt] is "right" and [wæt] is "wrong." The response must be a nonverbal response that reveals the child's underlying representation of the target form. A screen shot of a tablet-based speech perception assessment tool is shown in Figure 3–7.

Several specific conditions increase the validity of the mispronunciation identification task as a measure of a young child's speech perception abilities (Locke, 1980b). First, the test should examine the target sound in relation to the child's specific speech error. For example, if the child produces "rake" /ɹek/ → [wek], the test should contrast "rake" and "wake" to measure the child's perception of the phoneme /ɹ/. However, perception tests often contrast "rake" and "lake," even though /ɹ/ → [l] is an uncommon substitution pattern in English. Second, there

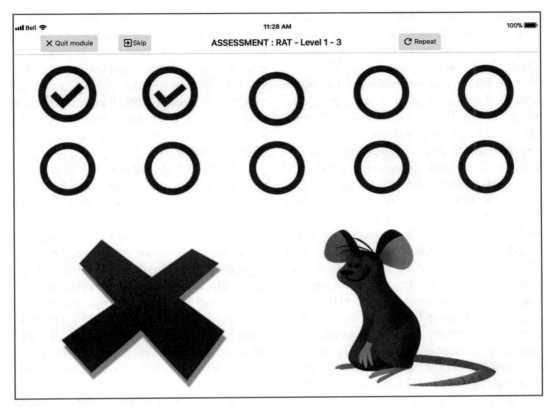

Figure 3–7. *Tablet-based mispronunciation task to assess perception of /ɹ/ in which the child touches the picture of the "rat" when [ɹæt] is heard and the X when any mispronunciation is heard. Check marks indicate completed trials and circles indicate uncompleted trials in assessment mode. Screen shot of SAILS shown with permission of the creators, Susan Rvachew and Alexandre Herbay.*

should be multiple trials targeting each of the child's error phonemes, as opposed to a single trial for each English consonant regardless of whether the child misarticulates each of these consonants or not. Third, there should be two types of nontarget items for a specific phoneme: stimuli that are similar to the target and the child's error production (such as [ɹek] versus [wek]) and control stimuli that are different from the child's error production (such as [ɹek] versus [mek]). The control stimuli confirm that the child understands the task and help to define the boundaries of the child's perceptual knowledge of the target. Finally, vocabulary items,

instructions given to the child, and type of expected response must all be appropriate for the child's age and cognitive abilities (Locke, 1980b; Vance, Rosen, & Coleman, 2009).

The SLP can present the stimuli to the child live-voice (the SLP produces the items during the session) or via recordings. Regardless of the way the stimuli are presented, the SLP must match the speech stimuli of the test to the dialect spoken by the child. There are several mispronunciation identification tasks now available for different dialects of English, specifically British English (McNeill & Hesketh, 2010; Vance et al., 2009), Australian English

(Claessen et al., 2009), and Midwestern North American English (Speech Assessment and Interactive Learning System [SAILS]; e.g., Rvachew, 1994, 2007).

Phonological awareness is the child's knowledge that spoken words are composed of smaller units, such as syllables, onsets and rimes, and individual phonemes (Gillon, 2005). Phonological awareness is a crucial prereading skill that emerges during the preschool period. Children with early speech delays often have difficulties learning to read, and individuals who are diagnosed with reading disability are likely to report they had difficulties with speech at a younger age. Consequently, it is important to assess phonological awareness in children with a current or prior history of SSD. There are a wide variety of tasks to assess phonological awareness, each involving spoken words rather than printed words. Commonly used tasks include identifying the first sound of a word (e.g., "What is the first sound in *cat?*" /k/), blending words or sounds (e.g., "What word do these sounds make when we put them together?" /s/ /ʌ/ /n/? *Sun*), and manipulating phonemes (e.g., "Say *spy* without the sss." *Pie*).

There are several standardized, norm-referenced tests of phonological awareness. For instance, the Comprehensive Test of Phonological Processing–Second Edition (CTOPP-2; Wagner, Torgensen, Rashotte, & Pearson, 2013) was normed on a U.S. sample of children ages 4 to 24 years. A range of phonological awareness tasks are included along with tests of short-term memory and rapid naming. The Preschool and Primary Inventory of Phonological Awareness ([PIPA; Dodd, Crosbie, McIntosh, Teizel, & Ozanne, 2000) consists of six subtests and measures syllable segmentation,

rhyme awareness, alliteration awareness, phoneme isolation, phoneme segmentation, and letter knowledge. It has a UK and Australian standardization sample of children ages 3;0 to 6;11 but may not be appropriate for American or Canadian children, as the ages of school entry and literacy instruction practices are different in these countries.

When testing children with SSD who are difficult to understand, the SLP will also consider the response mode. Tasks that use a nonverbal response such as pointing to the correct picture or tasks that require a yes/no response may be more appropriate for the child. The Phonological Awareness Test was developed by Bird, Bishop, and Freeman (1995) to investigate the emergence of literacy in children with speech impairments. It consists of three subtests: rime matching, onset matching, and onset segmentation and matching. Throughout the test, verbal responses are not required; on every trial, the child selects a picture that matches the sound that a puppet will like according to the verbal instructions provided by the tester. An example of the format used to test rime awareness is shown in Figure 3–8. The same procedure is used to test onset matching, except in this case the animal would prefer items that share the same first sound with its name. Many studies have shown that the responses of preschool-age children with SSD on this test are associated with later literacy outcomes (e.g., Bird et al., 1995; Peterson, Pennington, Shriberg, & Boada, 2009; Rvachew, 2007). The Silent Deletion of Phonemes Task (SDPT) also minimizes the impact of articulation difficulties and is appropriate for school-age children with SSD (Claessen, Leitão, & Barrett, 2010).

Phonological memory is often tested with a **nonword** repetition task, in which

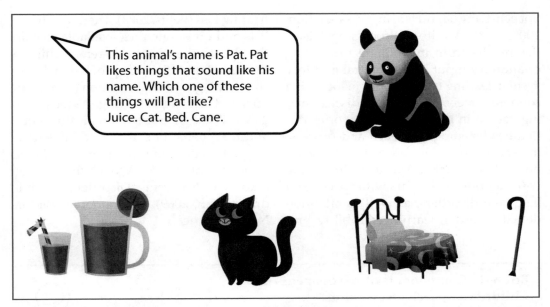

Figure 3–8. *Example of a rime matching task based on procedure used by Bird, Bishop, and Freeman (1995). Practice items with feedback are used to ensure the child understands the task. During test items, instructions to the child are repeated on each item while pointing to the response alternatives. A new animal with a different name is introduced for each rime that is tested. Illustrations by Edith Lebel.*

the child repeats "made-up" words that are not familiar to the child. Nonword repetition taps into many speech processes, including speech perception, encoding of the phonological representation, phonological memory, motor planning, and articulation (Coady & Evans, 2008; Rvachew & Grawburg, 2008). Nonword repetition tasks that are commonly used in English include the Nonword Repetition Test (Dollaghan & Campbell, 1998), the Children's Test of Nonword Repetition (Gathercole & Baddeley, 1996), and the Test of Early Nonword Repetition (Stokes & Klee, 2009). These tests have been used in many studies that included children with developmental language disorder. Young children or children with SSD, however, are likely to misarticulate speech sounds that are used to construct the difficult nonword stimuli for these tests. Therefore, Shriberg, Lohmeier, Campbell, Dollaghan, Green, and Moore (2009) developed the Syllable Repetition Task (SRT), which contains only one vowel (/ɑ/) and four consonants (/b/, /d/, /m/, /n/). Most children, even those with speech impairments, can pronounce these sounds correctly. The SRT contains eight 2-syllable items, six 3-syllable items and four 4-syllable items. Children with phonological memory difficulties should produce fewer errors on the short items compared with the longer items.

Auditory processing refers to "the perceptual processing of auditory information in the central nervous system and neurobiologic activity that underlies that processing and gives rise to electrophysiologic auditory potentials" (American

Speech-Language-Hearing Association, 2005, p. 2). Auditory Processing Disorder results from inadequate processing of auditory input by the central auditory system, leading to difficulties in localizing sounds, perceiving pitch, and discriminating speech in noise—in other words, difficulties listening to speech and processing speech in the presence of background noise (Hind, 2006). Auditory Processing Disorder often co-occurs with speech and language disorders, as well as attention deficit disorder, learning disability, and

hearing loss (Bellis, 2003). There are checklists and questionnaires available to help the SLP decide whether to refer a child to the audiologist, the only professional who should diagnose the condition (American Speech-Language-Hearing Association, 2005). These instruments typically probe auditory behaviors involved in listening skills, communication, and academic achievement. The SCAN-3C, the Test for Auditory Processing Disorders in Children (Keith, 2009), is commonly used in North America.

Box 3–4. Components of Assessments of Children's Speech: Key Points

- A standardized, norm-referenced single-word test of articulation/phonology is used to compare the child's performance with that of a normative group in a time-efficient and standardized manner.
- Two-way scoring classifies the child's productions as correct or incorrect.
- Five-way scoring classifies the child's productions as correct or an error of substitution, omission, distortion, or addition (SODA).
- Stimulability is the child's ability to correctly imitate a phoneme when given a model by the SLP.
- Examination of the oral-peripheral mechanism aims to determine if the structure and function of the articulators are adequate for age-appropriate speech production.
- Oral structure refers to the size, shape, and symmetry of the articulators.
- Oral function refers to the speed and precision of movement, range

- of motion, and coordination of the movements of the articulators.
- A continuous speech sample is more ecologically valid than a single-word test of articulation/phonology, and may reveal speech errors that are present in sentences but not in single words.
- Intelligibility is the degree to which the speaker is understood. This concept is related to, but different than, accuracy, which is the correctness of the articulation of the target.
- Language impairment often co-occurs in children with SSD, and at the very least a language screening measure should be administered.
- Phonological processing skills refer to the child's ability to construct, store, access, and manipulate phonological representations.
- Phonological processing skills are measured with tests of speech perception, phonological awareness, and phonological memory.

3.5 CONSIDERATIONS FOR DIALECT SPEAKERS, CHILDREN SPEAKING ENGLISH AS A SECOND LANGUAGE, AND MULTILINGUAL CHILDREN

SLPs are very likely to assess and provide intervention to children who are not monolingual speakers of the dominant local dialect of English. As of 2000, one in five school-aged children in the United States was not a native speaker of English (U.S. Bureau of the Census, 2000). The number of bilingual and multilingual children in the United States is also growing; 5.2 million bilingual children were attending American schools in 2005 (Goldstein & Fabiano, 2007). These students have a wide variety of native languages, including Spanish as the overwhelming majority with a smaller proportion speaking Asian languages such as Vietnamese, Hmong, Cantonese, and Korean (Office of English Language Acquisition, 2002). In Canada, the proportion of individuals speaking multiple languages at home is increasing; furthermore, approximately 20% of the population speaks a language at home that is not one of the official languages (i.e., English or French; Statistics Canada, 2012).

In addition, all English speakers use a **dialect**, which is a form of language spoken by a particular group of people sharing a geographic region, ethnic group, or social class. Dialects of the same language are differentiated from one another by pronunciation, vocabulary, or grammar. No dialect is superior to another, although the "standard" dialect of a language is promoted in the educational system and considered more prestigious than other dialects of the language (Adler, 1984). In North America, General American Eng-

lish is the dialect typically present in the media and promoted in educational settings. However, several English dialects are spoken in the U.S., including Eastern American English, Southern American English, Appalachian English, Ozard English, and African American English. All speakers of English use a dialect and use different **registers** of the dialect depending on whom they are communicating with, the topic of conversation, and the social setting. For example, speakers of English tend to use a formal register in writing and during formal speaking situations, such as a class presentation or an employment interview, but an informal register when talking to friends and family members. For readers who are interested in learning more about the pronunciation and vowel systems of English dialects in the U.S. and Canada, the Atlas of North American English (Labov, Ash, & Boberg, 2006) describes four major regions of distinctive varieties of English pronunciation across the U.S.: North, South, West, and Midland, as well as regional variability in pronunciation. Maps of ongoing sound changes within these regions are also provided in this excellent resource.

Practice 3–8

Think of how you would write an email message to your professor in comparison to how you would write a text message to a close friend. What are three differences in the register between your written communication to these respective communication partners?

Correctly identifying children who present with an SSD and require intervention can be challenging when the child is learning two or more dialects or languages. Ideally, the SLP would be proficient enough in each of the child's languages to assess the child's skills in all relevant dialects or languages. However, this is rarely the case, and standardized, norm-referenced tests of articulation/ phonology are not usually available for all the languages spoken by the child. Monolingual SLPs can work with interpreters, bilingual consultants, or bilingual communication disorders assistants (Langdon & Cheng, 2002). In addition, children learning English as a second language and multilingual children are exposed to English in different proportions and have different degrees of English proficiency. The timing of exposure to each of their languages also varies; simultaneous bilingualism refers to the acquisition of two languages from birth or shortly after, at the same time, while sequential bilingualism refers to the acquisition of a second language after the first language has been mostly or fully acquired. While the phonological development of bilingual children is similar to that of monolingual children in each of their languages, it is not identical (Goldstein, 2004; Goldstein, Fabiano, & Washington, 2005). In other words, bilingual children are not "two monolingual children in one." Like monolingual children, as they get older and with continued exposure to their languages, bilingual children will develop more precise perceptual, articulatory, phonological, and suprasegmental knowledge, eventually achieving adultlike pronunciation in each of their languages.

It may be challenging for the SLP to determine whether a bilingual child presents with an SSD or presents with speech errors due to influence from the other language(s) the child is learning (difference but not a disorder) or due to normal development (Yavas & Goldstein, 1998; Rvachew, Mattock, Clayards, Chiang, & Brosseau-Lapré, 2011). Goldstein and Fabiano (2007) described a five-step method to assess the speech abilities of second-language learners of English and bilingual children. SLPs also can draw on the growing body of data on cross-linguistic phonological development to help decide whether the child's speech abilities are within normal limits. The Multilingual Children's Speech website (McLeod, 2012), available at http://www.csu.edu.au/ research/multilingual-speech/home, provides information regarding the phonemic inventories (under the tab "Language") as well as assessment tools (under the tab "Speech Assessments") of many languages other than English.

SLPs should also be aware of how they view children and families from culturally and linguistically diverse populations. Cultural competence is a complex process that evolves over time and requires self-assessment of one's biases and assumptions about cultural variables. It encompasses beliefs, values, attitudes and behaviors toward individuals of various ages, gender identities, racial and ethnic origins, and levels of abilities (American Speech-Language-Hearing Association, 2017). Professionals must strive to provide appropriate services to all children and their families, as it is their right to receive assessments and interventions that are culturally appropriate (International Expert Panel on Multilingual Children's Speech, 2012). The American Speech-Language-Hearing Association has developed a series of checklists to help SLPs heighten their awareness of working with culturally and linguistically diverse populations (American Speech-Language-Hearing Association, 2010a, 2010b, 2010c).

Box 3–5. Dialect Speakers, Children Speaking English as a Second Language, and Multilingual Children: Key Points

- A dialect is a form of language spoken by a particular group of people sharing a geographical region, ethnic group, or social class. No dialect is superior to another.
- Simultaneous bilingualism refers to the acquisition of two languages from birth or shortly after at the same time. Sequential bilingualism refers to the acquisition of a second language once the first language has been mostly or fully acquired.
- Evaluating the speech abilities of children who are learning more than one linguistic code (dialects and/or languages) is challenging. Ideally, the SLP would be proficient in each of the child's linguistic codes.
- Cultural competence requires self-assessment of one's biases and assumptions about cultural variables that may influence how they interact with individuals from different cultural backgrounds, linguistic backgrounds, ages, gender identities, and levels of abilities.

Chapter 3 Study Questions

Pretend that you received the following referral from a family physician. Plan an initial assessment session to respond to this request. Use the materials in your school test library to guide your plan in addition to the information in this chapter. If time permits you may wish to role-play the initial assessment with a classmate.

Please assess this young boy (age 4;11) whose parents are concerned about his speech. History of otitis media since age 9 months but health history is otherwise unremarkable and he passed all Denver screenings. He is chatty and sociable but does mispronounce f, s, and r. His uncle is dyslexic and his older sister is receiving some support at school to help with spelling. His father is Spanish speaking but he and his mother speak English fluently.

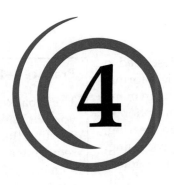

Diagnosis

- Explain why it is important to identify the underlying nature of the child's speech sound disorder (SSD).
- List five kinds of information that can be used to identify different subtypes of SSD.
- Explain why the classification of SSD into phonetic versus phonemic subtypes on the basis of the surface characteristics of the child's error types is not valid.
- Dodd (2014) described a model for differential diagnosis of SSD. List the four expected characteristics of this classification system. Identify the characteristics that have been supported by evidence. Compare and contrast the five diagnostic subtypes comprised by this model.
- Describe the clinical subtypes of SSD that are included in the Speech Sound Disorders Classification System (Shriberg et al., 1997, 2010). Include information about the clinical markers, the proximal causes, and the distal causes of each subtype.
- Compare and contrast the Psycho-linguistic approach to diagnosis with subtyping approaches. Describe some assessment tools that can be used when implementing this approach.
- Identify the best estimate of the prevalence of SSD in children aged approximately 5 years and in children aged approximately 8 years.
- Define comorbidity and list neuro-developmental disorders that are likely to be comorbid with SSD.
- Identify factors that predict good versus poor literacy outcomes for children with SSD.

An assessment, conducted as described in Chapter 3, will provide valuable information about the child's functioning in many domains, including articulation, phonology, oral-motor skills, language, hearing, auditory, and phonological processing. This is not the end stage of the assessment process, however. The population of children with a speech sound disorder (SSD) is **heterogeneous**: this means that these children differ from each other greatly even though they are joined by the common characteristic of poor speech accuracy relative to their age peers. Some children may be more similar to each other than they are different. These similarities within subgroups of children with SSD may indicate different subtypes that will respond differentially to specific approaches to intervention. Therefore, the assessment should lead to a **diagnosis**—a hypothesis about the underlying nature of the child's speech problem. The diagnosis should be revealed after interpreting the assessment information in relation to scientific evidence on the nature of SSDs. In some jurisdictions, speech-language pathologists (SLPs) are proscribed from claiming that they have diagnosed a disorder because this activity is part of the **scopes of practice** that are specifically reserved for certain medical practitioners. Nonetheless, it will not be enough to determine that the child's speech accuracy is below normal limits and recommend an intervention. In order to select the most effective intervention it is important to identify the specific subtype of SSD. A **conclusion** about the subtype of SSD is only possible because researchers have carefully examined the characteristics of children who share similar profiles of signs and symptoms. Four approaches to subtyping SSDs will be discussed in this chapter along with a brief overview of the relevant research.

Practice 4–1

Think back to a time when you felt unwell. How did you decide whether the problem was serious, requiring a visit to the doctor, or something that could be managed by applying over-the-counter remedies at home? Which symptoms (subjective indicators) and signs (objectively measured indicators) helped you come to a conclusion about the nature of your health problem?

4.1 CLASSIFICATION OF SPEECH SOUND DISORDERS

There are five kinds of information that are used to help classify subtypes of SSD in children. Different classification systems tend to focus on certain kinds of information more than others. All classification systems pay at least some attention to the **surface characteristics of the speech errors** produced by the child. Recall from Chapter 2 that when any given phoneme is misarticulated, the error might be a substitution, an omission, a distortion, or an addition. The types of error patterns in the child's speech may be typical or atypical. The child may produce a small number of errors or so many errors that the child's speech is virtually unintelligible. These differences in the types and frequency of misarticulations may be important indicators of different subtypes of SSD. This information will be revealed in the results of the articulation test, the phonological test, and the free speech sample.

Some classification systems also describe the **underlying speech processes** that are presumed to explain the speech errors that the child produces. Very broadly, the underlying speech processes that might be impaired were discussed in Chapter 1 in relation to Figure 1–1: processes for storing and accessing phonological representations in the lexicon, processes for planning and executing a speech utterance, and processes for abstracting and understanding phonological representations from heard speech. These processes will be assessed with the oral-motor assessment, auditory processing assessments, and various measures of phonological processing, including speech perception, phonological awareness, and phonological memory.

Causal-correlates of the SSD may be taken into account. These are known or hypothesized causes of impairments in the underlying speech processes that might explain the speech errors. There may be differences in the child's social or language environment that suggest inadequate exposure to the necessary language inputs, although most children receive at least grossly adequate linguistic experience. There may be structural impairments in parts of the articulatory system, or parts of the auditory system, or any of the neural mechanisms that are required for the function of these systems. Information relevant to these causal-correlates may be revealed in the case history, the family history, the hearing screening, or the oral-peripheral examination. In some cases, impairments in the structure and function of these speech-related systems can be caused by genetic mutations. Syndromes associated with genetic mutations can involve impairments that are so broad-based that they go beyond speech function. For example, speech, language, or cognitive delays can be associated with impairments in other systems such as the heart (as in Williams syndrome) or

the skin (as in Ehlers-Danlos syndrome). The diagnosis and management of these conditions require an interprofessional collaboration of all the professionals involved in the child's care.

The **developmental trajectory** of the speech problem, also called the **natural history**, may differentiate one subtype from another. The onset of the speech problem may be early in development or it may be late, as in after the age of 9 years when speech accuracy should have reached roughly adultlike levels. Furthermore, the onset of the SSD may be gradual or it may be sudden, as when caused by head trauma or an acute disease. The time taken to resolve may also be fast or slow. If a child with SSD achieves speech accuracy that is similar to age peers within two years or before the age of 6 years, the trajectory is called **short-term normalization**. If a child with SSD does not achieve speech accuracy that is similar to age peers before the age of 9 years, the trajectory is called **long-term normalization**. Some children have roughly normal speech development until the age of 6 years but common clinical distortions continue after that age, in which case they show a trajectory of **persistent speech errors**. These trajectories as described by Shriberg (1994) are illustrated in Figure 4–1.

Finally, the nature of the child's speech difficulties might be revealed by the child's response to intervention. Some signs and symptoms of different subtypes of SSD are not fully reliable indicators of any particular subtype. One problem is that SSD is usually a **neurodevelopmental disorder**, which is an impairment involving the development of the brain. Given that the brain is always changing as the child grows and learns, the presentation of the SSD will evolve as the child progresses toward normalization of the

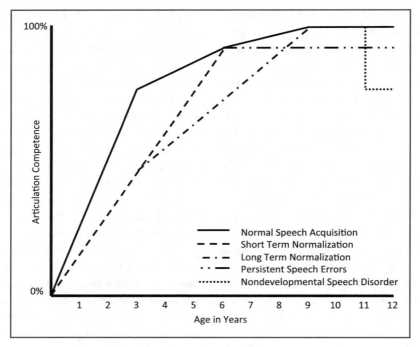

Figure 4–1. *Alternative developmental trajectories for the acquisition of articulation competence. Adapted from Shriberg (1994).*

overt speech errors. Second, some speech error patterns are characteristic of more than one subtype. Therefore if one subtype is hypothesized but the child does not respond well to the treatment, it is prudent to conclude that the child has a different subtype of SSD, which requires a different intervention.

Box 4–1. Classification of Speech Sound Disorders: Key Points

- A **diagnosis** is a hypothesis or conclusion about the nature of the speech sound disorder (SSD), derived from signs and symptoms as revealed by the assessment.
- The diagnosis serves to classify subtypes of SSD according to categories that are differentiated by unique profiles with respect to five kinds of information.
- The five kinds of information

considered when classifying subtypes of SSD are surface characteristics of the speech errors, underlying speech processes, causal-correlates, developmental trajectory, and response to intervention.

- Identifying the subtype of SSD for each child is important because the diagnosis should help to identify the intervention that will be the most effective treatment for the child.

4.2 LINGUISTIC CLASSIFICATION OF SPEECH SOUND DISORDERS

The most traditional practice in the history of speech-language pathology is to consider error types alone when classifying subtypes of SSD. It is assumed that different types of errors signal different underlying causes, which predict response to qualitatively different intervention approaches. Two approaches to subtyping that place primary importance on the surface characteristics of the child's speech will be considered in this section.

4.2.1 Phonetic versus Phonemic Disorder

It has long been assumed that distortion errors, which do not neutralize contrasts between words, reflect poor knowledge of articulatory gestures; therefore, these errors are taken as a sign of **phonetic disorder** (Gierut, 1998; Morley, 1957). On the other hand, substitutions and omissions are phonemic errors because they do collapse or neutralize contrasts between minimal pair words. These errors are thought to arise from a breakdown in linguistic knowledge, and are taken as a sign of **phonemic disorder** (Grunwell, 1981). These two subtypes of SSD are illustrated in Figure 4–2.

Many SLPs make the mistake of thinking that children with distortion errors should be treated with an approach that focuses on articulation, whereas children with phonemic errors must be treated with an approach that focuses on knowledge of phonemic contrast (Fey, 1992). However, there are three major problems with this approach. First, there are few children who present with only phonetic errors or only phonemic errors, especially throughout the complete trajectory of their SSD (Rvachew, Chiang, & Evans, 2007). As a related point, the SLP

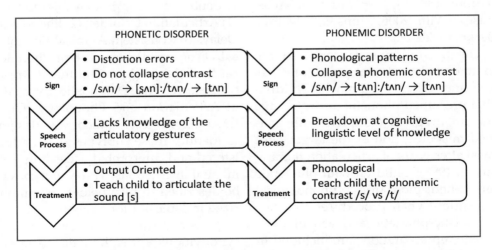

Figure 4–2. *Illustration of the reasoning used to suggest that there are two primary types of SSD: phonetic disorder and phonemic disorder. Research shows that this approach fails at all three levels of classification.*

may find it difficult to judge the child's phonological knowledge by listening to the child's speech errors alone. It can be hard to hear whether the child is producing a substitution "sun" /sʌn/ → [θʌn] or a distortion "sun" /sʌn/ → [s̪ʌn]. The child might appear to neutralize a phonemic contrast but actually produce a covert contrast that is not heard without careful listening. This would be the case if the child produced target /s/ as a stop with extra aspiration: "sun" /sʌn/ → [tʰʰʌn] versus "ton" /tʌn/ → [tʰʌn].

Second, research has shown that the type of error does not predict the impairment in underlying speech processes as reliably as suggested by Figure 4–2. Some children with phonetic errors have difficulties with acoustic-phonetic knowledge and articulatory-phonetic knowledge and phonological knowledge (Preston & Edwards, 2007; Shuster, 1998). Similarly, some children with phonemic errors have difficulties with acoustic-phonetic knowledge and articulatory-phonetic knowledge and phonological knowledge (Bradford & Dodd, 1996; Munson, Baylis, Krause, & Yim, 2006; Munson, Edwards, & Beckman, 2005).

Third, children's response to the recommended treatment procedures has not supported this approach. Children with a presumed phonetic disorder have made no progress (coupled with continued misperception of the target phonemes) after years of articulation therapy (Shuster, 1998). Children with phonemic errors benefit more from a phonological intervention when procedures that target acoustic-phonetic and articulatory-phonetic representations are included in the phonological intervention (Rvachew, Rafaat, & Martin, 1999).

4.2.2 Model for Differential Diagnosis

Subtype classification that focuses on the surface characteristics of the child's speech may be improved by also taking into account the consistency of the child's speech production (Dodd, 1995). Dodd (2014) describes a five-category model for differential diagnosis that is based on the types of errors observed in the child's speech and the consistency of the child's word productions over multiple repetitions. Dodd's classification system is expected to ensure exhaustive diagnosis: this means that every child with SSD will fall into one of the categories. Furthermore, the categories are expected to be mutually exclusive, which means that children can fit into only one category at a time. The categories are also meant to be universally applicable regardless of the child's age or language background. Finally, the child's classification should be developmentally stable even as he or she ages and the SSD becomes less severe. The five subtypes comprised by this model are: (1) Articulation Disorder, (2) Phonological Delay, (3) Consistent Atypical Phonological Disorder, (4) Inconsistent Phonological Disorder, and (5) Childhood Apraxia of Speech. The Diagnostic Evaluation of Articulation and Phonology (DEAP) (Dodd, 2014) test protocol was designed to identify these subtypes when administered and interpreted according to the manual instructions. These subtypes will be described in turn below and summarized in Table 4–1 for easy reference.

Articulation Disorder is roughly synonymous with phonetic disorder in that children with this subtype will typically produce a specific distortion error

Table 4–1. Model of Differential Diagnosis

Characteristics	Examples of Error Types
Articulation Disorder (12% of SSD cases)	
• Distortion errors	"sandbox" /sændbɑks/ → [ʂænbɑkʂ]
• Isolated substitution errors	"castle" /kæsl̩/ → [kæs̺l̩]
• Consistent across syllable positions	"octopus" /ɑktɪpʊs/ → [ɑktɪpʊʂ]
• Produced in imitative and spontaneous tasks	"spade" /speɪd / → [ʂpeɪd]
Phonological Delay (55% of SSD cases)	
• Predictable phonological error patterns	Fronting: "key" /ki/ → [ti] "egg" /ɛg/ → [ɛd]
• Patterns typical in normal speech development	Stopping: "face" /feɪs / → [peɪt] "zoo" /zu/ → [du]
• Produced in imitative and spontaneous tasks	Gliding: "race" /ɹeɪs/ → [weɪt] "lamb" /læm/ → [wæm]
Consistent Atypical Phonological Disorder (20% of SSD cases)	
• Predictable phonological error patterns	Backing: "toe" /to/ → [ko] "tunnel" /tʌnl̩/ → [gʌŋo]
• Patterns atypical in normal speech development	Gliding: "face" /feɪs / → [weɪt] "zoo" /zu/ → [ju] "race" /ɹeɪs/ → [weɪt]
• Co-occur with typical error patterns	"lamb" /læm/ → [wæm]
Inconsistent Phonological Disorder (10% of SSD cases)	
• Inconsistent production of words	"butterfly" /bʌɾɚflaɪ/ → ['bʌ'faɪ], ['bwʌ'faɪ]
• Higher accuracy in imitation than spontaneous	"umbrella" /ʌmbɹɛlʌ/ → [ˌbə'lɛˌlʌ], [bə'lɛˌlʌ]
• Phonemic paraphasia type errors	"helicopter" /hɛlɪkɑptɚ/ → ['hɑtˌdɑg], [ˌhɛ'pɑtɚ]
• More errors on long than short items	"kangaroo" /kæŋgəɹu/ → ['taɪ'nu], ['taɪn'du]
Childhood Apraxia of Speech (3% of SSD cases)	
• Groping	"pig" /pɪg/ → [eX]
• Verbal dyspraxia, possible oral apraxia	"snake" /sneɪk/ → [seɪX]
• Poor accuracy when imitating novel words	"duck" /dʌk/ → [dʌX] "helicopter" /hɛlɪkɑptɚ/ → [heitə]
• Unusual prosody in connected speech	

such as a dental distortion of the sibilants or derhotacized /ɹ/. Certain isolated substitution errors might also place the child in this subtype, such as /ð/ → [d]. The error should be consistent across syllable positions and produced in imitative and spontaneous elicitation tasks. Children with articulation disorder will tend to be older than the average child with SSD when diagnosed. In Table 4–1, the example involves dental distortion of /s/ in all contexts. It is assumed that these errors arise from a failure to learn the articulatory gestures that are required for accurate production of the phoneme or from a subclinical motor deficit that affects planning or execution of the articulatory movements. Approximately 12% of children with SSD will present with this subtype.

Children with **Phonological Delay** produce speech error patterns that are similar to those of younger children with normally developing speech, such as those listed in Table 1–6 in Chapter 1. About 55% of all children with SSD will fall into this category, covering a broad range of preschool ages from 3 to 6 years when diagnosed. The children's productions of these phonological patterns should be predictable, across multiple attempts at the same word, and in both imitative and spontaneous elicitation tasks. Predictable phonological error patterns may not be perfectly consistent, as in occurring in place of every target phoneme. Rather, the error, when it occurs, is predictable. For example, the child may front the velar phonemes (/k,g/ → [t,d]) but only in the coda position of syllables; furthermore, the error may occur for only 50% of the velars in the coda position, but whenever there is an error on these phonemes, the error is fronting. The example shown in Table 4–1 represents consistent fronting of velars, stopping of fricatives, and gliding of liquids in all word positions. Two potential causes have been put forward as hypotheses to explain this subtype of SSD, specifically "slow neurolinguistic maturation" or impoverished input.

The category of **Consistent Atypical Phonological Disorder** is diagnosed when the child produces predictable speech error patterns that do not typically occur in the speech of younger normally developing children. The child will usually produce the more typical kinds of error patterns at the same time. The example shown in Table 4–1 includes two predictable but atypical patterns (backing of velars and gliding of fricatives) as well as one pattern that commonly occurs in the speech of children with typical speech development (gliding of liquids). This subtype also occurs in preschool-aged children, although even younger children may be included, and this subtype occurs at lower frequency than Phonological Delay, affecting about 20% of children with SSD. Dodd (2011) hypothesized that these children have a specific problem abstracting linguistic rules from speech input but this has not been confirmed. In fact, the research suggests that children in this category are fundamentally similar to children with Phonological Delay but with a more severe disorder (Williams & Chiat, 1993). Furthermore, children with Phonological Delay and children with Consistent Phonological Disorder share a tendency to have difficulty with phonological awareness and a family history of speech problems (for further discussion, see Rvachew & Brosseau-Lapré, 2018).

> **Practice 4–2**
>
> List three error patterns that would be typical in a 3-year-old child and then list three error patterns that would be atypical in the speech of a child of any age. Consult the resources in Chapter 2 to confirm your answer.

Inconsistent Phonological Disorder is diagnosed after administering the Word Inconsistency Test from the DEAP (Dodd et al., 2006). The child is asked to name pictures to elicit the 25-word list three times during the same assessment, with other tasks interceding between elicitations of the word set. Children who show variable productions on at least 40% of the words meet the criterion for inconsistency. Furthermore, the inconsistent productions should represent multiple atypical productions of a word rather than alternations between a typical process and the correct production. For example, when attempting the word "vacuum," a child with delayed phonology might alternate between [bækjum] and [vækjum]—this kind of inconsistency does not indicate Inconsistent Phonological Disorder compared with the errors produced by a child classified in the Inconsistent Phonological Disorder subtype, specifically "vacuum" → [bækɒf], [bækɪf], and [bækhoʊ] (Dodd et al., 2005, p. 59). The vowel errors produced in each of these attempts at the word "vacuum" may also be particularly characteristic of Inconsistent Phonological Disorder. These highly unusual speech errors, in which some but not all of the intended speech sounds are retrieved during phonological planning, are referred to as **phonemic paraphasias**. Sometimes the child will retrieve a similar sounding but completely different word to the one that was intended, perhaps "vacuum" → ['vi,ɪ'kl] "vehicle." These types of errors are shown in the example in Table 4–1. Children with inconsistent phonological error patterns have also been shown to achieve higher accuracy in imitated than spontaneous productions of words. It is hypothesized that this disorder is caused by a breakdown in phonological planning. Phonological planning is closely related to phonological memory and therefore this diagnosis can be confirmed by administering the Syllable Repetition Task (Shriberg et al., 2009). Children with phonological planning and phonological memory deficits will make more errors when repeating longer items compared with shorter items (Rvachew & Matthews, 2017b; Shriberg, Lohmeier, Strand, & Jakielski, 2012). This subtype is diagnosed in approximately 10% of children with SSD. These children tend to be younger than average among children with SSD, and the disorder is inevitably severe or moderately severe.

Childhood Apraxia of Speech (CAS) is a rare disorder that arises from a deficit in motor planning. In addition to inconsistent speech errors, significant difficulties will be observed during the oral-peripheral mechanism examination. Specifically, groping while imitating movements, and difficulties attempting to sequence speech and nonspeech movements will be observed (that is, verbal dyspraxia and sometimes oral apraxia, as defined in Chapter 3). A striking characteristic associated with CAS is the inability to imitate novel words or nonsense words that are made of speech sounds that are accurately produced in spontaneous speech.

When the child is capable of producing connected speech, unusual prosody may also be noted. The example in Table 4–1 shows that the child often substituted a velar fricative for velar stops in the coda position of single-syllable words; however, this error did not emerge in the word "helicopter" because two complete syllables were deleted from this difficult word.

The research has generally supported the validity of this model of differential diagnosis in that it is possible to reliably classify children's error profiles at a given point in time using this framework (Broomfield & Dodd, 2004). Furthermore, this model appears to be useful for diagnosing subtypes of SSD among children who speak languages other than or in addition to English (Fox & Dodd, 2001; Holm, Dodd, Stow, & Pert, 1999; So & Dodd, 1994). When using this classification system with bilingual children or English Language Learners or speakers of another language, some adjustments are required to ensure appropriate classification of error patterns as typical or atypical for the language in question.

It has not been established that the resulting classifications reflect stable subtypes. In other words, when children are diagnosed at one age and then retested at a later age, they are likely to be reclassified into a new category (Dodd et al., 2017; Wright, 2017). It appears that the classifications may reflect a gradient of severity and age more clearly than qualitative differences in subtype. When retested, children often move from more severe to less severe subtypes. The exception to this rule is children with an Articulation Disorder who are likely to show long-term normalization. In particular, lateral lisps are atypical and persistent. **Cross-sectional** studies (in which groups of children of different ages are observed) and **longitudinal** studies (in which the same group of children is followed over time) show that this error pattern does not resolve without treatment.

Children with a Phonological Delay are likely to resolve their SSD within a few years, although the impact of intervention compared with "watchful waiting" has not been established for this subtype. Morgan et al. (2017) reported that 70%

Box 4–2. Linguistic Classification of Speech Sound Disorders: Key Points

- Phonetic errors maintain phonemic contrast, whereas phonemic errors neutralize a phonemic contrast. Therefore, distortion errors are often treated with articulation therapy, compared with substitution errors, which may be treated with a phonological approach.
- Research does not support the assumptions of the phonetic-phonemic distinction: children

with phonetic errors and children with phonemic errors often have the same kinds of impairments in underlying speech processes.
- The five-category Model of Differential Diagnosis takes into account consistency of within-word production in addition to the types of errors produced by the child. See Table 4–1.)

of 4-year-olds with Phonological Delay achieved resolution of the SSD before age 7 years; in contrast, only 40% of children with atypical speech errors showed this trajectory of short-term normalization. Children with Consistent Atypical Phonological Disorder are very likely to change to Phonological Delay as time progresses. Inconsistent Phonological Disorder is severe and persists at least over the short term. Further study is required to understand how this disorder evolves in children over the longer term when they receive an appropriate intervention.

4.3 SPEECH DISORDERS CLASSIFICATION SYSTEM

The **Speech Disorders Classification System (SCSD)** was developed by Shriberg and colleagues as a framework that reflects past research and supports future research into the nature of speech disorders. At the most overarching levels there are many possible ways to categorize humans on the basis of their speech competence, as described in the many versions of this framework (Shriberg, 1994; Shriberg, Austin, Lewis, McSweeny, & Wilson, 1997; Shriberg et al., 2010). Only those subtypes that pertain specifically to the **pediatric** (child) population will be discussed here, as shown in Figure 4–3;

furthermore, the figure shows subtypes for children with a primary developmental SSD. This means that nondevelopmental disorders that have their onset after age 9 years have been excluded, as have secondary SSD associated with a known impairment, outside the psycholinguistic system directly, that causes the speech disorder (for example, hearing impairment or craniofacial disorder).

Practice 4–3

Working in small groups, attempt to create a tree diagram to show relationships among speech disorders that might be differentiated according to the following categories: child (pediatric) and adult disorders; normal or normalized speech competence; speech difference (foreign accent), speech delay, and speech disorder; primary speech disorders and secondary speech disorders; phonetic, phonological, and motor speech disorders. You may add additional categories if you wish and leave out categories that don't fit in your scheme. Compare and contrast the different models that are created within your class. Does your model account for all of the different cases of speech disorder that you can think of?

SPEECH DISORDERS CLASSIFICATION SYSTEM (Pediatric, Developmental, Primary Subtypes)							
Speech Delay			Speech Errors		Motor Speech Disorder		
SD-Gen	SD-OME	SD-DPI	SE-/s/	SE-/r/	MSD-AOS	MSD-Dys	MSD-NOS
Genetic	Otitis Media with Effusion	Developmental Psychosocial Involvement	/s/	/r/	Apraxia of Speech	Dysarthria	Not Otherwise Specified

Figure 4–3. Speech Disorders Classification System.

The SCSD framework is essentially a medical model that is intended to link signs and symptoms of the disorder to the **etiology** (that is, the cause or origin of the disorder). For each subtype, a proximal cause and a distal cause is hypothesized. The **proximal cause** is the underlying speech process that explains the types of speech errors that are produced by the child. The **distal cause** is the origin of the impairment in the underlying speech process. The proximal and distal causes interact with environmental inputs over time; these interactions account for commonalities and individual differences in the developmental trajectory of the SSD that is seen in children with the same subtype.

4.3.1 Speech Delay

Speech Delay is actually a set of three subtypes that pertain to children with many substitution and omission errors that impact speech intelligibility. The proximal cause of all three subtypes of Speech Delay is related to impaired phonological representations. Two processes might explain these impaired phonological representations. Some children might have an auditory-perceptual impairment that makes it difficult to transform acoustic input into phonological representations when listening to speech. Other children might have a problem with phonological memory processes that interfere with the storage and retrieval of phonological representations when perceiving and producing speech. When the Speech Delay is especially severe, the child will have both kinds of processing problem—difficulty with auditory-perceptual encoding and difficulty with phonological memory.

These children with pervasive phonological processing difficulties will inevitably have language impairment in addition to speech impairment. Regardless of severity, however, children diagnosed with Speech Delay are expected to achieve short-term normalization with appropriate interventions. The three subtypes in this group are Speech Delay–Genetic (approximately 60% of all children with SSD), Speech Delay–Otitis Media with Effusion (about 30% of all children with SSD), and Speech Delay–Developmental Psychosocial Involvement (about 12% of all children with SSD).

The difference between the three Speech Delay subtypes is at the level of the distal cause. The most frequently occurring subtype, **Speech Delay–Genetic**, is hypothesized to be heritable. There is good evidence that a large number of children with SSD have a heritable disorder linked to a family history of problems in speech, language, and or reading development (Lewis et al., 2006). Furthermore, there is evidence for an overlap between the genetic basis of SSD and reading disability (Eicher et al., 2015). Behavioral, neuroimaging, and genetics studies indicate that the shared proximal cause in speech and reading disorders involves difficulties with phonological processing (Larrivee & Catts, 1999; Pennington & Bishop, 2009; Preston et al., 2012, 2014).

Shriberg (1994) observed that about a third of children with Speech Delay have histories of **otitis media with effusion (OME)** before the age of 3 years. OME means that there is fluid in the middle ear space. This fluid can cause a hearing loss of mild or moderate severity regardless of whether there is an infection. When OME starts at a young age it is more likely to occur repeatedly or last over a long period of time, which is called chronic OME. Chronic OME starting in infancy may be a risk factor for speech and language delay, although a direct causal link has not been established (Bennett & Haggard, 1999; Roberts et al., 2004). The severity of middle ear disease varies widely among young children and the course of language development varies significantly as well. There is little doubt that the amount of hearing loss experienced by a child as a result of OME is one factor that explains individual differences in speech and language development (Feldman et al., 2003), even if OME by itself does not cause speech and language impairment. OME may also interact with other factors, including environmental inputs (Vernon-Feagans, 1999; Yont, Snow, & Vernon-Feagans, 2003). One study observed an interaction between genetic risk and middle ear disease: specifically, poorer vocabulary skills were associated with a history of middle ear disease but only when genetic risk for speech delay was high (McGrath et al., 2007). Nittrouer and Burton (2005) found that children with the joint risk factors of low socio-economic status and OME had significant difficulties with speech perception and phonological awareness tasks.

In the final category, some children with Speech Delay have been observed to have **Developmental Psychosocial Involvement**, in that they were observed to be either aggressive or shy and withdrawn during their speech therapy sessions (Hauner, Shriberg, Kwiatkowski, & Allen, 2005). Hauner et al. suggested that heritable differences in temperament might be associated with genetic factors that cause speech delay. Another hypothesis is that poor social interactions deprive the child of speech inputs that support speech and language development, thus causing a delay. However, it is also possible that poor speech intelligibility itself causes frustration with the social environment, which in turn causes the child to act out or withdraw. The explanation for the association between psychosocial issues and Speech Delay is not clear, but there is research showing that children with speech problems are at risk for mental health problems. The risk of psychiatric problems is even more elevated if the child has a language disorder at the same time as the Speech Delay (Baker & Cantwell, 1987). Behavioral disorders, attention deficit disorders, and anxiety disorders are all unusually common in children with speech disorders compared with children who do not have communication impairments.

Practice 4–4

Imagine that a 4-year-old child is listening to her preschool teacher present a lesson on jungle animals: elephant, giraffe, gorilla, hippopotamus, gazelle. The child has a problem with auditory-perceptual encoding of speech input and some problems with phonological memory as well. How will these difficulties affect the child's learning in this situation? What kinds of speech errors will you expect if the child tries to name the animals during class activities?

4.3.2 Speech Errors

Some children show a trajectory of normal speech accuracy through approximately age 6 years but persistent speech errors thereafter. In other words, the child shows the same speech competence as any other child during the preschool period. Furthermore, no issues with speech intelligibility arise during the child's development. However, during the period 6 through 9 years of age, when distortions of the sibilants and/or rhotics should resolve, the typical pattern of progressively greater speech accuracy and acceptability does not occur. Rather, the child plateaus with a pattern of persistent distortions of one or more late developing phonemes. Persistent speech errors are associated with long-term normalization by definition. The cause is hypothesized to be environmental in origin, but in the form of a practice effect: it is speculated that the child may have mislearned the articulatory gestures for the phoneme at a very young age, before achievement of the physical maturity required to produce the sound correctly; then, having produced the sound incorrectly over many years, the misarticulation becomes resistant to change. There is no experimental evidence to support this claim. There is some evidence based on acoustic analysis to suggest that these errors are different from those produced by children who have residual distortion errors after a history of early speech delay. When children have persistent speech errors after having an earlier history of speech delay, it is possible that the distortion errors have the same cause as the speech delay itself. Some older children with distortion errors have been shown to have difficulties with auditory-perceptual encoding and phonological processing, as in the case of younger children with speech delay (Preston & Edwards, 2007). Other older children with distortion errors have been shown to have motor speech disorders associated with significantly reduced tongue strength (Dworkin, 1980; Dworkin & Culatta, 1980) or deficits in nonspeech and speech motor praxis (Redle et al., 2015). In any case, the child's distortion errors should be treated with an approach that addresses the proximal cause.

4.3.3 Motor Speech Disorders

Motor Speech Disorders (MSDs) involve processes for producing a spoken utterance: (1) planning the series of overlapping vocal tract gestures required to produce the sounds and syllables in the utterance (motor planning); (2) planning the muscle movements that will result in those vocal tract gestures (motor programming); and (3) sending and executing commands to the relevant muscles in order to produce the planned utterance (execution). Motor Speech Disorders are rare, occurring in less than 5% of cases of SSD, and complex, associated with long-term normalization or persistent SSD. Three subtypes are proposed: MSD–Apraxia of Speech (AOS) (a disorder of motor planning and/or programming), MSD-Dysarthria (a disorder of motor execution), and MSD–Not otherwise specified (in which case, the motor involvement is not specifically or uniquely apraxia or dysarthria). Here, the discussion will focus on Childhood Apraxia of Speech.

MSD-AOS is also called Developmental Verbal Dyspraxia in some jurisdictions and Childhood Apraxia of Speech in others. Childhood Apraxia of Speech (CAS) is defined by the American Speech-Language-Hearing Association (2002) as "a neurological childhood (pediatric) SSD in which the precision and consistency of movements underlying speech are impaired in the absence of neuromuscular deficits" (pp. 3–4). The cause of this SSD appears to be genetic, but the exact nature of the genetic cause cannot typically be determined for any given child. Lewis, Freebairn, Hansen, Taylor, et al. (2004) investigated the family pedigrees of children with CAS, or speech-language impairment, or speech delay without language impairment. These researchers found **familial aggregation** of CAS and related diagnoses, that is, clustering of speech and language deficits in families, going back three generations. Familial aggregation was high in all three groups, although highest in the CAS group. In this study, the authors suggested that CAS is associated with an accumulation of multiple commonly occurring genetic risk factors. However, some children with CAS have been found to have specific mutations in a particular gene that is known to be very important in speech development: these are the rare cases of speech disorder linked to an inherited mutation of the *FOXP2* gene (Graham & Fisher, 2015; Vargha-Khadem, Watkins, Alcock, Fletcher, & Passingham, 1995). More recently, it has been found that unusual mutations in other genes that are involved in early brain development are associated with CAS; in these cases the mutations are de novo, which means that they arose in the children without being inherited from the parents (Eising et al., 2018).

Speech errors in apraxia arise from miscoordination of the timing among multiple articulatory gestures, resulting in distortions and single feature substitution errors, such as oral/nasal and voiced/voiceless confusions. Inconsistency in sound production will appear in that the child might produce a given phoneme in one word, even a word where the sound is not expected, but fail to produce it in another word where it is expected. For example, a 9-year-old with CAS was observed to produce "watch" /watʃ/ → [waʃ], "splash" /splæʃ/ → [tæs], "sheep" /ʃip/ → [sip], and "basket" /bæskət/ → [baxtet]. However, within-word inconsistency as revealed by the Word Inconsistency Test is not a reliable indicator of CAS (Murray, McCabe, Heard, & Ballard, 2015). In fact, Murray et al. found that CAS could be reliably diagnosed by two procedures—an oral-mechanism examination and a test that involved naming pictures to elicit polysyllable words. CAS was reliably diagnosed by measures of lexical stress match when producing the polysyllable words, overall phoneme accuracy, syllable segregation, and an inability to sequence [pataka]. The errors in the production of lexical stress reflect the characteristic of **unusual prosody** that is commonly reported for CAS; these issues with prosody arise from the challenge of coordinating duration, loudness, and pitch cues. Syllables might be segregated by a noticeable pause or by the insertion of an extra sound, usually a nasal. Murray et al. observed the problem with syllable segregation in the polysyllable word task. However, this problem with syllable segregation can also be observed by administering the Syllable Repetition Task (Shriberg et al., 2009, 2012). The child is asked to repeat sequences of syllables such as "bada" and "banada." If the child inserts a sound into four or more of the 18 items (e.g., "banda," "bananda"), it is almost certain that the child has CAS (Rvachew & Matthews, 2017b). These errors are just as likely to occur on the short items as the long items when the child has CAS. Shriberg et al. refer to these errors as transcoding errors because they arise during the process of transcoding the phonological plan into a motor plan.

Children with apraxia have particular difficulty imitating words, especially if the adult is trying to teach the child to produce a new word or to produce a learned word in a new way. Children with apraxia frequently perseverate, which means that once they have produced a word in a particular fashion, it will be very hard for them to correct the error or change that production even when given an imitative model and other supports for greater accuracy.

CAS can be differentiated from another motor speech disorder, dysarthria, which involves more pervasive effects on phonation, resonance, articulation, and prosody secondary to paresis, weakness, or abnormalities of tone in the muscles. Children with dysarthria will typically produce very slow single syllable repetition rates and have difficulty prolonging a vowel. Guidelines for differentiating CAS and dysarthria on the basis of maximum performance tasks have been published by Thoonen, Maassen, Gabreels, and Schreuder (1999).

Box 4–3. Speech Disorders Classification System: Key Points

- The Speech Disorders Classification System (SCSD) defines subtypes that link signs and symptoms to proximal and distal causes.
- Three types of developmental SSDs are proposed in the SCSD: Speech Delay, Speech Errors, and Motor Speech Disorders.
- SD-Genetic, SD–Otitis Media with Effusion, and SD–Developmental Psychosocial Involvement are three subtypes of Speech Delay that are thought to share the same proximal cause involving impairments in phonological representations.
- The Speech Error subtypes involve persistent distortions of sibilants or rhotics.
- All of the Motor Speech Disorders are rare but the most common is Childhood Apraxia of Speech, a disorder in which the precision, consistency, and sequencing of speech motor movements are impaired.

4.4 PSYCHOLINGUISTIC APPROACH

The psycholinguistic approach to diagnosis shares the goal of identifying the speech processing deficits that account for the surface characteristics of the child's speech. The assumption remains that it is important to understand these underlying deficits in order to select a treatment approach that is best suited to the child's unique needs. This approach differs from Dodd's (1995) model and Shriberg et al.'s (2010) framework in that no predetermined system of subtypes is specified. Importantly, there is no expectation that all children with SSD can be classified into a small set of discrete, mutually exclusive categories. Each child is considered as an individual with a unique profile. The profile of deficits is determined by testing underlying processes that are hypothesized to be important while listening to or producing speech. The difficulty for the SLP is that many models exist to generate hypotheses about the important underlying speech processes (Baker, Croot, McLeod, & Paul, 2001; Maas, 2016). An additional problem is that the technologies that are used to assess the underlying processes are not always available for clinical use. However, most of the models propose that speech impairments are caused by breakdowns in input processes, phonological representations, or output processes. Some clinical measures have been developed in these three domains.

4.4.1 Speech Perception

Word identification tests are useful to assess the child's knowledge of the acoustic-phonetic cues that define phonological categories. It is important that such tests target phoneme categories that are relevant to the child's speech sound errors. The test stimuli should be highly variable exemplars of the target words. Often, children with SSD can identify words accurately when presented with clearly produced live-voice exemplars of the target words. For example, a speech perception deficit may well account for the error "sick" /sɪk/ → [θɪk] in a child who does not distinguish these sounds in speech. This child may be able to identify the words "sick" and "thick" when presented live-voice by the SLP. The child might differentiate these words perceptually on the basis of duration, however, because /s/ is longer than /θ/. Focusing on this unreliable cue will not help the child to produce the sound with correct tongue placement to achieve the sibilant spectral characteristic of /s/. Therefore, variable natural

speech or synthetic speech that varies the duration and spectral characteristics of the fricative is necessary for a valid test of the child's perceptual knowledge of this contrast (Rvachew & Jamieson, 1989). Many studies have shown that children with SSD have difficulty perceiving speech sound contrasts that they misarticulate (Hearnshaw, Baker, & Munro, 2018; Hoffman, Daniloff, Bengoa, & Schuckers, 1985; Hoffman, Stager, & Daniloff, 1983; Kronvall & Diehl, 1952; Rvachew, Ohberg, Grawburg, & Heyding, 2003).

One interesting aspect of this research is that these speech perception deficits have been observed in children with phonological delay (Hearnshaw et al., 2018), in children with persistent speech errors (Shuster, 1998), and in children with CAS (Maassen, Groenen, & Crul, 2003). However, the research shows that a speech perception deficit is not a necessary cause of SSD in that many children with speech errors do not have a speech perception deficit relative to children with typical speech (Rvachew & Grawburg, 2006). Furthermore, a speech perception deficit may co-occur with speech errors while not being causal: Zuk, Iuzzini-Seigel, Cabbage, Green, and Hogan (2018) found that speech perception deficits in children with CAS were specifically associated with language impairment; that is, children who had CAS but normally developing language skills did not have difficulty with a speech discrimination task. Therefore, they concluded that poor speech perception is not a core deficit in CAS, but rather reflects language impairment that sometimes co-occurs with the speech impairment. Altogether, these findings support the psycholinguistic approach by reinforcing the importance of identifying each individual child's profile of strengths and weaknesses. It is not possible to assume by diagnostic label alone that any given child will have deficits in input processes or output processes exclusively.

4.4.2 Phonological Awareness

It is commonly assumed that children who produce predictable patterns of phonological error in their speech have a breakdown at the level of phonological representations. Many tasks tap the growing sophistication of the child's phonological knowledge as experience with language increases. Tests of phonological awareness are frequently used by SLPs because they reveal the child's knowledge of the smaller phonological units that make up words; knowledge of the small units that can be combined and recombined to form words is important for speech accuracy and the organization of the lexicon. Furthermore, the child's performance on these tests is predictive of reading acquisition, an important part of the SLP's scope of practice. Finally, phonological awareness tests are readily available and easy to administer in the clinic. Relatively poor phonological awareness skills in children with SSD compared with children with typical speech is a consistent finding (Anthony et al., 2011; Holm, Farrier, & Dodd, 2007; Larrivee & Catts, 1999; Nathan, Stackhouse, Goulandris, & Snowling, 2004a; Raitano, Pennington, Tunick, Boada, & Shriberg, 2004; Rvachew & Grawburg, 2006; Rvachew et al., 2003). These studies also show that the phonological awareness deficit will be considerably worse if the child with SSD has a co-occurring language delay. However, even when there is SSD with no co-occurring language problem, the child is at risk for significant difficulties with phonological awareness (Rva-

chew et al., 2003). One possible reason for poor phonological awareness skills is that some children abstract poor quality phonological representations from speech input (Claessen, Heath, Fletcher, Hogben, & Leitão, 2009; Claessen & Leitão, 2012; Munson et al., 2006). Other children may have poor phonological awareness skills because they have difficulty accessing and manipulating phonological representations (Ramus, Marshall, Rosen, & Van der Lely, 2013).

4.4.3 Nonword Repetition

Tests of nonword repetition are traditionally thought to measure the capacity of short-term phonological working memory. In fact, it has become clear that this task reflects many aspects of speech processing (Moore, Fiez, & Tompkins, 2017; Rvachew & Grawburg, 2008). The child must encode the phonetic information in the nonword as presented, retrieve those same units from long-term memory while constructing a plan for production of the nonword, and then execute a motor plan to produce the nonword accurately. Poor performance on tests of nonword repetition has been associated with developmental language disorder in many studies, but interestingly, nonword repetition correlates closely with articulation test scores in children with language disorders and children with typical language (Colledge et al., 2002; Gray, 2006).

Performance on tests of nonword repetition is impacted by many factors, including the developmental difficulty of the speech sounds used to construct the nonwords. Therefore, a special Syllable Repetition Task has been developed for use with children who have SSD, in which the items are composed exclusively of early developing speech sounds (Shriberg et al., 2009). The child's performance on this task can be scored to reveal deficits in auditory-perceptual encoding, phonological memory, or transcoding (Shriberg et al., 2012). This test is useful to identify children who will benefit from a treatment approach that targets phonological planning deficits versus a treatment approach that targets motor planning deficits (Rvachew & Matthews, 2017b).

Practice 4–5

Download the Syllable Repetition Task from the Waisman Center Phonology Project (http://www2 .waisman.wisc.edu/phonology/ pubs-tech.html). In pairs, administer the test to each other and score the test using the reference data in Lohmeier and Shriberg (2011).

4.4.4 Multisyllable Repetition

When conducting the oral-peripheral mechanism examination, the child is asked to repeat [pata] or [pataka] as fast as possible. This task may seem similar to nonword repetition, but there are important differences. During nonword repetition, many different items are presented and thus the task challenges phonological planning: the child must select and order a new arrangement of phonemes each time. During the [pataka] task, the SLP allows the child many trials to learn the sequence; once the sequence is learned, the child tries to repeat it quickly. The challenge is in motor planning and execution. Rvachew and Brosseau-Lapré (2018) reported that 18% of preschoolers with SSD failed to repeat at least one

of [pata] or [pataka] with expected rate, rhythm, and accuracy. This rate of failure is higher than would be expected for diagnosis of CAS on a clinical caseload: poor multisyllable repetition rate by itself does not imply a motor speech disorder. Typically, children with CAS will not be able to sequence the syllables at all and will demonstrate other signs of a motor speech disorder such as syllable segregation and unusual prosody. However, the common finding of slow repetition rates (see also Bradford & Dodd, 1996; Dodd & McIntosh, 2008) indicates that delays in the acquisition of speech motor control may play a role in some children's SSD.

4.4.5 Undifferentiated Lingual Gestures

Electropalatography (EPG) is used to examine tongue movements while speaking by showing the pattern of tongue contacts with the palate over time. Studies using this technology show that children gradually gain control of the different parts of the tongue (tongue tip/blade, lateral margins or sides of the tongue, and tongue dorsum). The ability to control the different parts of the tongue independently is achieved by approximately 6 years of age. EPG shows that when the older child is producing alveolar sounds (e.g., /n,t,s/), the lateral margins of the tongue make contact with the palate first and then the tongue tip and/or blade is raised to the alveolar ridge while the tongue dorsum remains lowered; the movement to close the vocal tract is back-to-front and then, to open the vocal tract, the movement is front-to-back (Gibbon, 1999). Importantly, lateral bracing, whereby the sides of the tongue remain in contact with the back of the palate, is maintained throughout speech except for certain sounds (such as /l/). Active and continuous bracing of the tongue during speech suggests that lateral bracing provides essential stability to the tongue, permitting the fast and precise movements that are used during speech production (Gick, Allen, Roewer-Després, & Stavness, 2017).

In contrast to the normal course of development for tongue gestures, some children with SSD do not learn to control the different parts of the tongue precisely and independently. These children with SSD produce **undifferentiated lingual gestures** when they are speaking: they raise the entire tongue to make contact across the whole palate at once when producing a lingual stop; if the closure is released front-to-back, a [k] will be perceived; if the closure is released back-to-front, a [t] will be perceived. The same child attempting fricative sounds (e.g., /s,ʃ/) will likely produce a lateral distortion. This problem with the production of differentiated tongue gestures during speech articulation will usually be associated with persistent speech errors or atypical errors such as backing. Undifferentiated lingual gestures are associated with a trajectory of long-term normalization. Not all children with lateral lisps produce undifferentiated lingual gestures, however (Goozée et al., 2007).

It is important to know that undifferentiated lingual gestures may underlie certain atypical speech patterns. Furthermore, the importance of lateral bracing in normal speech production is essential when conducting articulation therapy. Unfortunately, however, the tools used to confirm that children are producing these imprecise tongue gestures during speech are not typically available in the speech clinic. EPG requires that a custom-made artificial palate be constructed for each child, and therefore the procedure is expensive, even when the equipment is available. More recently, relatively inexpensive ultrasound equipment has become available for clinical use that provides some information about tongue movements during speech. Ultrasound does not show the pattern of tongue contacts with the palate, however, so this technology does not provide all of the information that is required. Nonetheless, ultrasound combined with careful observation of the child while speaking will provide some information about whether the speech errors have an underlying basis that is articulatory in nature.

Practice 4–6

Produce the following disyllables while thinking carefully about where each part of your tongue is throughout the movement: /ata/, /asa/, /ana/, /ala/, /aɹa/, /aʃa/, /aka/. Consider: (1) the position of your tongue in relation to your lower jaw; (2) the way that each part of your tongue makes contact with the top of your mouth; (3) the timing of those contacts as you move into and out of the consonant. Now say multisyllable words such as "stationary" and "assistant" quickly. How important is **lateral bracing** to your ability to say those words quickly?

4.4.6 Tongue Strength

Children with lateral and frontal lisps have also been shown to have reduced tongue strength in some studies (Dworkin, 1980; Goozée et al., 2007), but not all (Dworkin & Culatta, 1980; Fairbanks & Bebout, 1950). Reduced tongue strength has also been observed in some children with CAS (Murdoch, Attard, Ozanne, & Stokes, 1995; Robin, Somodi, & Luschei, 1991). Significantly low tongue strength cannot be detected reliably without special equipment, however, and therefore the SLP risks underdiagnosis or overdiagnosis of difficulties with tongue strength using the methods that are typically employed during the oral-peripheral mechanism examination. The scientific studies on this topic strongly suggest that low tongue strength is reliably associated with slow monosyllable repetition rates, which are easily measured by the SLP in the clinic. Slow monosyllable repetition rates when measured reliably in school-aged children are a good indicator of dysarthria (Thoonen et al., 1999).

4.5 EPIDEMIOLOGY OF SSD

This chapter has focused on diagnosis, that is, identifying SSD and subtypes of SSD in an individual child and understanding the factors associated with that child's speech problem. Some researchers are especially interested in describing SSD in populations of individuals, that is, the **epidemiology** of SSD. Epidemiologists ask certain kinds of questions about how health conditions are distributed in a population of individuals. For example, it is important to know the **prevalence** of SSD in the population: that is, what is

---

Box 4–4. Psycholinguistic Approach: Key Points

- Using the Psycholinguistic Approach to diagnosis, the SLP attempts to discover each child's unique profile of strengths and deficits in underlying speech processes.
- Different tests are administered to assess input processing, phonological processing, and output processing.
- Deficits in any of these areas may be proximal causes of the child's speech errors. Other deficits may be related factors but not direct causes of the speech errors.
- Tests of speech perception can be used to assess perceptual knowledge of the acoustic-phonetic cues associated with the phoneme contrasts that the child misarticulates.

- Phonological awareness tests tap the child's knowledge of the small phonological units that make up words.
- Nonword repetition can be used to assess auditory-perceptual encoding, phonological memory and planning, and transcoding.
- During the oral-peripheral mechanism examination, it is routine to assess monosyllable and trisyllable repetition rates to differentiate apraxia from dysarthria.
- When the specialized equipment is available, differentiated versus undifferentiated lingual gestures can be observed and tongue strength can be assessed.

the proportion of people at any one time who have SSD? It may also be important to understand the distribution of SSD: in other words, is SSD more likely in some parts of the population than others if divided by age or social circumstances or geography or other such variables? Epidemiologists also study the determinants of health conditions: specifically, what are the factors that are causally associated with variations in the distribution of SSD? Finally, epidemiologists study the natural history of health conditions at the population level; in the case of SSD, the time course of the disability from first diagnosis through resolution is of interest, including any secondary disabilities that might arise from the speech disorder itself.

Epidemiology research is critical to public health practice, which is focused on preventing health problems and maximizing health in the population (Law, Reilly, & Snow, 2013). SLPs who work in public health settings engage in three kinds of prevention. Primary prevention is concerned with preventing the occurrence of speech and language difficulties by targeting causal factors. For example, exposure to passive tobacco smoke increases the risk of otitis media. Therefore, SLPs and audiologists can educate the population about the risks of smoking with respect to child hearing and the possibility of subsequent speech and language difficulties. SLPs can also encourage adoption of public policies that would reduce those risks. Secondary prevention is concerned with the provision of targeted early interventions to people who are at risk of developing a health problem or in the early stages of a health problem. Secondary prevention is strongly associated with screening pro-grams to identify people who might be at risk and thus require an early intervention to avoid the consequences of living with an undetected health problem. Universal neonatal hearing screening is promoted as a secondary prevention program because early intervention is essential to achieving normalized speech in the short and long term by children with hearing impairment (Ertmer & Nathani Iyer, 2012). Tertiary prevention aims at preventing unnecessary secondary impacts of a health problem. For example, successful treatment of speech problems prior to school entry may prevent the subsequent appearance of reading difficulties (Nathan, Stackhouse, Goulandris, & Snowling, 2004b). Public health planning to target resources efficiently at these three levels of prevention requires good quality epidemiology research.

4.5.1 Prevalence of SSD

The process of determining the prevalence of SSD in the population is complicated. Any such study employs a series of steps, roughly as follows: (1) identify some part of the population for study such as all the pupils registered to a given school board or all the babies born in a certain hospital during a certain time period; (2) administer a relatively inexpensive screening procedure to identify children who are likely to have speech problems versus those who are not likely to have speech problems; (3) test a random sample of the children who failed the screen and a matched sample of children who passed the screen, using a longer set of diagnostic tests to confirm the presence or absence of SSD in those children; and (4) estimate the prevalence of SSD for the entire population using the data obtained from the direct testing administered in the third step, after statistical adjustments for screening errors. It can be seen that researchers can make many different decisions at each of these steps. For example, the screening tests vary a great deal: some researchers test children directly, others test children over the phone, and others screen the children via parent questionnaires. The criteria used to define SSD vary greatly as well, especially regarding the inclusion or exclusion of distortion errors in the coding of children's speech errors. Therefore, it is not surprising that as many as 100 different estimates have been obtained with no consensus as to the correct estimate for the prevalence of SSD in the population (Shriberg, Tomblin, & McSweeny, 1999). One estimate for the prevalence at school entry is 6%, arrived at by calculating the average of all the estimates that varied between approximately 2% and 25% (Law, Boyle, Harris, Harkness, & Nye, 2000).

Rvachew and Brosseau-Lapré (2018) took a different approach, reasoning that the best estimate should be associated with the most satisfactory methods overall. After reviewing certain studies in detail, two studies with sensible procedures for the kindergarten-aged population yielded estimates of approximately 11% to 12% having SSD (Beitchman et al., 1986; McLeod & Harrison, 2009). This estimate includes children who have speech problems alone (~6%) and those who have combined speech and language problems (~5%).

Another well-designed study found that 18% of children aged 8 years produced persistent speech errors (Roulstone, Miller, Wren, & Peters, 2009). In this study any type of speech errors heard in connected speech were counted, including substitution, omission, and distortion errors of any type. The children in this study were part of a population-based longitudinal follow-up study and therefore the children who had speech errors at age 8 years (the **cases**) could be compared with children who did not (the **controls**) at ages 2, 5, and 8 years. The case–control comparisons revealed that the cases and controls did not differ with respect to social class or maternal age, but there were more boys among the cases (60%) than controls (51%). At age 2 years the case and control groups both tended to make many speech errors, and therefore this variable did not predict the child's speech status at age 8 years. At age 5 years the higher number of speech errors produced by the cases was striking in comparison to the controls.

A tendency for boys to be more likely to have SSD than girls has been reported in other studies. Campbell et al. (2003) found that speech delay was 7.71 times more likely in a child who had these three risk factors: male sex, mother not graduated from high school, and family history of stuttering, articulation, and/or language disorder. This estimate of risk comes from a large population-based sample (639 participants) with exceptionally good experimental procedures and thus this is likely to be a reliable estimate of risk due to these factors. However, it is possible that the strength of the maternal education risk factor is specific to the United States. The male sex and family history risk factors may be indicators of distal causal factors.

Practice 4–7

As a class project, investigate the prevalence of different neurodevelopmental diseases. Each student or group of students should choose a developmental condition that you have heard of (for example, Autism Spectrum Disorders, Craniofacial Disorders, Down syndrome, and others that you are interested in). Research the prevalence of this condition via internet search. Find the prevalence for the population of children as a whole. Decide on a best estimate for the prevalence either by taking an average of multiple estimates or by taking the best estimate from a trusted source. Be sure to identify prevalence and not incidence from the sources that you consult. With the help of your instructor, make a bar chart that shows the prevalence estimates for each developmental condition, including SSD, in descending order from most to least prevalent. What does the chart tell you about the prevalence of SSD relative to these other conditions?

4.5.2 Comorbidity

Comorbidity is defined as the presence of another health problem that co-occurs with the primary health problem. Here, three neurodevelopmental conditions that co-occur with SSD will be discussed: (1) developmental language disorder; (2) reading and/or spelling disability; and (3) stuttering. It should be noted that mental health and behavioral disorders are also comorbid with SSD, as briefly described in subsection 3.4.1 and discussed in greater depth in Rvachew & Brosseau-Lapré (2018).

Developmental Language Disorder involves difficulties with receptive and expressive vocabulary, morphology, and syntax (Bishop, Snowling, Thompson, Greenhalgh, & CATALISE-2 consortium, 2017) and these may all co-occur with SSD. One population-based study found that one-third of the children identified as having SSD also had developmental language disorder (Shriberg et al., 1999). Clinic-based samples find much higher overlap between these two communication disorders. For example, Cantwell and Baker (1987) reported that two-thirds of children assessed at a speech-language clinic had comorbid speech and language disorder. This discrepancy might be explained by the fact that children with language disorders are more likely to receive treatment if they also have a speech disorder (Zhang & Tomblin, 2000). However, the estimate of comorbidity between speech and language disorders may be underestimated in some studies because persistent speech errors are often excluded from consideration. Kindergarten children with many distortion errors are likely to experience long-term persistence of the speech disorder (Roulstone et al., 2009) and they may have significant difficulties with the production of morphosyntax (Haskill & Tyler, 2007); therefore it is not clear that it is reasonable to exclude this group from the definition of speech delay when the number of speech errors is unusually high. Taken together, these studies suggest that it is very common for children with SSD to have comorbid developmental language disorder. These children with SSD are at risk for other comorbidities that are common to the language-impaired population, especially in the mental health and academic domains.

Reading Disability is diagnosed when the child does not achieve grade level reading despite high-quality literacy instruction. Reading is assessed with tests of word recognition (accuracy in oral reading of printed words), nonword decoding (accuracy in oral reading of printed nonwords), reading comprehension (ability to answer questions about a printed passage), and reading fluency (ability to read a printed passage quickly, smoothly, and accurately). Children with reading disability usually have especially poor nonword decoding skills, reflecting an underlying impairment in phonological processing. Some children have a specific reading comprehension deficit that reflects poor oral language comprehension skills. Other children have difficulties in multiple areas, showing poor word reading and reading comprehension simultaneously. Children with developmental language disorder are twice as likely to have reading disability as children with normally developing language skills (Catts, Fey, Zhang, & Tomblin, 2001; Puranik, Petcher, Al Otaiba, Catts, & Lonigan, 2008). Children with SSD do not have significantly elevated risk of reading disability (Catts, 1993) unless there is comorbid language disorder (Lewis, Freebairn, & Taylor, 2000) or the SSD persists past the age of school entry (Nathan et al., 2004a). Children with SSD are at heightened risk of spelling disorder even when language skills are within normal limits (Lewis et al., 2000).

Stuttering is one of the Childhood Fluency Disorders (American Speech-Language-Hearing Association, 2018). The primary characteristic in childhood is an excessive number of repetitions and prolongations of speech sounds and syllables while speaking. Sasisekaran (2014) reviewed three kinds of studies that illuminate the role of phonology in stuttering, with the following conclusions: (1) phonetic complexity and syllable stress patterns in words contribute to the occurrence of dysfluencies in speech; (2) children who stutter seem to have phonological planning deficits; and (3) it is not clear whether preschoolers who stutter are more likely to have SSD than preschoolers who do not stutter. In fact, several small sample studies suggested that children who stutter eventually achieve age-appropriate speech accuracy during the preschool period. On the other hand, surveys of school SLP caseloads suggest a high level of comorbidity. For example, Blood, Ridenour, Qualls, and Hammer (2003) found in a sample of 2,628 children in grades 1 through 12 that 33% of children who stuttered had a co-occurring articulation disorder and 12% had a co-occurring phonological disorder. This finding may reflect the particular criteria for providing services to children in those schools, located in the United States. Alternatively, children whose fluency disorder persists into the school years may be more likely to have a comorbid SSD.

4.5.3 Short- and Long-Term Outcomes

Children with SSD can experience different kinds of outcomes over the short and the long term. First, there are outcomes that are specific to the speech disorder (that is, speech accuracy and acceptability). Second, there are outcomes in other domains that are related to the speech disorder (such as literacy skills). Third, there are outcomes that may be consequences of having the speech disorder when young (for example, vocational outcomes and life satisfaction). Researchers can study groups of children who have been diagnosed with SSD at a young age, and then follow them for years to determine these outcomes. The results will depend upon the age of the children at diagnosis and at follow-up. The type of speech disorder will also play a role: specifically, these studies usually compare children who have SSD alone with those who have a comorbid language disorder.

When diagnosis and intervention begin at a young age, the probability that the child will achieve normalized speech accuracy in the short term appears to be relatively good. For example, Webster, Plante, and Couvillion (1997) treated 45 children at an average age of 3 years for remediation of their phonological delay. They found that 66% of these children achieved normalized speech 3 years later. It is possible that early intervention is particularly effective. Alternatively, 3-year-olds may be at greater risk of overdiagnosis compared with older children, or children diagnosed at this age may be most likely to fall into the Phonological Delay subtype. In any case, it is possible that some younger children might resolve their phonological errors without direct intervention (Glogowska, Roulstone, Enderby, & Peters, 2000).

When children are diagnosed and treated just before or after school entry, the probability that the child will achieve normalized speech accuracy in the short term is not as good. Shriberg and Kwiatkowski (1994) defined short-term normalization as achieving age-appropriate speech within two years of diagnosis or before 6 years of age. They followed 54 four-year-old children whose SSD was severe on average. Only 18% of these children achieved short-term normalization. Severity of the SSD certainly plays a role. Dodd et al. (2017) followed 93 children from 4 to 7 years of age and found that 58% of the children achieved normal speech production skills, but these children, as a group, had less severe speech impairment compared with the group followed by Shriberg and Kwiatkowski (1994). Within the group followed by Dodd et al. (2017), short-term normalization was most likely for the children with Phonological Delay (67%), less likely for children with consistent atypical error patterns (45%) and least likely for children with inconsistent errors (0%).

A few studies have followed children for longer periods to trace the time course of speech normalization into the school-age period. When children are referred as preschoolers due to concerns regarding speech and language function, as many as 30% will have ongoing difficulties with speech accuracy and language (Baker & Cantwell, 1987) as well as problems with reading acquisition and social-emotional issues (Glogowska, Roulstone, Peters, & Enderby, 2006; Lewis et al., 2000) when assessed 3 to 5 years later.

Johnson et al. (1999) also found that diagnosis at school entry was highly stable, in this case following the children into young adulthood. Of those children who had speech delay at 5 years, 44% still had speech errors at age 19 years. Considering children who had speech or language problems at school entry, 49% had speech errors as adults compared with 17% of the control group.

The primary consequence of persistent speech errors appears to be in the domain of literacy skills (Lewis et al., 2000). Children with SSD as preschoolers are very likely to have spelling disorder in third grade (30% for children with SSD only and 58% for children with SSD and a language disorder). Children with speech and language disorder as preschoolers have a 46% chance of reading disability in third grade. These children who have a greater likelihood of reading problems in third grade are also more likely to have a family history of speech, language, or reading disability.

Adults who were diagnosed with speech and/or language delay at school entry tend to choose occupations that require lower levels of reading or writing competency, a choice that may impact employment and earnings potential over the long term. Nonetheless, these adults reported similar life satisfaction to individuals who have never had speech or language problems (Felsenfeld, Broen, & McGue, 1994).

Epidemiology studies have implications for the prioritization of speech and language services. Rvachew and Rafaat (2014) reviewed these studies and concluded that immediate speech therapy should be provided upon diagnosis of SSD when the following conditions were met: (1) child age between 4 and 6 years inclusive; and (2) family history of speech, language, or fluency disorder; or (3) comorbid language disorder; or (4) significant impact of the SSD on activities of daily living. In the absence of these risk factors, waits for service could be longer.

Box 4–5. Epidemiology of SSD: Key Points

- Among 5-year-olds, the prevalence of SSD is approximately 11%, comprising 6% with SSD alone and 5% with speech and language disorder.
- Among 8-year-olds, approximately 18% have persistent speech errors.
- Language, reading, and spelling disorders are known to be frequently comorbid with SSD.
- It is not clear if stuttering and SSD are comorbid in the preschool population, but these two conditions co-occur frequently on school SLP caseloads.
- A large proportion of children who are treated for SSD as preschoolers continue to produce speech errors into adulthood.
- Children with a preschool history of SSD are more likely to have reading difficulties in third grade if the SSD persists into the school-age period and/or if there is comorbid language disorder and/or if there is a family history of speech, language, or reading disability.
- Despite ongoing weaknesses in literacy skills that impact vocational choices, adults who had a history of SSD report good life satisfaction.

Chapter 4 Study Questions

Question 1: Each characteristic listed below pertains to one of the five subtypes in Dodd's (2014) Model of Differential Diagnosis. Put the letter associated with the appropriate subtype next to each relevant characteristic. Note that characteristics marked (*) are associated with more than one subtype.

Subtypes: (a) Articulation Disorder, (b) Phonological Delay, (c) Consistent Atypical Phonological Disorder, (d) Inconsistent Phonological Disorder, (e) Apraxia of Speech.

Characteristics:

1 _____ Mix of typical and atypical but predictable phonological error patterns.

2 _____ Greater accuracy in spontaneous speech than in imitation.

3 _____ Approximately 10% of children with SSD will present with this subtype.

4 _____ Word productions may be highly dissimilar to the target (phonemic paraphasias).

5 _____ Approximately 55% of children with SSD will present with this subtype.

6 _____ Poor phonological awareness and a family history of speech problems.*

7 _____ Consistent in imitative and spontaneous tasks.*

8 _____ Repeated productions of the same word are inconsistent.

9 _____ A rare disorder that arises from a deficit in motor planning.

10 _____ Groping when imitating new words or nonspeech movements.

11 _____ Predictable phonological error patterns.

12 _____ Higher accuracy in imitated than spontaneous productions of words.

13 _____ Make more errors on longer items compared with shorter items.

14 _____ Approximately 3% of children with SSD will present with this subtype.

15 _____ Arise from a failure to learn the necessary articulatory gestures.

16 _____ Speech error patterns that are similar to those of younger children with normal speech.

17 _____ Approximately 12% of children with SSD will present with this subtype.

18 _____ Approximately 20% of children with SSD will present with this subtype.

19 _____ Caused by a breakdown in phonological planning.

20 _____ May be caused by "slow neurolinguistic maturation" or impoverished input.

21 _____ Unusual prosody in connected speech.

22 _____ Distortion error or isolated substitution error.

23 _____ Consistent across word positions.

Question 2: Each characteristic listed below pertains to one of five subtypes in Shriberg et al.'s (2014) Speech Disorders Classification System (Framework for Research in Speech Sound Disorders, 2012). Put the letter associated with the appropriate subtype next to each relevant characteristic. Note that characteristics marked (*) are associated with more than one subtype.

Subtypes: (a) Speech Delay–Genetic, (b) Speech Delay–Otitis Media with Effusion, (c) Speech Delay–Developmental Psychosocial Involvement, (d) Persistent Speech Errors, (e) Motor Speech Disorder–Apraxia of Speech.

Characteristics:

1 _____ Approximately 12% of children with SSD will present with this subtype.

2 _____ The children achieve short-term normalization with appropriate interventions.*

3 _____ Syllable segregation errors are a good indicator of this subtype.

4 _____ Approximately 30% of children with SSD will present with this subtype.

5 _____ This subtype is a disorder of motor planning and/or programming.

6 _____ This subtype is associated with a trajectory of long-term normalization.*

7 _____ This subtype is associated with persistent speech errors.

8 _____ Approximately 60% of children with SSD will present with this subtype.

9 _____ This subtype is heritable due to commonly occurring genetic risk factors.*

10 _____ This subtype is sometimes caused by specific mutations in the *FOXP2* gene.

11 _____ The proximal cause involves difficulties with phonological processing.

12 _____ This subtype may be associated with aggressive or shy and withdrawn behavior.

13 _____ The child may perseverate when attempting to produce a word several times.

14 _____ The child with this subtype might distort the sibilant or the rhotic sounds.

15 _____ This subtype is associated with fluid in the middle ear space causing mild hearing loss.

16 _____ This subtype is related to impaired phonological representations.*

17 _____ Speech movements are imprecise in the absence of neuromuscular deficits.

18 _____ Speech errors reflect mistiming and miscoordination of multiple articulatory gestures.

Treatment Planning

Learning Objectives

- Differentiate the norm-referenced approach, medical approach, and ICF framework to the process of deciding whether a child requires speech therapy.
- Given assessment data and a diagnosis, use the flow chart shown in Figure 5–1 to decide whether to recommend speech therapy for a child.
- Identify the components of a service delivery model.
- Quantify cumulative intervention intensity after identifying the dose, the dose frequency, and the total intervention duration.
- Describe six evidence-based strategies to ensure an efficient and effective service delivery model.

- Differentiate basic, intermediate, and specific treatment goals.
- Differentiate vertical, horizontal, and cyclical goal attack strategies.
- List seven factors that may impact the likelihood that a potential treatment goal will be achieved. Discuss the impact of those factors.
- Identify error patterns in a speech sample that would be candidates to target as a potential stabilize goal, extend goal, or expand goal.
- Differentiate specific goal from instructional objective. Define the three components of an instructional objective.
- Explain why it is important to document the child's treatment progress.
- Differentiate stimulus generalization from response generalization.

In the United States, speech therapy is the most frequent type of speech-language intervention provided to preschool-age children (ASHA, 2011). Children with speech sound disorders (SSDs) represent the highest proportion of clients seen by speech-language pathologists (SLPs) practicing in schools (Schooling, 2003). In typical clinical practice, treatment planning decisions may occur in two phases and may be made by two different SLPs. In the first phase, the SLP will conduct an initial speech-language assessment by gathering information about the child's communication skills and functioning in a number of domains for the purpose of making a diagnosis. The information gathered during the initial assessment is also used to determine whether the child needs services. In a second phase, once the child is receiving intervention, an SLP will select intervention goals and decide which treatment approach is most likely to help the child achieve those goals. In other words, reaching a diagnosis and making decisions about treatment options are not the same process. Several important treatment planning decisions follow the initial assessment (described in Chapter 3) and the diagnosis (discussed in Chapter 4): specifically, should the child receive speech therapy, and if so, who should provide the intervention, and at what intensity?

The purpose of this chapter is to describe treatment planning processes and principles that are generally applicable to children with SSD of various ages, with diverse profiles of communication strengths and weaknesses. Chapters 6, 7, and 8 will provide detailed information about specific intervention approaches.

5.1 DECIDING WHETHER TO PROVIDE AN INTERVENTION

A child who produces speech errors is not automatically eligible for speech therapy. Even when the child's speech is unintelligible, there are many options for providing a service. The diagnosis itself does not lead in a straightforward way to a treatment recommendation. The SLP must synthesize child- and context-related information to decide how to intervene. There are three basic perspectives on how to decide whether a child should receive speech therapy. In this section, these perspectives are described, with a summary shown in Table 5–1. Subsequently these perspectives are combined to form a recommended protocol for deciding when to provide a speech intervention.

5.1.1 Norm-Referenced Approach

The frequently used **norm-referenced approach** for deciding whether a child should receive speech therapy relies heavily on standardized test scores. Using this approach, the child's performance on a norm-referenced test is compared with those of a reference group of similar children; if the child's standard score or percentile rank falls significantly below a mandated minimum, the SLP would recommend intervention (Spaulding, Plante, & Farinella, 2006). The typical cut-off score for receipt of service would be a standard score of 80 or a percentile rank of 10 (~1.25 standard deviations below the mean), although this criterion varies by service provider. From this perspective, children scoring at the low end of the normal distribution receive services because the discrepancy between the child's performance and the average performance of other children is so great as to constitute a risk to the child. The goal of this approach is to avoid providing services to children who will "catch up" to their peers without intervention, at least by the age of 4 years with respect to speech intelligibility and 9 years with respect to speech accuracy. Even if there were unlimited resources

Table 5–1. *Three Perspectives for Deciding Whether to Provide Speech Therapy*

Characteristics of Approach	Criteria to Recommend Treatment
Norm-Referenced Approach	
Consider the discrepancy between the child's performance and the average performance of other children because a child scoring at the low end of the normal distribution may not "catch up" and may be at risk of poor social or academic outcomes.	Child scores more than 1.25 standard deviations below the mean on a norm-referenced test of articulation or phonology (standard score of 80 or percentile rank 10).
Medical Approach	
Make decision based on medical diagnosis which is assumed to indicate the nature and severity of the child's speech impairment and the prognosis in the absence of treatment.	Child has speech disorder indicated by (1) persistence of phonological processes beyond the expected ages; (2) presence of atypical speech errors; (3) variable production of a phoneme over time rather than gradual improvement toward adultlike levels of consonant accuracy; and (4) mastery of later developing sounds alongside persistent misarticulation of earlier developing sounds.
International Classification of Functioning, Disability, and Health (ICF) Framework	
Consider the impact of the speech impairment on participation after taking contextual (personal and environment) factors into account.	Provide treatment if significant activity limitations and/or participation restrictions occur when the speech impairment interacts with child-related factors (age, temperament, and coping style) or environment factors (physical environment and resources, social network and attitudes of people in that network).

for providing speech therapy, there are costs to recommending these services if they are not necessary. First, the child may be stigmatized if given a diagnostic label. Second, the child is prevented from engaging in other educational or leisure activities while attending speech therapy. However, if the child is not making much progress without intervention, there are considerable risks to the child's well-being. These include the possibility of bullying or poor social relationships with peers. Furthermore, the child may not learn to read as well and as quickly as classmates. Preventing these negative outcomes should be weighed against the cost of providing intervention to the child.

In clinical practice, a common means of determining eligibility for speech therapy services is to compare the child's performance with normative data regarding the acquisition of specific phonemes. One problem in using phoneme-based standards is that data related to the age of acquisition of phonemes are difficult to interpret and vary considerably from one study to another. Another problem with these phoneme-based standards is that they are not sensitive to the child's actual risk of persistent speech delay. For example, some service providers require that a child produce three or more consonants in error in order to receive a service; furthermore, the provider may require that the delay exceed the expected age of acquisition by a specified amount of time such as a full year or more. Many children with significant delays who are unlikely to "catch up" to their peers will be denied speech therapy when these kinds of phoneme-based criteria are used. The expected ages of acquisition, as reported in Chapter 2, are the ages at which 90% of children produce a given consonant correctly. Smit et al. (1990) showed that children's accuracy does not change after the 90th percentile age has been reached; for example, 90% of children produced /dʒ/ accurately between 6 and 7 years, and they observed virtually no further growth in accuracy in older children. Therefore, there is no reason to expect a child to acquire phonemes spontaneously after reaching the 90th percentile age for acquisition of the sound. Another problem in using phoneme-based standards is that this criterion does not take into account

the specific type of speech errors produced by the child. For instance, a 5-year-old child could be mispronouncing /s, z, ʃ, dʒ/ and would not qualify for intervention based on the age of acquisition alone. Yet, if the child is stopping these fricatives (that is, producing them consistently as [t, d]), the child is using a phonological process that should be suppressed by the age of 3 years.

In short, a percentile cut-off score is preferred over phoneme-based standards when applying a norm-referenced approach. The 10th percentile cut-off is recommended because the research indicates that young children who score at or below the 10th percentile on standardized articulation tests face significant risks of poor psychosocial and/or literacy outcomes in the future (the research evidence to support this standard is presented in full in Rvachew and Brosseau-Lapré, 2018). Different service providers will set their own criteria to determine eligibility for service, however, and depending upon the mandate of those providers, those criteria may be justifiable. For example, in some cases school boards will require that a child with an SSD obtain an even lower score on an articulation test to qualify for in-school service; children with less severe SSD will be referred to private providers. SLPs in private practice often provide service to children whose standardized test scores are as high as the 16th percentile and this is also justifiable given that this score is the margin between performing within the average range and below normal limits.

Regardless of these variations in the exact standard, the general idea behind the norm-based approach has value. It is sensible to provide treatment to children who will not "catch up" without treatment and to avoid treating those who will "catch up" without special support.

However, it is important to use normative standards that are consistent with this goal. Furthermore, there may be additional information, besides the child's score on a standardized measure of articulation or phonology that helps to identify the child's risk of experiencing poor outcomes as a consequence of poor speech intelligibility or accuracy.

> **Practice 5–1**
>
> Look at Table 2–6 (Recommended Ages of Acquisition by Phoneme or Cluster) and at Table 2–9 (Expected Age Ranges for Occurrence of Phonological Patterns). Find two more examples of a specific speech error that should no longer be present in the speech of a child age 4 years 6 months according to data on the use of phonological processes but whose phoneme has not yet reached the recommended age of acquisition.

5.1.2 Medical Approach

The medical approach to deciding whether the child should receive speech therapy focuses on the diagnosis of impairment as an indicator of the underlying cause of the child's speech difficulties. The assumption behind the medical approach is that the clinical diagnosis itself predicts the child's developmental trajectory and identifies the child's needs (for further discussion, see Bishop, 2014). Therefore, children with different diagnoses will be entitled to receive different types and intensities of services. In particular, speech disorders that are secondary to medical diagnoses are sometimes automatically eligible for support by insurers and services from tertiary care providers (that is, health care

from specialists, usually working in a hospital). However, a medical diagnosis such as cleft palate does not identify the nature or severity of the speech and language difficulties that will be experienced by any individual child (Stackhouse & Wells, 1993). In fact, approximately half of this population will achieve normal speech and language functioning after the initial surgery; the remainder will require additional therapeutic interventions of varying intensity to achieve a good outcome (Blakeley & Brockman, 1995). Therefore a diagnosis of secondary versus primary SSD does not specifically indicate the child's need for speech therapy services.

Among those children receiving services from primary care providers (e.g., health units, schools), it is common to differentiate those diagnosed with a speech disorder from those with speech delay. It is often assumed that children who are following the normal sequence of speech development at a slow pace will eventually catch up to their peers and achieve intelligible speech without intervention. Therefore, children with speech delay as defined in Chapter 4 may be denied speech therapy or at least direct therapy from an SLP. It has been shown that some children with outward symptoms of speech delay have underlying difficulties with phonological processing that put them at risk for reading impairment. The underlying cause of the child's speech difficulties cannot be assumed from the diagnosis and in some cases cannot be determined (Baker, Croot, McLeod, & Paul, 2001). Therefore, the SLP must seek additional information about the impact of the speech delay on the child's functioning at home and in school.

It is generally agreed that children with a speech disorder, especially when severe, should be recommended for speech therapy. Stoel-Gammon and Dunn (1985) identified characteristics of disordered phonological development that clearly indicate a need for speech therapy. These include (1) persistence of phonological processes beyond the expected ages; (2) presence of atypical speech errors; (3) variable production of a phoneme over time rather than gradual improvement toward adultlike levels of consonant accuracy; and (4) mastery of later developing sounds alongside persistent misarticulation of earlier developing sounds (this is referred to as **chronological mismatch**).

The research evidence does not confirm that there are fundamental differences between children with speech delay compared with children with a speech disorder. As seen in Chapter 4, the frequency of atypical speech errors is related to the child's age and the severity of the child's SSD rather than differences in the cause of the deficit. It is our recommendation to refer children on the basis of norm-referenced test scores below the 10th percentile for all children with SSD, making no distinction between speech delay and speech disorder. This does not mean, however, that all children with SSD will benefit from the same types of intervention or will respond as well to speech therapy. Clearly, children with different profiles of underlying deficits and different patterns of overt speech errors will respond optimally to different treatment approaches. These issues are addressed in Chapters 6 through 8.

5.1.3 International Classification of Functioning, Disability, and Health Framework

The International Classification of Functioning, Disability, and Health (ICF) provides an interdisciplinary and interna-tional framework to describe health issues that challenge how we view disability (World Health Organization [WHO], 2001). The World Health Organization defines *health* as "a state of complete physical, mental, and social well-being and not merely the absence of disease or infirmity" (WHO, 2006). The International Classification of Functioning, Disability, and Health for Children and Youth (ICF-CY; WHO, 2007) was later developed specifically for individuals from birth to 17 years, but based on the same structure as the ICF.

The **ICF-CY approach** to assessment includes a description of the impact of the disability on the child's activities limitations and participation restrictions. The approach considers the child's personal factors such as age, temperament, and coping style, and environmental factors such as the physical environment, the child's social network, and attitudes of the people in the network. These factors may serve as either barriers or facilitators of the child's performance (McCormack, McLeod, Harrison, & McAllister, 2010). The framework aims to describe the child's individual functioning as an interaction between the SSD and contextual factors in order to identify interventions to maximize the child's functioning in daily life.

To decide whether the child should receive intervention in accordance with the ICF framework, it is necessary to assess the impact of the child's SSD on participation in everyday activities. The presence of participation restrictions and activity limitations cannot be predicted from standardized test scores alone, but should be determined directly, by observing the child in different environments and gathering information from the child and the child's parents and teachers. The FOCUS described in Chapter 3 is a tool that may facilitate this process for preschool-aged children (Thomas-Stonell, Oddson, Robertson, & Rosenbaum, 2010). The assessment of participation restrictions and activity limitations differentiates between **capacity** and **performance**, while taking into account a variety of contextual factors. For example, a child might be diagnosed with dysarthria that is associated with mildly distorted fricatives (this is a description at the level of impairment in body structure and function). The child might achieve good intelligibility during standardized testing (indicating excellent capacity) but become only moderately intelligible when talking with friends at the end of the school day (an indicator of performance). Although fluctuating intelligibility causes some activity limitations, the child experiences few participation restrictions because he is gregarious and sociable and a talented soccer player (personal factors), and is supported by a large family that is active in the sports club and their church, environments that are welcoming to their son despite his speech disorder (environmental factors). This is the kind of case in which the diagnosis (dysarthria) might suggest a high priority for treatment, but the impact of the speech difficulties in terms of activity limitations and participation restrictions suggests that direct speech therapy might not be required.

5.1.4 Recommended Protocol for Deciding When to Treat

Figure 5–1 shows a flow chart to facilitate the process of deciding when a child should be referred for speech therapy. The flow chart incorporates elements from the norm-referenced approach, the medical approach, and the ICF framework. The

first step in the process is an assessment that includes all of the required elements described in Chapter 3. The SLP must derive a standard score from at least one norm-referenced measure of articulation accuracy to compare the child's performance to an appropriate normative reference group. For most children, using a single-word, norm-referenced test of articulation/phonology will be perfectly adequate. There are other children for whom a single-word test is not appropriate, specifically older children or children who are less intelligible in conversation than in single words. In these cases, a measure of speech accuracy in conversation such as Percentage of Consonants Correct (PCC) may be a better choice. After calculating the percentage of consonants articulated correctly from a sample of connected speech (as described in Shriberg and Kwiatkowski 1982), PCC can be compared with an appropriate normative reference group to determine if the child's score is less than 1.25 standard deviations below the mean (Austin & Shriberg, 1997).

Once the SLP has conducted the initial assessment and scored the speech-language tests, it is time to make a decision about whether the child should receive an intervention. The protocol shown in Figure 5–1 focuses on children for whom the primary difficulty is in the area of phonology. Many children with SSD have concomitant language disorders, and may qualify for SLP intervention services based on their performance on norm-referenced tests of language alone. This possibility is not incorporated into the flow chart. The first question is, did the child score at or below the 10th percentile on the norm-referenced test of articulation accuracy? If so, the child can be deemed to have an SSD, but it is necessary to refine this judgment further. Therefore, the SLP should

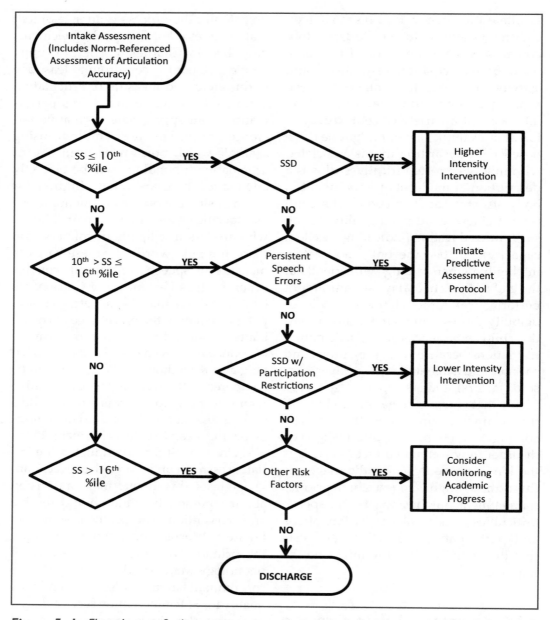

Figure 5–1. *Flow chart to facilitate treatment recommendations. SS = standard score (on a standardized measure of articulation accuracy); SSD = speech sound disorder with delay or disorder profile including motor speech disorders. Predictive assessment protocol described in text and in Smit et al. (1990). See text for application guidelines. Used with permission from Susan Rvachew.*

scan the scoring sheet of the articulation test to determine if the speech errors produced by the child are primarily phono- logical in nature. Essentially if the child would meet the criteria for speech delay, consistent atypical phonological disorder, or inconsistent phonological disorder, as defined in Chapter 4, then the child would remain in the SSD category; following the arrows on the flow chart, the child would then be recommended to receive a higher-intensity intervention. More details about variations in intensity of intervention for children in this category will follow in section 5.2.1 of this chapter.

Alternatively, the child's errors might be of the type called common clinical distortions (Shriberg, Austin, et al. 1997), such as labialized or derhotacized liquids or dentalized or lateralized sibilants. A predominance of these distortion errors would place the child in the Speech Errors category. Children whose standardized test score is between the 10th and the 16th percentile might also present with common clinical distortions and fall into the speech errors category. In any case, this finding should lead the SLP to initiate the **predictive assessment protocol** (Smit, Hand, Freilinger, Bernthal, & Bird, 1990). This protocol mandates repeated monitoring of the child's speech accuracy at regular intervals in order to determine if the child is making progress without treatment. If the child is making progress, treatment may not be necessary. Furthermore, it is harmful to the child's self-esteem to begin treatment before the child has the maturity to correct the error, even with treatment. However, it is important to treat errors that are unlikely to self-correct and which draw attention to the acceptability of the child's speech. Therefore, distortion errors are typically not treated before the age of 7 years, except in the case of lateral distortions which do not self-correct without treatment (Wright, 2017) and therefore should always be treated as soon as they are detected. Between 7 and 9 years, treatment will be delayed if the distortions are declining in frequency; or treatment can

be initiated if they are persistent without an improving trend. The changing state of the child's dentition may also be taken into account during this period. Participation restrictions might lead to a treatment recommendation even in the case of improving speech accuracy, however, so there is some flexibility in the application of the protocol. Finally, at age 9 years, intervention is warranted if there are any distortion errors remaining in the child's speech.

Some children scoring between the 10th and 16th percentiles on the norm-referenced measure of speech accuracy may present with a mild speech delay. In these cases, the SLP should consider whether there are participation restrictions that would warrant an intervention. Many publicly funded agencies may not be mandated to provide services to children with mild speech delay, especially if there are no co-occurring language or literacy difficulties. Nonetheless, children with mild SSD in the absence of other communication impairments are at risk for participation restrictions and anxiety disorders. If the agency mandate is based on the ICF framework, intervention could be recommended on the basis of these secondary impacts. Private SLPs could also provide services to children with mild SSD. The child could possibly also receive services through a university speech and language clinic.

If a child scores above the 16th percentile on the norm-referenced measure of articulation/phonology, does not present with persistent speech errors, and does not present with participation restrictions, it would be appropriate to discharge the child from service under most circumstances. Rarely, however, it would be prudent to maintain the child on the speech therapy caseload, especially if the child presents with risk factors for academic difficulties or poor psychosocial outcomes. In particular, if the child has a family history of speech, language, or reading disability or has received intervention in the past for speech and language difficulties, the SLP might consider monitoring the child's progress over time, implementing preventative interventions when necessary. When it becomes clear that the child's prognosis is good and there are no further risks for future success in school, the child can be discharged from the service.

Once a decision has been reached as to whether to provide intervention to the child, additional questions arise before intervention can be initiated. These decisions concern the effective use of resources, or more specifically, the choice of who should deliver the intervention, in what setting, and how often.

Practice 5–2

Consider the case of a boy age 5;1 who received speech and language therapy between the ages of 2;0 and 4;0. He was recently reassessed and scored at the 12th percentile on the Goldman-Fristoe Test of Articulation–Third Edition (GFTA-3). The parents report they are concerned about their son's upcoming entry to kindergarten in a few months and note that he is not easily understood by his preschool teachers. The parents add that their son seems aware of his speech difficulties and is more reluctant to speak to unfamiliar children and adults. Apply the flow chart shown in Figure 5–1 to decide whether this child should be referred for intervention.

Box 5–1. Deciding Whether to Provide an Intervention: Key Points

- According to the norm-referenced approach, a child whose speech accuracy performance falls significantly below a mandated minimum would be referred for intervention.
- According to the medical approach, intervention should be reserved for children diagnosed with a speech disorder as differentiated from a speech delay.
- The ICF framework considers participation restrictions, activity limitations, and the child's personal and environmental factors to identify interventions to maximize the child's functioning in daily life.
- Taking into account all three perspectives to deciding whether to provide an intervention, we recommend intervention for children with SSD who score below the 10th percentile rank on a norm-referenced test of articulation/phonology. Children who scored above the 10th percentile rank may also be referred for intervention if they present with other risk factors, participation restrictions, or persistent speech errors.

5.2 SERVICE DELIVERY OPTIONS

The flow chart presented in Figure 5–1 suggested that children with SSD may be recommended to receive different intensities of speech therapy depending on the severity and the underlying nature of their speech deficit. In order to ensure that each child on the caseload receives the optimum amount of speech therapy, the SLP will need to organize resources in the most efficient way possible. For example, a child with a severe phonological disorder might be scheduled to receive several sessions of speech therapy weekly, from the SLP and a communication disorders assistant. The child with a lateral lisp might receive one brief session per week from the SLP, following up with daily practice at home supported by a computer program. The child with a mild phonological delay might receive weekly group therapy from the SLP. Children who have recently been discharged from direct therapy might still receive services in the classroom with consultation support to the teacher. These different options for organizing service providers in different locations at varying intensities of service are called **service delivery models** (Cirrin et al., 2010). Whenever a child is recommended for speech therapy, it is necessary to decide where the child will receive intervention, who will provide it, and at what intensity. These recommendations are necessarily individualized to take into account the unique needs of each client. Furthermore, the child and the child's family should be invited to participate in the decision-making process, in keeping with a **client-centered approach**. Shared decision making helps the child and family to engage fully with an intervention that will lead to realistic outcomes that they value. In the school environment, school personnel must be involved in this process to ensure that an inclusive service delivery model is designed to provide services in the **least restrictive environment** in order to facilitate the child's inte-

gration into the school community and to support academic success (American Speech-Language-Hearing Association, 1996). The service delivery model that is designed through this shared decision-making process should also be evidence based. Research supports some general principles for the design of service delivery models and for caseload management that will be discussed in this section.

5.2.1 Intensity of Intervention

Warren, Fey, and Yoder (2007) identified several variables that are used to quantify treatment intensity. These are described in Table 5–2. **Dose** is the number of teaching episodes per therapy session. Dose is the aspect of treatment intensity over which the SLP has the most control. For example, a young school-age child might be receiving speech therapy because he misarticulates the [ʃ] sound. During the first session, the SLP asks the child to put a token in a box each time he hears her make an [ʃ] sound while he listens to her read a story; if the child hears 100 [ʃ] sounds in a 15-minute session, the dose is 100 even if the SLP had to prompt him to notice some of the sounds. During the next session, the child practices saying [ʃ] while looking in a mirror; if the child says [s] on 10 attempts and [ʃ] on 10 attempts while receiving feedback from the SLP, the dose is 20. It is more important to count dose than the number of minutes of therapy because the child may not be practicing throughout an entire speech therapy session. Depending on the clinician and the child, many minutes out of the entire duration of the therapy session could be taken up by manipulating materials, writing notes, and having a conversation with the child that is not related to the task. To

Table 5–2. *Quantifying Treatment Intensity*

Variable	Definition
Treatment intensity	Quality and quantity of service provided in a given period of time
Dose	Number of properly implemented teaching episodes per session
Dose form	Task or activity within which the teaching episodes are delivered
Dose frequency	Number of sessions per unit of time (e.g., day/week/month)
Total intervention duration	Time period over which the intervention is provided (e.g., 5 days or 12 weeks or 9 months)
Cumulative intervention intensity	Dose × Dose frequency × Total intervention duration

cope with high caseload sizes, SLPs often treat children in small groups. Group therapy can be effective as long as the dose for each child is sufficiently high, and it may be more effective to see children individually for short periods of time than seeing a few children together for a longer period of time. Williams (2012) concluded that a minimum of 50 trials per session is required to achieve a good outcome in phonology therapy. However, Murray, McCabe, and Ballard (2014) found that dose is often as low as 30 trials per session in clinical practice. As will be seen in Chapter 7, dose for children with apraxia of speech should be as high as 100 practice trials per session. The next variable, **dose form**, is important because the task or activity in which the speech practice is embedded may influence the dose. A drill activity in which the child practices [ʃ] repeatedly with verbal feedback may be efficient, leading to a high dose, unless the child becomes bored and refuses to engage or makes many mistakes due to fatigue or inadequate motivation. A drill-play activity such as saying [ʃ] to put dolls to sleep may be more motivating but there will be many fewer practice trials and thus a lower dose. The SLP will need to find the right balance. Most children are willing to maintain a high dose as long as they receive a clear indication that their speech is improving in a fun context.

Dose frequency is the number of speech therapy sessions per unit of time. Even if different children receive the same amount of therapy, the treatment schedule can vary. If you have attempted to learn a new skill as a teenager or adult, such as playing a musical instrument, learning another language, or playing a new sport, you probably would agree that more practice makes perfect. You may also agree that practicing the skill only once per month for a few hours may not lead to as much learning as practicing twice per week for short periods of time. Similarly, cramming for exams is never the best policy: **distributed practice** is always more effective. There are many options to distribute treatment sessions, however: treatment could be provided in one-hour sessions once per month, or 30-minute sessions twice per week, or 15-minute sessions once per day. Although few studies have systematically investigated the impact of different treatment schedules on outcomes, shorter periods of frequent treatment may be more effective than infrequent sessions spread over a long period of time (Allen, 2013; Barratt, Littlejohns, & Thompson, 1992). This may be especially true when periods of treatment are broken up by periods without treatment that allow the child to consolidate learning; in other words, an optimum treatment schedule for many children might be to attend 6 weeks of twice-weekly sessions, a 12-week break, followed by another 6 weeks of twice-weekly intervention, another 12-week break, and so on. This kind of schedule is known as **block treatment**. There is no solid research that has identified the best length of treatment block or the ideal length of break period for this kind of treatment schedule. However, there is good evidence that children make satisfactory gains during the break periods (McKercher, McFarlane, & Schneider, 1995). Therefore, it is perfectly acceptable to treat a child for a block of therapy and then schedule a break even if the child has achieved only 40% to 75% correct production on the treatment goals (Olswang & Bain, 1994).

Total intervention duration is the time period over which the treatment sessions are distributed, and when multiplied by the dose frequency, determines the amount of intervention that is provided. The general rule regarding the **amount of intervention** a child should receive is that more is better, but too much is a waste of resources. Jacoby, Levin, Lee, Creaghead, and Kummer (2002) used the ASHA National Outcome Measurement System (NOMS) to research the average amount of intervention that is associated with gains in communication skills in preschool children. The participants were children ages 3 to 6 years who were receiving intervention for primary speech and language impairment in a pediatric hospital. The outcomes for the children were reported using the functional communication measure of the NOMS, as rated by the child's SLP. A change of two or more levels in functional communication that reflect the child's speech intelligibility with various communication partners was considered to be a reasonable amount of progress. The SLPs completed the functional communication assessments at the initial intake, at regularly scheduled progress reports, and when the child was discharged from intervention. Jacoby et al. (2002) drew three general conclusions from the data. First, there was a trend for children who began therapy with more severe deficits to require more units of therapy to achieve a functional gain. Second, younger children required fewer units of therapy to make a functional gain compared with older children. Third, the amount of improvement observed was significantly correlated with the amount of therapy received. Specifically, an improvement of more than two levels on the functional communication measure required at least 20 hours of intervention. Nationally, the ASHA NOMS project also found that for preschoolers, the amount of intervention associated with no change, one level, or at least two levels of change on the articulation functional communication measure was approximately 11 hours, 15 hours, and 21 hours (American Speech-Language-Hearing Association, 2009).

Overall, 20 or more hours of speech therapy are required to obtain a clinically significant functional outcome. However, this recommendation is highly dependent on interactions between the child, the family, the clinician, and the treatment program. Some children achieve great outcomes with less than 20 hours of intervention, while others, unfortunately, fail to make a clinically significant improvement even after years of speech therapy. While it is difficult to predict how much intervention a specific child will require to achieve the desired communication goals, the NOMS data demonstrate that interventions lasting less than 10 hours are not likely to impact the child's speech intelligibility in daily communication contexts.

The **cumulative intervention intensity** is the multiplication of the variables discussed thus far, such as 50 practice trials per session × 2 sessions per month × 6 months. In this example, the cumulative intervention intensity would be 600. Ideally, cumulative intervention intensity would be varied so that each child receives just the right amount to achieve his/her speech goals, and indeed some researchers have shown that this is an efficient and effective way to organize speech therapy services (Blakeley & Brockman, 1995). This level of individualization is achieved by first providing treatment at a low intensity, reassessing the child to document the rate of progress, and then gradually increasing the intensity of service provision if the child is not on track to achieve age-appropriate speech at school entry or adultlike speech accuracy by age 9 years. When implemented at a school level, gradually increasing the intensity of service to meet the needs of individual children as required is called **response-to-intervention** (Justice, 2006). However, this type of service provision is regrettably rare. Very often service providers or insurers will limit the number of hours of speech therapy that each child can receive

each year to an arbitrary amount. In this case, it is important to remember that the dose remains under the control of the SLP. It is often feasible to double the dose during each session, thus significantly increasing the cumulative intervention intensity at no extra cost.

Practice 5–3

Pretend you have been diagnosed with an ear infection. The doctor prescribed antibiotics to be taken, two 100 milligram capsules twice per day for 14 consecutive days. In this example, what are the dose, dose form, dose frequency, total intervention duration, and cumulative intervention intensity?

5.2.2 Intervention Agents

One way to increase the dose frequency and therefore the cumulative treatment intensity for a given child is to involve other **intervention agents** in the rehabilitation program, such as SLP assistants, parents and other caregivers, or teachers. In particular, parents spend time with their child every day and have the opportunity to implement practice at home. Research has shown that home programs substantially improve the effectiveness of speech therapy that is provided by an SLP, especially when the total amount of therapy provided by the SLP is less than 20 hours (Schooling, 2003). Most studies investigating the effectiveness of speech-language intervention involved direct intervention from the SLP supplemented by parents completing homework at home. These studies have found that parents can be effective intervention agents when they receive highly structured and standardized training from the SLP prior to implementing intervention at home (e.g., Eiserman, Weber, & McCoun, 1995; Sommers et al., 1964). Some home programs are given directly to the parents to carry out with very little input from the SLP beyond monitoring the child's progress at longer intervals, such as every 6 to 12 weeks. Sometimes parents are provided with structured training so that they can continue the speech therapy program after discharge or during the transition between one service provider and another (Rvachew & Brosseau-Lapré, 2015).

Speech-language pathology assistants may also be involved to increase the dose frequency depending upon the complexity of the child's intervention program. The SLP assistant must be trained and supervised in accordance with the relevant guidelines, and the tasks assigned to the assistant must be consistent with the scopes of practice as specified by the employer and professional association. Typically an SLP assistant is permitted to implement a carefully documented treatment plan that is developed by the supervising SLP (American Speech-Language-Hearing Association, 2013). Assistants have been shown to be effective for teaching vocabulary (Boyle, McCartney, Forbes, & O'Hare, 2007) and in the delivery of phonological awareness interventions (Ehri et al., 2001). Although it is common for SLP assistants to implement articulation therapy programs, it can be difficult for individuals who do not have SLP training to provide effective feedback (Gardner, 2006) and the effectiveness of SLP assistants for articulation and phonology therapy has not been established. In summary, the best service delivery model for an individual child is the configuration of resources that best meets the child's needs, using evidence-based strategies to ensure efficiency and effectiveness, as outlined in Table 5–3. To provide an appropriate service, it is best to focus on the child's progress toward a well-defined goal and adjust the delivery of services to ensure that the child maintains a trajectory toward achieving the goal. Clear goal setting from the beginning of the child's speech intervention is perhaps the most important element. We now turn to treatment planning for the individual child.

Box 5–2. Service Delivery Options: Key Points

- A service delivery model specifies where the intervention will be provided, who will provide it, and at what level of intensity.
- Cumulative intervention intensity is a primary determinant of treatment outcomes.
- Between 12 and 20 hours of intervention are required for most children with SSD to show a functional improvement in speech outcomes, although there is considerable variability in the required amount of intervention to achieve the child's communication goals.

5.3 INTERVENTION GOALS

Detailed information about the child's phonological knowledge is required in order to plan intervention. Time invested to conduct an in-depth initial assessment as described in Chapter 3 will allow the SLP to construct a treatment plan for the

Table 5–3. *Evidence-Based Strategies to Ensure an Efficient and Effective Service Delivery Model*

1. **Increase dose** to at least 50 and ideally 100 practice trials per session.

2. Plan **short individual sessions** with high dose per child rather than long group sessions with low dose per child.

3. In accordance with **distributed practice**, distribute speech practice over several short sessions throughout the week rather than one long session per week.

4. Supplement direct therapy by the SLP with a structured **home program** in which the parent is supported by training and feedback to ensure completion.

5. Use a **block treatment** approach in which the child receives frequent sessions over a short intervention duration to ensure rapid onset of progress followed by a longer break to allow consolidation of learning before the next block of treatment is implemented.

6. Use a **response-to-intervention** approach, in which the intensity of the intervention is gradually increased until the child has achieved the optimum rate of progress; all children are receiving the most effective and efficient service for their individual needs; and no child is receiving more service than is required to achieve the desired outcome.

child. Oftentimes, the initial assessment, even when many tests are given, will not provide sufficient information for effective goal selection. A deep phonological analysis of the child's speech may be required for those children with the most complex or severe phonological disorders, as described in detail in Rvachew and Brosseau-Lapré (2018). The selection of treatment goals will be more straightforward for those children who present with persistent speech errors or speech delay and may be accomplished by examining their articulation or phonological test protocols to identify commonly occurring error patterns or clinical distortions. According to Kahmi (2014), selecting intervention goals is one of the most important roles of the SLP. There are many factors to consider when selecting goals for a child with SSD as outlined in this section.

5.3.1 Types of Goals

An important aspect of planning intervention for a child is to select three types of goals: basic or long-term goals, intermediate or medium-term goals, and specific or short-term goals (Fey, 1992; McCauley, Fey, & Gillam, 2017). These three types of goals are summarized in Figure 5–2.

For children with SSD, the **basic goal** is usually to achieve intelligible speech, but this may require a global reorganization or expansion of the child's phonological system. For children with persistent speech errors, the long-term goal may be to achieve adultlike speech accuracy or social acceptability of the child's speech. In addition to achieving intelligible speech, a long-term goal for children with SSD may include prevention of reading and spelling impairment and other nega-

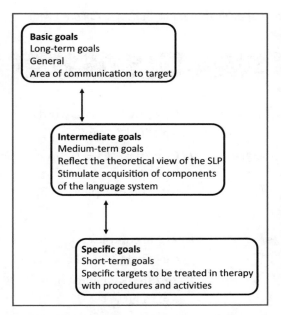

Figure 5–2. *Three types of intervention goals. Used with permission from Françoise Brosseau-Lapré.*

tive consequences of the underlying difficulties with phonological processing.

Intermediate goals can be achieved in the medium term and reflect the SLP's theoretical view of speech development and disorders. Intermediate goals should be selected to stimulate the child's acquisition of the language system rather than to teach specific targets (Fey, Long, & Finestack, 2003). Usually, there are several intermediate goals associated with each basic goal. If the basic goal is to reorganize the child's phonological system, intermediate goals could be selected to stimulate the child's acquisition of phonological categories. These categories might be at the segmental or prosodic level of the phonological hierarchy. Segmental goals could

be features (e.g., voicing) or sound classes (e.g., fricatives). Prosodic goals could be stress patterns (e.g., strong-weak-strong three-syllable words), or syllable structures (e.g., complex onsets meaning syllable-initial clusters). The number of intermediate goals selected for any given child will be determined by the individual characteristics of the child and the service provider. The SLP will typically plan to treat as many goals as might be achieved in the period between mandated progress reports. This period might be six months in a hospital setting, nine months in a school setting, or four months in a university clinic.

The **specific goals** are the phonological units that will be treated in therapy with planned procedures and activities. Sometimes the intermediate goal and the specific goal are the same phoneme. More typically, several specific goals are associated with one intermediate goal. Note also that the total intervention duration may be shorter than the period of time that passes between progress reports. Therefore the SLP may expect the child to suppress fronting of velars between September (intake) and March (first progress report), which is the period during which the intermediate goal is expected to be achieved. However, the child is entitled to receive only six treatment sessions, provided weekly in October and November. During these sessions the specific goal is to practice the phoneme /k/. It is hoped that the intermediate goal will be achieved as a consequence of generalization from the specific goal (/k/) to other members of this phoneme class (/g, ŋ/). Table 5–4 presents other example sets of basic, intermediate, and specific goals.

Table 5–4. *Examples of Basic, Intermediate, and Specific Treatment Goals for Children with SSD*

Basic Goal	Intermediate Goals	Specific Goals
Example 1		
Speech 80% intelligible to a stranger	1. Fricatives	1. C_1 = /f,v/ in CVC words e.g., "fall," "van"
	2. Consonant clusters	2. C_1 = /b,p/, C_2 = /l/ in CCV words e.g., "blue," "play"
Example 2		
Adultlike accuracy and acceptability of speech articulation	1. Mastery of /s/	1. /s/ in complex codas e.g., "bats," "walks"
	2. Mastery of /ɝ,ɚ/	2. /ɝ/ in disyllabic words e.g., "cherry"
	3. Mastery of /ɹ/-clusters	3. /kɹ,gɹ/ word onset clusters, 1-syllable words e.g., "green," "cry"
Example 3		
Kindergarten-level emergent literacy skills	1. Implicit awareness of subsyllabic units	1. Match CVC words with shared onsets or shared rimes e.g., "Which words go together? pan, ball, fan, nose"
	2. Knowledge of letter sounds	2. s, m, p, l, t, g, a, e e.g., "Here is a picture of tea and a picture of moon. Which picture goes with the letter t?"

Practice 5–4

Pretend that you are creating a 9-month treatment plan for a 10-year-old girl who presents with a persistent dental distortion of all the sibilant consonants. What will be your basic, intermediate, and specific treatment goals? Imagine that your school year (total treatment period) is divided into three blocks (fall, winter, and spring terms), each allowing approximately eight weeks of treatment.

5.3.2 Goal Attack Strategies

Once the SLP has identified basic, intermediate, and specific goals for the child, the next step is to decide how to address the goals over time. The way that goals are targeted over time in therapy is called goal attack strategy. Fey (1992) identified three categories of goal attack strategies: vertical, horizontal, and cyclical. When using a vertical goal attack strategy, the SLP targets only one goal at a time; the child must achieve a predetermined level of production accuracy before the SLP will advance to a new goal. The criterion for advancing from one goal to another can vary broadly depending upon the likelihood that the child will regress after the SLP moves on to a new goal. For example, the child could be required to master the target before a new goal is introduced (that is, achieve at least 90% correct production of the target). Alternatively, the SLP could set a criterion that is less stringent, such as customary production (that is, at least 50% correct production of the target).

An alternative is the horizontal goal attack strategy, in which the SLP targets multiple specific goals simultaneously during each therapy session. While this goal attack strategy may increase the time needed for the child to achieve the predetermined level of production accuracy for each specific goal, it may decrease the total amount of time it takes the child to achieve all the specific goals. The goals might be related to each other (for example, several fricative sounds, /f,s,ʃ/) or unrelated (such as one fricative, one liquid, and one velar stop, /s,l,k/). In either case, the SLP will set specific criteria to discontinue working on the set of goals and advance to a new set. Again, the criteria to advance to new goals or schedule a treatment break may be stringent or lenient. The SLP might continue practice with /f,s,ʃ/ until mastery is achieved and then introduce liquid phonemes as a new goal. With another child, the strategy might be to schedule a treatment break after the child achieves between 40% and 70% correct production across the set /s,l,k/, monitoring for continued and spontaneous improvements over time.

A cyclical goal attack strategy has become an increasingly popular choice because it is intended to stimulate gradual acquisition of speech sound targets as presumably seen in normal development (Hodson, 2011). The SLP targets multiple intermediate goals in a given cycle, but only one specific goal is targeted during any one treatment session. Specific goals are targeted for a predetermined period of time, and new goals are introduced in a fixed sequence whether or not the child made progress with the goal. The sequence of intermediate goals is cycled with new specific goals until the targeted structures are observed in conversational speech. These three goal attack strategies are summarized in Figure 5–3.

5.3.3 Selecting Goals

There are several factors to consider when selecting specific goals for speech therapy. Considering these factors will help the SLP answer three questions about potential intermediate and specific intervention goals: (1) Is the child likely to achieve this goal spontaneously, in other words, without treatment? (2) Is the child likely to achieve this goal at this time with treatment? and (3) Will the achievement of this goal effect substantial change toward the achievement of the basic goal? Some factors that the SLP would consider are related to the characteristics of the phonological units themselves. These factors include the frequency and/or functional

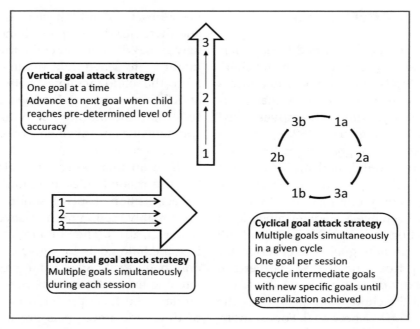

Figure 5–3. *Goal attack strategies. Used with permission from Françoise Brosseau-Lapré and Susan Rvachew.*

load of the phonemes in the language and the order of emergence of the units in normal development. Other factors are related to the individual child, such as the child's age, motivation, attentional skills, stimulability, consistency of production, and phonological knowledge of the potential target. Both types of factors will be discussed in turn.

The roles of **input frequency and functional load** on the order of emergence and acquisition of a phoneme vary from one language to another. For instance, functional load is the best predictor of the age of emergence of phonemes in English (Stokes & Suredran, 2005). Phonemes that have high functional load are involved in many minimal pairs in the language and are thus early developing. Phonemes that create few minimal pairs could disappear from the language with almost no cost and therefore have low functional load and tend to develop late. This is the rea-

son that /ð/ is a late developing phoneme in English, even though it occurs very frequently (in the word "the," for example). In contrast, /s/ has high frequency and high functional load in English. The phoneme /s/ emerges at earlier ages in the phonetic repertoire of English-speaking children (although the age of mastery may be late due to the difficulty of articulating the sound correctly). The phoneme /s/ plays an important role in the production of grammatical morphemes such as plural, possessive, and third person singular "-s." The phoneme also plays an important role in the accurate production of complex onsets and codas, such as in the words "stop" and "box." Targeting the phoneme /s/ in English is therefore common, as it can have a broad impact on the child's intelligibility.

SLPs often consider the **developmental order** of emergence of potential phoneme targets. However, as seen in

Chapter 2, different studies report different ages of acquisition for the same phonemes. It is also unclear whether treatment goals should be selected and ordered on the basis of the age of emergence of a phoneme or the age of mastery of the phoneme. In general, it is expected that "earlier developing" phonemes will be easier for the child to learn, with or without intervention, but there is ambiguity in the application of developmental norms to the selection of intervention goals. First, it is not always clear which developmental norms to use when predicting relative ease of learning for candidate phoneme goals. Second, it is not always clear whether it is better to begin therapy with earlier developing or later developing phonemes. Traditionally, SLPs have selected phoneme targets in order from early to late developing with the expectation that earlier developing phonemes will be easier to acquire and thus the child's self-esteem will be enhanced and speech intelligibility will be impacted faster. Some researchers recommend beginning therapy with late developing phonemes, with the justification that generalization to untreated sounds will only occur when more difficult phonemes are taught (Gierut, Morrisette, et al. 2001). However, this hypothesis was unsupported by a randomized controlled trial: Rvachew and Nowak (2001) found that early developing phonemes were easier for children to learn and resulted in the acquisition of untaught difficult sounds.

As you will see in Chapters 6, 7, and 8, the choice and implementation of a specific intervention approach should take into account intrinsic factors that are individual to the child, such as the child's age and the nature and severity of the child's SSD. In terms of goal selection, intrinsic factors often considered by the SLP include **stimulability**, that is, the child's ability to correctly imitate a pho-

neme when given a model. Assessment of stimulability was described in Chapter 3. If the child is successfully able to produce a specific sound in response to the adult's model and cues, it indicates that the child is able to physically produce the target speech sound. It may also indicate that the child is able to perceive the difference between his or her errored productions and the adult's model and adjust articulatory gestures required for the correct production of the target phoneme. Therefore, stimulability targets several domains relevant for learning to produce new speech sounds, such as the child's attention, motivation, speech perception skills, and motor learning. Several studies have shown that children who are stimulable for the production of a phoneme are more likely to master this phoneme than children who are not stimulable (e.g., Miccio, Elbert, & Forrest, 1999; Sommers et al., 1967). Rvachew et al. (1999) found that treatment outcomes were best for treatment targets when the child was stimulable and had good perceptual knowledge for that target. Overall, studies suggest that it is best to ensure that children are stimulable for treatment targets and that they have good perceptual knowledge of those targets before those sounds are selected as specific goals in a phonological intervention (Rvachew, 2005).

Inconsistent correct production of a phoneme that is usually produced incorrectly by the child is also traditionally viewed as a positive predictor of a good treatment outcome. One assumption is that children who inconsistently produce the target phoneme correctly are able to physically produce the required articulatory gestures. However, inconsistency is an ambiguous predictor of treatment outcome, since it does not mean that the child has good underlying phonological knowledge of the phoneme. For example, consider a child who produces /ʃ/ as [s] almost all the time, but with the occasional correct production. The child does not necessarily have an adultlike representation of this phoneme and therefore would not have a clear /ʃ/ target to aim for. Researchers have shown that good underlying phonological knowledge of a target sound predicts changes in production accuracy (e.g., Rvachew, 2006; Tyler, Edwards, & Saxman, 1990).

Sometimes a child who is heard by the adult to collapse a phoneme contrast in a consistent fashion actually produces the two contrasting sounds differently in a way that is so subtle it is called a **covert contrast**. For example a child might produce /s/→ [s] with a high frequency fricative sound on average; at the same time /ʃ/ is produced [sʲ], resulting in a slight lowering of the average frequency of the [s] in this context. Even this small difference, hard for the adult listener to detect, indicates phonological knowledge of a contrast between the alveolar and the alveopalatal sibilants. This level of phonological knowledge of the contrast indicates a greater likelihood of acquiring the contrast even though the child is not clear on all the phonetic differences between these phonemes.

These extrinsic and intrinsic factors are listed in Table 5–5 along with information about their predictive significance. This table highlights the factors to consider when choosing treatment goals but does not provide any clear guidelines

Table 5–5. *Factors That May Predict Outcomes for Potential Treatment Targets*

Factor	More likely to acquire	Less likely to acquire
Input frequency	High frequency in the language, e.g., /s/ in English	Low frequency in the language, e.g., /ʒ/
Functional load	Large information loss when merged with other phonemes, e.g., /m/	Small information loss when merged with other phonemes, e.g., /ð/
Developmental order	Early developing, e.g., /b/	Late developing, e.g., /ɹ/
Stimulability	Stimulable in words when provided with an imitative model	Unstimulable even when provided with phonetic placement assistance
Inconsistency	Target /s/ occurs in conversational speech as [s] 40% and [s̠] 60%.	Target /s/ occurs in conversational speech as [s̠] 100%.
Perceptual knowledge	The child perceives, e.g., [sit] and [ʃit] to be different words.	The child perceives, e.g., [sit] and [ʃit] to be the same word.
Underlying phonological knowledge	A covert contrast between e.g., /t/→ [t] and /k/→ [t] is apparent upon acoustic analysis.	Productions of e.g., /t/→ [t] and /k → [t] are identical with overlapping acoustic characteristics.

about how to make choices among the many alternatives that may be present in the speech of children with moderate and severe disorders. These factors could lead SLPs to make different decisions for the same child: consider a child who misarticulates but is stimulable for /s/, a frequently occurring phoneme with high functional load. One SLP might choose to not treat it, reasoning that the child will acquire it on the basis of spontaneous practice alone; another SLP might decide to treat the sound, reasoning that it will help the child achieve quick and substantial progress toward improved intelligibility. The factors in this table guide the information-gathering process but do not structure decision making. There are a number of different protocols for choosing treatment goals for children with multiple speech errors. One will be presented in this chapter, based on guidelines to promote progressive change in a child's phonological system, as proposed by Grunwell (1992).

There are several important features of Grunwell's guidelines that contribute to the power of this approach to target selection. The first is that the targets are selected after a deep analysis of the child's phonology so as to effect broad change across the entire system. Second, there is no reason to worry about whether the targets will be too easy or too difficult for the child because three targets are selected that represent a range of difficulty levels and therefore the child is sure to learn at least one of them. Third, the targets cover different aspects of the child's phonology, including feature contrasts, phonemes, and syllable structures—in short, multiple levels of the phonological hierarchy. Therefore, the child should experience learning that will interact among the goals to produce more change across the pho-

nological system than would be achieved if individual targets were selected one at a time. The proposed target selection strategies are based on normal developmental mechanisms of change, described as *stabilization* of variable patterns; *destabilization*, which increases variability, a process essential for change, in particular innovation or the introduction of a new pattern; and *generalization* of a known pattern to new contexts. Therefore three types of goals are selected for the child: a variable pattern in the child's speech is selected for stabilization (**stabilize goal**); a context-specific pattern is targeted so that the child learns to generalize correct production of a phoneme from one context where it appears to a new context (**extend goal**); and a syllable structure or phoneme that is consistently absent from the child's speech is selected as a goal that will force a significant change in the child's phonological system (**expand goal**). These goals are described with examples in Table 5–6. Another principle that can be incorporated into the goal selection framework is **use of strengths to support needs**: this means that new phonemes are treated in the context of stable syllable structures and new syllable structures are taught by incorporating phonemes that are reasonably well established in the child's system (Bernhardt, Stemberger, et al. 2006).

The three goals that are selected using these guidelines can be targeted with any of the possible goal attack strategies—vertical, horizontal, or cyclical. It is also possible to combine a horizontal and cyclical approach. Taking the goals listed in Table 5–6, one specific goal for each of the intermediate goals could be taught during each session for a specified period, such as six weeks: for example, l-clusters (stabilize goal), initial /k/ (extend goal), and /tʃ/ (expand goal) would be taught

Table 5–6. *Guidelines to Select Goals to Achieve Progressive Change*

Pattern Type	Example of Goal
Stabilize Goal	
Variable pattern	Liquid clusters may be reduced or simplified:
	blue → [bwu], black → [bæk], clay → [tjeɪ], play → [peɪ]
	crayon → [tjejã], break → [bweɪk], green → [dɹin], grow → [do]
Extend Goal	
Context-specific pattern	Velars are produced correctly in coda but fronted in onset:
	black → [bæk], lake → [leɪk], dog → [dɑg], peg → [pɛg]
	carrot → [tɛɚwʌt], cake → [teɪk], gate → [deɪt], get → [dɛt]
Expand Goal	
Consistent pattern	Affricates are deaffricated and fronted (no affricates):
	cheese → [siz], chocolate → [sɑtwɪt], jump → [zʌmp]
	patch → [pæs], peach → [pis], catch → [tæs], page → [peɪz]

in each session, one 60-minute session per week for six weeks; at the end of the treatment block, treatment on these specific goals would stop regardless of the level of progress. In the next block, /ɹ/-clusters (stabilize goal), initial /g/ (extend goal), and /dʒ/ would be initiated. Regardless of the goal attack strategy that is selected, there is a good probability that the child will experience early success during treatment sessions and experience a significant reorganization of the phonological system over the course of the treatment program with these varied goals.

Box 5–3. Goals and Goal Attack Strategies: Key Points

- Three types of goals are selected for each client: basic goals, intermediate goals, specific goals.
- The specific goals may be targeted using a vertical, horizontal, or cyclical goal attack strategy.
- When choosing goals, consider characteristics of the potential speech sound or syllable structure goals, that is, frequency of the phonological unit in the language, functional load, and developmental order of acquisition.
- When choosing goals, consider the child's knowledge of the potential goal, that is, stimulability, consistency of production, and underlying phonological knowledge as revealed by perceptual knowledge or covert contrast.
- Choose three goals for each treatment block: a stabilize goal, an extend goal, and an expand goal.

5.4 MONITORING TREATMENT PROGRESS

Treatment planning is a dynamic process. It will never be possible to select and order all the treatment goals prior to the onset of treatment and be sure that the plan will unroll exactly as expected. It is essential to monitor the child's performance and update the plan continuously as treatment progresses and the child's phonological knowledge changes. A monitoring plan provides information to ensure that the treatment plan is adjusted as necessary to meet the child's needs; otherwise the child might spend too long practicing a goal that has been achieved or the SLP might fail to substitute new goals when it should be clear that the child is not progressing. Monitoring the child's progress is also necessary in order to be accountable to the child, the child's family, and the service provider. Everyone involved in providing speech therapy and resources to support the speech therapy program will want to be sure that the service is effective and efficient.

Olswang and Bain (1994) recommend that the SLP collect data to answer three questions: (1) Is the child responding to the treatment program? (2) Is significant and important change occurring? (3) Is treatment responsible for the change? In order to know if the child is responding to treatment, it is necessary to have clearly planned instructional objectives and to document the child's achievement of those objectives. Significant and important change occurs when the child's success during treatment sessions has an impact on speech performance in other contexts; in other words the SLP must document generalization learning. Finally, it can often be assumed that the child's speech

improvement is due to the treatment if the SLP is adhering to the principles of evidence-based practice. In some cases it is even possible to collect data in the clinic that confirms the causal link between the treatment and the child's progress. Each of these points will be discussed in turn.

5.4.1 Instructional Objectives

One way to document the child's progress is to keep track of whether the child is succeeding at the small steps in the pathway toward achievement of the specific goal. When the SLP writes a lesson plan for each session, there will be at least one **instructional objective** that the child is expected to achieve that takes the child a little bit closer to the specific goal at the end of the treatment block. Demonstration 5–1 provides an example of how to construct and order instructional objectives. In this example, the instructional objectives are ordered to teach the child to produce /tʃ/ over six weeks (the expand goal from Table 5–6). The example demonstrates that the instructional objectives are ordered to progress toward the specific goal in very small steps. Furthermore, each instructional objective has three components: (1) a **do** statement, (2) a **condition**, and (3) an **accuracy** statement. The "do" statement is an objective description of what the child will do during each practice trial. These practice trials might be embedded in an activity (such as linking train cars together), but this activity is not important to the instructional objectives. Activities must be differentiated from objectives. A badly written lesson plan might give the impression that the goal of the first session is to play with trains when the actual goal is to learn to keep the lips rounded while sequencing a stop and a fricative to

How to Construct and Order Instructional Objectives

This demonstration shows a sequence of instructional objectives for an imagined block of 6 sessions, scheduled to occur once per week. The specific goal is spontaneous production of /ʧ/ in the onset position of single syllable words. Each instructional objective is constructed to contain a *do*, condition and **accuracy** statement. The sequence of statements leads to the terminal objective in small steps, assuming about 100 practice trials within a drill-play format. Achievement of each objective as planned during the session permits transition to the new objective in the next session.

Session	Instructional Objective
1	*Produce* [t] – [s] *or* [t] – [ʃ] *with lips rounded* throughout while looking in mirror and simultaneously hearing the co-produced model [t] – [ʃ], with lip rounding observed **over 10 consecutive trials** to progress to the next step.
2	*Produce* [ʧ] *sound* with tongue blade between teeth to facilitate tongue retraction while observing and hearing the co-produced model [ʧ], with **accurate production on 8/10 trials** required to progress to the next step.
3	*Produce* [ʧ] *sound* after observing and hearing the prior model [ʧ], with **accurate production on 8/10 trials** required to progress to the next step.
4	*Produce* [ʧu] *syllable* after observing and hearing a prior model [ʧu], with **accurate production on 8/10 trials** required to progress to the next step. *Produce* [ʧ] *syllables with various vowels* after observing and hearing a prior model, with **accurate production on 8/10 trials** required to progress to the next step.
5	*Produce* [ʧ]*-initial words with various vowels* after observing and hearing a prior model, with **accurate production on 8/10 trials** required to progress to the next step.
6	*Produce* [ʧ]*-initial words with various vowels* while naming pictures, with **accurate production on 8/10 trials** required to progress to the next specific goal.

make an affricate. The instructional objective also describes the conditions under which the child will complete the task and should be focused on the teaching procedures that the SLP will use to help the child achieve the objective that is described in the "do" statement. For example, in Demonstration 5–1, the SLP co-produces the target during some sessions, models the target during others, and finally shows the child a picture to stimulate a spontaneous response in the last session of the treatment block. The level of accuracy that indicates achievement of the objective is stated so that the SLP knows when to transition to the next, more complex instructional objective in the sequence. The last instructional objective in the sequence is the same as the specific goal, so this is called the **terminal objective**. When the child achieves the stated accuracy level for the terminal objective, a new specific goal can be introduced. In the example shown in Demonstration 5–1, the SLP might introduce the voiced affricate /dʒ/, in the onset or coda position of syllables,

to help the child make progress toward the intermediate goal, which is acquisition of the affricate sound class. The development of a sequence of instructional objectives is based upon a **task analysis**, which requires good knowledge of the phonetic and phonological properties of the goals that the SLP wants the child to achieve.

The child's achievement of the instructional objectives can be documented by keeping detailed notes of the child's performance after every practice trial. Sometimes this kind of record keeping is recommended or even required, but most experienced SLPs recognize that it is difficult to maintain a natural interaction with the child and remain alert to the child's needs for precise feedback if the record keeping system is too detailed or complex. Therefore the child's performance relative to the stated accuracy expectation might be estimated by informal observation across the session. Alternatively, a brief probe could be administered at the end of the session to determine the child's accuracy across a group of 10 practice trials. A **probe** is a quick test that is custom-made specifically to document the child's progress toward the treatment goals. These probes can also be given at the beginning of a treatment session to confirm that the child has maintained gains from the last treatment session and to ensure that the child has not spontaneously learned the task that the SLP has planned to practice during that session.

Treatment progress is usually documented in the child's chart, often using a **SOAP note** format, in which information is structured to include *s*ubjective and *o*bjective observations, *a*ssessment data, and a *p*lan for future treatment. Continuing with the example shown in Demonstration 5–1, a SOAP note for session 6

Practice 5–5

In small groups, brainstorm a task analysis for learning to ride a bicycle. Write a series of instructional objectives for teaching a child to ride a bicycle. Divide up the steps among group members so that each group member has a chance to write the instructional objectives in proper form with a do statement, condition, and accuracy statement. Check each other's instructional objectives to ensure that they each have the correct structure.

could be: (S) mother reports that the child completed homework practice three times in the past week and had no difficulty imitating the "ch" words; (O) child named a group of 10 pictures of "ch" words five times while playing Snakes 'n Ladders; fronting [s] and deaffrication [ʃ] were heard; he was able to produce a correction when the error was pointed out to him but no spontaneous self-corrections were observed; (A) session end probe administered via spontaneous picture naming, 9/10 correct productions; (P) switch specific goal to word-final /dʒ/ next session.

5.4.2 Generalization

The notes written in the child's chart might indicate that excellent progress is occurring during treatment sessions. This is not to say that the basic goal is being met, however. Sometimes children achieve perfect speech accuracy for the specific goal during speech therapy sessions while speaking with the SLP but no appreciable change occurs in other contexts. In other words, treatment progress specifically does not mean that important and significant change is occurring.

The SLP must document **stimulus generalization**, which means transfer of learning from the therapy context to other contexts such as the classroom, the playground, and the home environment. There are three ways to gather information about the child's use of treatment targets in nonclinic environments. Direct observation may be used by way of a variety of strategies: the SLP could go into the classroom and take note of the child's speech; a colleague could converse with the child at lunch and record accuracy of the target

sound; or the family could send a recording from home. More informally, parents, teachers, and peers could provide reports of their impressions of the child's speech accuracy with respect to the therapy target. Regardless of the method used, it is important to be sure that the child has generalized use of the target phoneme or prosodic structure to these other environments and that the child remembers to maintain accuracy when the SLP is not present.

It is also necessary to document **response generalization**, that is, transfer of learning from the treatment goal to other aspects of the child's phonology. Table 5–6 identifies three error patterns that could be targeted with three specific goals in the first treatment block: word-initial /l/-clusters, word-initial /k/, and word-initial /tʃ/. Before progressing to the second block it would be wise to probe for generalization of learning to word-initial /ɹ/-clusters, word-initial /g/, and word-final /dʒ/. If the child was acquiring all of these specific goals without direct treatment, a treatment break might be in order. On the other hand, the child might also have difficulty with /s/-clusters. If the child's progress with the treated liquid clusters does not generalize to untreated /s/-clusters, it will be necessary to introduce this structure as a new goal for direct treatment.

Figure 5–4 illustrates different categories of response generalization using an example of a child who is taught to produce /ʃ/. This child demonstrates generalization of the correct production of /ʃ/ in the word "shoe," targeted in therapy, to the untreated word "shell." The child also demonstrates generalization to another word position not targeted in therapy, in this case the coda position in the word "brush." Within-class generalization is observed when the child transfers learning the fricative /ʃ/ to another fricative not targeted during the intervention (e.g., /s/). Finally, the child demonstrates generalization to a more complex linguistic unit when she correctly produces /ʃ/ in the carrier phrase, "where is the ___?" during a structured intervention activity designed by the SLP to prompt production of the target phoneme in phrases.

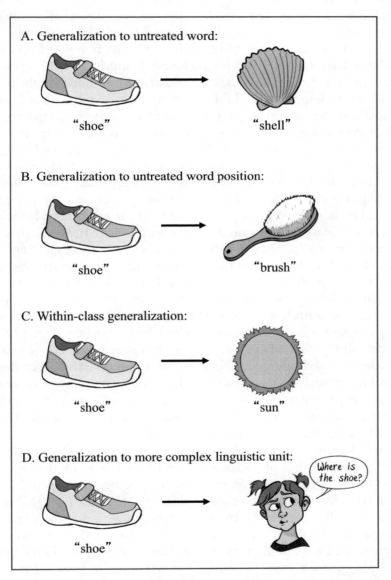

Figure 5–4. *Different categories of response generalization. Used with permission from Françoise Brosseau-Lapré and Ellen Graham-Platt.*

5.4.3 Evidence-Based Practice

When a child receives speech therapy, it is inevitable that the child's speech intelligibility or speech accuracy will improve, either quickly or slowly. It is difficult to be certain that the improvement in the child's speech was caused by the speech therapy intervention, however. Besides the fact that the child is getting older, there are other influences in the child's life. Furthermore, the parents may have made other efforts to improve the child's speech in addition to consulting with the speech therapy service. Even when the speech therapy program has played a role in the child's growing speech competence, it might be due to the specific factors in the program (e.g., the particular treatment procedures used by the SLP) or it might be a general effect related to the common factors in the intervention (e.g., a nonspecific motivational effect of drawing attention to the child's speech problem and praising the child for speaking more clearly). One way to increase confidence that the speech therapy program is responsible for changes in the child's speech behavior is to use an evidence-based approach. This means integrating clinical experience with the best research evidence to choose treatment approaches that are known to work for children who are similar to the client.

An effective treatment approach will be supported by specific kinds of evidence. First there will be basic science evidence that explains why the treatment procedures might achieve the goals of the treatment approach. Second there should be high-quality research that demonstrates **treatment efficacy**. As a related point, the associated research reports should describe the children who were treated in the studies very explicitly so that the

SLPs can match the treatment to similar clients on their caseloads. There are many indicators of research quality, but the most important for treatment efficacy research is randomized control of extraneous variables that might impact the child's outcome. In the most common type of randomized controlled trial, the children in the study will be randomly assigned to the different treatment options that are being compared. For example, a new treatment approach might be compared with no treatment, with a sham treatment (which is not expected to have any effect), or with an old treatment that is typically used in clinical practice. It would be exciting if 4-year-old children with moderate speech delay made greater improvements in speech accuracy after six weeks of a new treatment in comparison to the control condition, the sham treatment, or usual care. It would be even more exciting if there were **treatment effectiveness** research showing that the new treatment was also effective when implemented in typical clinical environments and not only in a laboratory clinic by researchers. If an SLP decided to use this new treatment with a 4-year-old child with moderate speech delay and that child made good improvements in speech accuracy, there would be good reasons to assume that the treatment played a role in the child's progress.

It may be possible to document the child's response to the new treatment more specifically by probing the child's rate of progress for treatment targets compared with other speech sounds that were not treated. Continuing with the example shown in Table 5–6, the SLP might choose to treat /l/-clusters during the first treatment block. If /l/-clusters and /ɹ/-clusters were mastered but /s/-clusters continued to show a pattern of inconsistent reductions and simplifications, it would be reasonable to think that the treatment program was responsible for this pattern of results.

In some cases there may be no good quality research to guide the selection of a treatment approach. It will be particularly important to determine whether the child is responding to the treatment procedures that the SLP chooses to use for rare cases. Even in the clinical environment it is possible to implement single subject experiments with randomization to document whether the child is benefit-ing from the treatment or to observe the child's response to one treatment approach in comparison to another (Rvachew & Matthews, 2017a).

The implication is that there are many approaches and treatment procedures to choose from and the choice must be individualized to suit the unique needs of each child. These approaches and procedures are described in the final three chapters of this book with evidence-based guidelines for selecting procedures in relation to child needs.

Box 5–4. Monitoring Treatment Progress: Key Points

- Progress monitoring provides essential information for continuous updating to the treatment plan and for documenting treatment outcomes for accountability purposes.
- Achievement of instructional objectives, structured to move the child in small steps toward the specific goal, indicates that the child is responding to the treatment program.
- Direct observation of the child in a variety of environments or reports from family, peers, and teachers provides information about stimulus generalization, that is, transfer of learning from therapy to other speaking situations and environments.
- Probes can be constructed to test for response generalization, that is, transfer of learning from the specific goal that is practiced in therapy to other phonological structures, indicating that significant and important change is occurring.
- Evidence-based practice means combining clinical experience with the best research evidence to choose and implement effective treatment approaches and procedures.

Chapter 5 Study Questions

Consider the following hypothetical case and answer the questions below.

Case history: A girl age 3;6 is brought by her mother for assessment because her speech is unintelligible. The mother needs to return to work but the child is too shy to speak at child care because no one understands her, even when she asks to go to the bathroom. Her birth and health and developmental history is otherwise unremarkable.

Speech assessment results: Receptive language skills are within normal limits. Phonology test score is at the first percentile, with the following patterns observed: consonant voicing in all syllable positions (consistent); velar fronting in the syllable onset position (consistent); gliding of labial fricatives in the onset position (consistent); fronting of palatal fricatives in all syllable positions (consistent); stopping of affricates in all syllable positions (inconsistent); gliding of liquids in all syllable positions (inconsistent); reduction of liquid clusters (inconsistent); reduction of /s/-clusters in onset position (consistent) and in coda position (inconsistent).

Questions:

1. Explain why you would recommend treatment for this child from the perspective of the norm-referenced approach.

2. Explain why you would recommend treatment for this child from the perspective of the medical model.

3. Explain why you would recommend treatment for this child from the perspective of the ICF-CY.

4. Explain why you would recommend treatment for this child using the flow chart in Figure 5–1.

5. Describe an appropriate service delivery model to provide treatment to this child. In your selected model, identify the three essential components.

6. Imagine that this child is rationed to two half-hour treatment sessions per week over an eight-week block by your service provider. You find that she is capable of accomplishing an average of 100 practice trials during each treatment session. What is the cumulative intervention intensity? Show your calculation.

7. Select three treatment goals for this child using the guidelines shown in Table 5–6. Include the basic goal, the intermediate goal, and the specific goal for each of the three goals.

8. Remember that you have been rationed to two half-hour treatment sessions per week over an eight-week block. What would be the best goal attack strategy in this situation: vertical, horizontal, or cyclical? Justify your answer.

9. Pick one of your specific goals. Write the first three instructional objectives for the achievement of this goal.

6

Input-Oriented Approaches

Learning Objectives

- Describe the primary goal of input-oriented approaches to phonology intervention.
- Identify the characteristics of children who are most likely to benefit from focused stimulation procedures to remediate phonological delay.
- Describe the therapeutic context that is used for implementing focused stimulation techniques.
- List and give examples of six focused stimulation techniques that can be used to help a child acquire

phonological knowledge of target words or phonemes.
- Identify the context in which ear training should be used.
- List and describe the four ear training techniques.
- Explain the rationale for including dialogic reading as a home program component of an intervention for a preschool-aged child with phonological delay.
- Define eight dialogic reading techniques and give examples.

The treatment procedures that the speech-language pathologist (SLP) chooses to use when intervening to improve a child's speech intelligibility will be determined largely by the nature of the underlying problem as discussed in Chapter 4 and the treatment goals that are derived from the process described in Chapter 5. When a child is unable to correctly produce the expected word shapes and speech sounds, the natural inclination is to begin by targeting articulatory gestures. For some children, there are many reasons to delay direct speech practice and begin with an **input-oriented approach**. An input-oriented approach targets children's **acoustic-phonetic representations**, that is, their knowledge of the acoustic characteristics of sounds and words—this knowledge underpins their ability to abstract a sound-based representation of words from spoken language input for word recognition and language comprehension. The rationale for using an input-oriented approach, the associated therapeutic procedures, and expected outcomes are derived from the basic science on early speech development as described in detail in Rvachew and Brosseau-Lapré (2018). A brief summary will be provided here.

6.1 RATIONALE FOR THE INPUT-ORIENTED APPROACH

Recall that even before the emergence of babbling, the infant is learning about speech by listening. The infant learns to recognize prosodic patterns, word shapes, phones, and sound sequences that are used in the ambient language. The infant acquires detailed acoustic-phonetic representations for words long before accurate production of those words is mastered.

Certain children need to begin their therapeutic journey at this listening stage of speech development. In particular children who are very young (that is, at an early stage of phonological or language development) and children who have specific difficulties with auditory or phonological processing will be good candidates for the procedures described in this chapter. These procedures are designed to provide children with varied, concentrated, and focused speech inputs with the goal of improving their acoustic-phonetic representations for words, syllables, and speech sounds. Detailed acoustic-phonetic representations provide the child with more accurate targets for speech production and help the child use feedback to acquire greater accuracy and precision in speech production. A

larger store of acoustic-phonetic representations will force successive reorganizations of the lexicon. Consequently, the child will gradually develop adultlike phonological knowledge. Specifically, the child will develop **implicit** knowledge of phonemes and phoneme classes and how these units are used to form and contrast meaningful words. Implicit knowledge emerges before the child has conscious metalinguistic access to it. For example, an important advance in phonological knowledge can be seen when a child's error pattern transitions from inconsistent ("cat" /kæt/ → [dæt], "pickle" /pɪkəl/ → [pɪpo], "crane" /kɹeɪn/ → [tʃeɪn]) to consistent ("cat" → [tæt], "pickle" → [pɪto], "crane" → [tweɪn]), revealing a new understanding of /k/ as a phoneme regardless of the word it appears in or the syllable position it occupies. The implication is that the SLP can intervene before the child is ready for the structured drill practice procedures described in Chapter 7 or the explicit metalinguistic procedures described in Chapter 8.

Three input-oriented procedures will be described: focused stimulation, ear training, and dialogic reading, each composed of a group of techniques applied in a specific context. In each section of this chapter, the children who will benefit from the procedure will be described, the techniques will be listed and defined, and the research evidence to support the efficacy of the treatment procedure will be briefly discussed.

6.2 FOCUSED STIMULATION

Focused stimulation techniques are especially appropriate for the following groups of children: (1) children who are very young, i.e., between birth and 3 years of age; (2) children who have lower levels of language development, with limited expressive vocabularies and mean length of utterance; (3) children who are very shy or otherwise unwilling to talk freely with the SLP or engage in articulation drill practice; (4) children whose error patterns are highly inconsistent and therefore the therapy targets are words rather than specific phonemes or word shapes; (5) children who are unstimulable for their potential speech sound targets; and/or (6) children who demonstrate poor auditory or phonological processing skills. Focused stimulation procedures may be adopted as the only therapeutic procedure for the child. More typically, focused stimulation will be combined with other input-oriented procedures or with phonological procedures as described in Chapter 8.

Focused stimulation procedures are used in the context of carefully planned play interactions between SLP and child (Fey, Long, & Finestack, 2003). The play activities are designed to feel like unstructured play but are in fact carefully structured in advance to provide many models of the target words to the child. Notice that it is important to identify target words that will be presented during the play activity. The play activity, the environment, and the treatment procedures are also combined in such a way that the child will have opportunities to hear and produce the target words. However, the SLP does not put any explicit pressure on the child to produce speech. The primary goal is to strengthen the child's acoustic-phonetic representation of the target words. Initially, the SLP's focus should be on dose (how many times did I say each target word?) and salience (did I get the child's attention when I said the target words?). When the child begins

to produce the target words voluntarily, the SLP should switch focus to providing appropriate feedback that will help the child monitor the similarities and differences between the child's production and the SLP's production of the target words.

Practice 6–1

In small groups, consider the child who produced the speech sample presented in Demonstration 1–1. Imagine that you want the child to begin producing CVCV words in which the two consonants do not share the same place of articulation. Select three target words that can be used coherently in the context of a single activity. Describe the activity and the associated materials and explain how you would implement it so the toddler would have many opportunities to hear those words.

The focused stimulation techniques that are used during these planned activities are listed and defined in Table 6–1. The first two techniques serve to provide many models of the target words using a speaking style that increases the salience of the speech input to the child. Critically, there is no expectation in the early period of this intervention that the child will attempt to say the words. Rather, the goal is for the child to listen to the target forms. Needless to say, having a clear sense of the target words is a critical first step, for the SLP and the child. The selected target words should be appropriate to the child's language and phonological skills. The second step is to design a play activity that will encourage repeated modeling of those target words. Third, while playing with the child it is important to use

Table 6–1. *Focused Stimulation Techniques for Phonological Intervention*

Technique	Description
Model Many Exemplars of the Target Word	
Slow rate	Use a slow rate of speech and a child-directed speaking style without distorting the phonetic content of the target word.
Model	Repeatedly present the target word, in the context of natural language input, without prompting the child to say the words.
Encourage the Child to Attempt Production of the Target Words	
Time delay	Use completion prompts in which you pause for insertion of the target word but wait longer than is typical for the child to respond.
Question	Ask a question (which may or may not include the target word) in order to prompt the child to produce the target word.
Highlight Relationship Between Child and Adult Production of Target Word	
Recast	After the child attempts the target word, immediately repeat some of the child's words while correcting or modifying the target form.
Expansion	After the child attempts the target word, immediately repeat some of the child's words while adding details.
Imitation/ feedback	After the child produces the target form correctly, immediately respond by imitating the child's correct use of the target form.

parallel talk to coordinate speech inputs with the child's focus of attention. Parallel talk is a kind of running commentary about what the child is doing or attending to. Research has shown that learning from speech input is enhanced when there is joint attention—this means that the child should be shifting gaze between the play materials and your face while you are talking about the play activity (Conboy, Brooks, Meltzoff, & Kuhl, 2015). Therefore it is important to position yourself and the play materials to facilitate joint attention during the focused stimulation session. Finally, while providing this speech input it helps to **talk slowly**, using the exaggerated pitch contours that parents use when talking to babies and young children (sometimes called motherese,

or infant-directed speech). Controlled studies have shown that children with language impairments learn more from speech when it is presented at a slow rate (Weismer & Hesketh, 1996).

When the child begins to feel capable of approximating or achieving correct production of the target words, the child will begin to attempt those targets with increasing frequency. At this point it is appropriate to begin using the prompting techniques described in Table 6–1. An indirect type of prompt is a **completion prompt** in which an expectant pause signals an opportunity for the child to finish the SLP's sentence or phrase, most likely one that has reoccurred frequently during the activity. When playing with young children who have communication disorders, it may be necessary to use longer pauses than you might think is natural when you say, for example, "and now comes the big bad . . . " A more direct prompt is a **question** to elicit the target word: "I see the wolf over there. Who is coming to blow down the house?" These prompts for production of the target forms are a key component of focused stimulation when it is used for grammar facilitation with older children (Proctor-Williams, 2009). When using focused stimulation to remediate phonological delay, it is best to delay the introduction of production prompts until after the child has acquired clear acoustic-phonetic representations of the target words. The child's willingness and ability to spontaneously attempt the words and achieve close approximations is one indication that the child is ready to respond to these prompts.

When the child attempts a target word, the SLP should respond in a way that helps the child notice whether her/his production attempt was similar or dissimilar to the adult target. Three possible responses are defined in Table 6–1. Notice that none of these responses involves a direct correction or evaluation of the child's production attempt. Rather the SLP should recast, expand or imitate the child's response while maintaining the play interaction. For example, if the target word is "bus," and the child says [ʌ bʌ], the SLP can respond "yes, a bus" [ˌjɛs ʌ ˈbʌs] (**recast**) or "the bus is big" [ðə ˈbʌs ɪz ˌbɪg] (**expansion**). Even if the child says the target word correctly [ʌ bʌs], it is helpful to immediately **imitate** the word so that the child can evaluate the match to the adult form, "I see the bus" [aɪ ˌsi ðə ˈbʌs]. Notice that the SLP does *not* use **telegraphic speech**—that is, ungrammatical speech such as "bus go" [ˈbʌs go]—when responding but nonetheless provides

opportunities to compare child and adult forms of the word "bus" in the context of natural dialogue, "the bus is going" [ðə ˈbʌs ɪz ˌgoɪŋ]. Demonstration 6–1 presents a small amount of data from a real case to motivate the selection of three target words for a single session, followed by a demonstration of how to implement focused stimulation techniques to model the target words for the toddler.

> **Practice 6–2**
>
> The hypothetical treatment session shown in Demonstration 6–1 includes all the focused stimulation techniques defined in Table 6–1. Try to identify the techniques that the SLP is using in utterances marked with superscripts before referring to the key at the bottom of the demonstration.

We have described focused stimulation as a treatment approach that should be implemented by the SLP with young children. Often, however, young children are treated with indirect service delivery methods such as home programs or consultation with parents and child care workers. Focused stimulation techniques can be learned and implemented successfully by parents and child care personnel, especially when the therapy goals are simple, but only when those individuals receive structured training and follow-up support. In some jurisdictions, the amount of time required for adequate training and support of parents or child care staff exceeds the ration for publicly funded direct treatment to the child! Involvement of families and school personnel should be considered to be an adjunct to high-quality SLP service provision rather

Application of Focused Simulation Techniques with Boy Aged 2;5

A. Speech Sample		B. Phonotactic Analysis	C. Goals
more	[moʌ]	Vowel repertoire	Stabilize goal
mummy	[mʌmʌ]	ʌ (o)	2-syllable words:
duck	[dʌ]	Consonant repertoire	CV_1CV_1
puzzle	[pʌ]	m p (b) (d)	CV_1CV_2
puppy	[pʌ]	Word shape repertoire	Extend goal
me	[m:]	V CV (CVCV) (C)	Labial → glide
meow	[ʌ]	Prominent patterns	[wʌ]
house	[ʌ]	Labial C Central V	Expand goal
boy	[bʌ]	1-syllable words	[i, u, æ, ɛ, ʊ...]

D. Focused stimulation with speech-language pathologist (SLP) and child (C)

SLP: Let's play a bedtime game—3 babies go to bed. I have 3 beds, 3 babies, 3 mummies, and 3 puppies too. I am going to set these on the table.[a]

SLP: We need 1 baby for each bed. 1 baby...2 babies...3 babies. Each baby has a puppy, 1 puppy...2 puppies...3 puppies. Their mama will tell them "bedtime!" 1 mama...2 mamas...3 mamas...Now we're ready to play.[b]

SLP: You take baby. Mama says "Bedtime baby!"

C: [Puts baby in bed.]

SLP: Baby is sleeping zzzzz. Oh-oh! Puppy comes. Woof-woof. What happens?[c]

C: Wawa. [picks up the baby]

SLP: [wʌwʌ][d]

SLP: Mama comes, "bad puppy" she says, "bad..."[e]

C: [pʌ]

SLP: Puppy. [f] Bad puppy. [walks puppy off the table]

C: [be:] [puts baby in bed]

SLP: Baby is sleeping zzzzz.[g]

Key: [a]model; [b]slow rate; [c]question; [d]imitation; [e]time delay (completion prompt); [f]recast; [g]expansion.

than a replacement for it, especially when improved speech accuracy and intelligibility is the goal of the intervention. That being said, Girolametto, Pearce, and Weitzman (1997) conducted a randomized controlled trial of focused stimulation in which mothers of late-talking toddlers were taught focused stimulation techniques, specifically: (a) child-oriented techniques to establish joint attention; (b) interaction promoting techniques to foster balanced turn-taking in nonverbal and verbal routines; (c) language modeling techniques applied incidentally in the natural environment to highlight relationships between language content, form, and use; and (d) focused stimulation techniques to teach 20 specific vocabulary items selected individually for each child. The training program was highly structured and included eight parent group sessions and three home visits. After 4 months, large and significant differences were observed between the treated and untreated groups on a variety of language and phonology outcomes. The co-occurring increase in phonetic repertoire, syllable shape repertoire, and expressive vocabulary size was not unexpected given that young children are known to learn "words, not sounds." Child care workers can also be taught to apply language facilitation techniques and will maintain the use of those techniques over time, especially when the children are responsive, i.e., show improvements in language skills when their child care workers provide good inputs (Girolametto, Weitzman, & Greenberg, 2003). If the speech and language targets are complex or the children have severe communication disorders, parents and child care workers may have difficulty implementing and maintaining these techniques. In most cases, direct SLP services to the child are essential

along with ongoing supports to parents and child care workers who can augment the speech therapy program (Fey, Cleave, & Long, 1997; Flowers, Girolametto, Weitzman, & Greenberg, 2007).

Box 6–1. Focused Stimulation: Key Points

- Focused stimulation is meant to strengthen acoustic-phonetic representations of words.
- Focused stimulation techniques are used in the context of structured play activities.
- The SLP provides many models of the target words to the child at a slow rate.
- The SLP responds to child attempts with recasts, expansions, or imitations.
- Children should implicitly compare their own productions with the adult forms.

6.3 EAR TRAINING

The purpose of **ear training** is to help the child develop an internalized auditory model of the phoneme to serve as a target for the child's productions. Therefore, ear training should be started prior to implementing the output-oriented procedures described in Chapter 7. Ear training, like focused stimulation, is an input-oriented intervention procedure in that the goal is to strengthen acoustic phonetic representations for speech, but in this case the target is at the level of the phoneme. Therefore, the child who will benefit from ear training will be older with a more mature underlying phonological system than was described for focused stimulation. Specifically, the techniques described in Table 6–2 are best used with children aged approximately 4 through 6 years. Older children with phonological delay or persistent speech errors and difficulties with auditory or phonological processing may also benefit from ear training; however, the activities should be modified to involve more complex speech inputs and age-appropriate themes. Nonetheless the principles of the intervention approach would be similar, especially with respect to the requirement that the child make explicit judgments about target sounds as presented in varied speech inputs.

Ear training techniques, as described by Van Riper (1978), should be implemented altogether during one session whenever a new phoneme target is introduced. Four activities, each lasting 2 to 10 minutes, should be planned in order as listed in Table 6–2. A first and crucial step is to identify the phoneme target for the child. **Identification** primarily involves labeling the target phoneme, typically with a child-friendly name; however, school-aged children can be taught the letter or letters that are associated with the sound. For example, "we are going to listen for [s], the snake sound" or "we will work on the sound [k] that goes with the letter 'c' as well as with the letter 'k.'" The SLP also models the new sound and then, using age-appropriate language, describes it: What does it sound like? What does it look like? How do you make it? What does it feel like when you make it? Later in the therapy program the SLP will use the same vocabulary used in this identification process to describe the child's productions; for this reason it is important to find descriptors that are meaningful to the child. An example of identification

Table 6–2. Ear Training Techniques Summarized from Van Riper (1963)

Technique	Description
Identification	SLP identifies the target for the child by briefly demonstrating the auditory, visual, articulatory, and tactile-kinesthetic properties of the sound.
Isolation	Child signals when he or she hears the target; SLP produces the target against a background of other speech sounds in isolation, words, phrases, and sentences.
Stimulation (auditory bombardment)	SLP presents the target to the child in a variety of different ways. Word lists, storybooks, and recorded materials may be used as inputs. Amplification is advised.
Error detection[a]	SLP produces words with correct and incorrect articulations of the target, mimicking the child's error. The child identifies each word as correctly or incorrectly produced by producing a unique motor response for correct and incorrect productions.

[a]Van Riper referred to this step in the program as "discrimination," but other terms such as "error detection" and "phoneme identification" are more accurate labels because discrimination usually involves judging the similarity of pairs of stimuli rather than making judgments about individual stimuli presented one at a time.

is shown in Demonstration 6–2, which focuses on /f/ as the target phoneme.

Practice 6–3

In pairs, select one of the following commonly misarticulated consonants: /k,g,f,v,θ,ð,s,z,ʃ,ʒ,tʃ,dʒ, l,ɹ/. Given your sound, write scripts for introducing this target to a child aged 4 years and to a child aged 6 years. Consult a practicing SLP as well as online or other published sources to get ideas for labeling and describing the target phoneme that you have chosen. Share your scripts with your classmates.

The second technique, **isolation**, involves presenting the child with a variety of speech sounds, some similar and others very different from the target. Specifically, the SLP: (1) makes sure the child cannot see her face; (2) produces a variety of sounds, syllables, words, and sentences, using varied intonation; (3) helps the child to signal when the target sound is produced. Speech input should be planned before the session to make sure that the child hears sounds that are very different from and similar to the target. When presenting sentences, it should be clear that the child is responding to the target sound. For example, if the target sound is [ʃ] and the SLP says "I see a ship," the child might respond to the word "see" or "ship"; therefore, it would be better to present "I went on a ship" and "I see a boat" separately. An example of an isolation activity is shown in Demonstration 6–2.

The third technique, **stimulation**, is commonly used in speech therapy practice and shares some characteristics with focused stimulation except that books may be used more often than toys with these older children. This technique is also referred to as **auditory bombardment**. The goal is simply for the child to hear many good exemplars of the target phoneme. Amplification may be used while presenting the speech input, which may come in the form of word lists, poems, or stories that are loaded with words containing the target phoneme. When using amplification, it is important to not introduce distortion by speaking too loudly or overemphasizing the target sound. Speaking slowly with amplification is the best strategy to ensure that the child can hear the speech input; when possible and where prosodically natural, prolonging the sound slightly may be helpful and will be more effective than adding loudness. The example shown in Demonstration 6–2 suggests a well-known commercial picture book, but it is common for the SLP to create stories specific to the child's target and interests, and speech therapy stories may be purchased specifically for this purpose.

Finally, an **error detection** task caps the ear training session. Now that the child has an improved representation of the target phoneme, the child should be able to identify well-produced exemplars of the target and mispronunciations of the target, especially mispronunciations that are similar to the child's own error sound. The SLP must present minimal pair words that contrast the target with the child's error and ask the child to identify the correct and incorrect exemplars, using clear motor responses that are associated with the two words. The minimal pair may be constructed of a target word that contains the target phoneme and the nonsense word that results when the child's substitution or distortion is used. For example, if the child's error is a lateral lisp, the SLP

Technique	Identification
Materials	Large mirror
Positioning	SLP and child sit side by side in front of large mirror.
Script/stimuli	We are going to listen to the sound /f/ today. Watch me make it, [f]. I put my bottom lip up and under my top teeth like this, [f]. Then I blow air out gently, [f]. Do you hear the sound of the wind blowing, [f]? The sound [f] goes with the letter "f." (Draw lowercase 'f' on the mirror with dry erase pen.) The letter "f" looks a bit like a fishhook. The sound [f] is at the beginning of the word "fish." [f], [fːɪʃ] (draw a fish, mouth to left). We catch it with a fishhook (draw an "f" shaped fishhook in its mouth).

Technique	Isolation
Materials	Paper fish
Positioning	Child sits with fish in right (or preferred) hand; SLP sits behind child.
Script/stimuli	We are going to play a listening game. Listen for the [f] sound. If you hear me say the [f] sound, hold up the fish. [f], [m], [z], [f], [bi], [fu], [mu], [pe], "feet," "soot," "white rabbit," "funny clown," "pea pod," "kick it," "sun down," "barbecue fork." (If the child does not respond when an /f/ item is said, repeat the item close to the child's right ear. Reinstruct if the child responds to an item that does not have the /f/ sound in it.)

Technique	Stimulation
Materials	"One Fish, Two Fish, Red Fish, Blue Fish" by Dr. Seuss
Positioning	Child and SLP sit side by side with book between them.
Script/stimuli	I will read the book to you. Have you heard this one before? Next week if you remember some of the words, you can help me read it. Today I want you to listen carefully while I read. I will move my finger along the words as I read. Notice how I will say the /f/ sound when my finger finds the letter "f." One fish...

Technique	Error detection
Materials	Paper cut-outs of 10 fish; felt-tip pen or crayon.
Positioning	SLP and child sit side by side at a table.
Script/stimuli	We are going to play a game where you get to catch these fish and take them home to play games with your mom. When I say "fish," draw a fishhook on the mouth and put it in your notebook. I am going to try to trick you sometimes. If I say the word the wrong way, if I forget to put the windy /f/ sound on the word, that means the fish gets away. Give it back to me. You will have another chance to catch it later.

might produce a series of "words" that represent "sock" and "not-sock" like this: [sɑk], [sɑk], [ɬɑk], [sɑk], [ɬɑk], [ɬɑk], [sɑk], [ɬɑk], [sɑk]. The child puts the "sock" on the boy's foot when said correctly and a spaceboot on the monster foot when said incorrectly. Notice that the child is not expected to produce any speech during this activity. Also notice that the child is instructed to "do" something with the socks or spaceboots in response to the SLP's productions. There is no expectation of a verbal response on the part of the child. If the SLP says "sock" → [sɑk], and the child repeats [[ɬɑk], this exchange will create confusion and make it difficult for the child to judge whether the SLP said the word "sock" with the correct acoustic-phonetic form. Also, if the SLP says "sock" → [sɑk] and the child answers "that was wrong," prompting the SLP to correct, "no that was right," some very confused conversations will occur. Rather, the idea is that the SLP will say "sock" → [sɑk], the child will listen quietly, and then choose a sock to put on the boy's foot. The SLP may respond, "That sock makes his foot warm" in order to reinforce the relationship between the lexical item "sock" and the acoustic-phonetic form [sɑk]. Another example of an error detection task is shown in Demonstration 6–2.

If the child is having difficulty with the error detection task, it is advisable to continue with error detection tasks alongside production therapy. The first few minutes of each therapy session could be devoted to error detection, using different kinds of speech inputs. It is important to be aware that the child may achieve excellent performance with these error detection tasks and yet have a poor underlying acoustic-phonetic representation for the target phoneme. This happens when the SLP cannot mimic the child's speech error

exactly. For example, adults often hear children substitute [w] for /ɹ/; if these children are presented with words such as "white" and "right," they may have no difficulty identifying these words. This happens because the children are producing a distortion that is midway between [w] and [ɹ], and SLPs typically cannot produce this exact error; therefore, children have no experience learning to listen for the acoustic cue that differentiates /w/ and /ɹ/ from their own specific distortion. One way to help these children with persistent /ɹ/ errors learn the boundary between [ɹ] and [ɹʷ] is to present recordings of children's /ɹ/ productions, some correct and some incorrect. A therapy program that does this is the Speech Assessment and Interactive Learning Program, as described in Rvachew and Brosseau-Lapré (2010). This program has been shown in nonexperimental studies, single subject experiments. and randomized control trials to markedly improve the efficiency of speech therapy, even when only 45 to 60 minutes of input is provided.

> **Box 6–2. Ear Training: Key Points**
>
> - Ear training should be used when the target is individual phonemes.
> - Ear training techniques are identification, isolation, stimulation, and error detection.
> - The SLP should contrast the target with other sounds in varied contexts.
> - The SLP should not allow the child to watch the SLP's face when presenting the speech input.
> - Ear training has been shown to improve the efficiency of speech therapy.

6.4 DIALOGIC READING

Research shows that vocabulary size is associated with speech perception skills (Tsao, Huei-Mei, & Kuhl, 2004; Werker, Fennell, Corcoran, & Stager, 2002), underlying phonological knowledge (Munson, Kurtz, & Windsor, 2005), and phonological awareness (Metsala, 1999; Walley, Metsala, & Garlock, 2003). Furthermore, there are trade-offs between skill levels in these areas: a child with deficits in speech perception and production skills but average vocabulary size will have poorer phonological awareness skills than would otherwise be expected (Rvachew & Grawburg, 2006). Individual differences in vocabulary learning are jointly and independently determined by intrinsic differences in language processing speed and the amount of language input that the child receives (Hurtado, Grüter, Marchman, & Fernald, 2014). Altogether, this research suggests that it is valuable to teach parents to provide high-quality inputs to their children to enhance vocabulary learning, especially when they have or are at risk for speech, language, and literacy delays (Rvachew & Brosseau-Lapré, 2018). Shared reading is a powerful context for providing high-quality language input and for teaching vocabulary and phonological awareness skills (Weizman & Snow, 2001). We recommend that parents of children with phonological delay be taught to use evidence-based shared reading techniques, even if their child's vocabulary skills are within normal limits.

Dialogic reading prompts were developed by Whitehurst et al. (1988) to improve the oral language skills of 2- to 3-year-old toddlers when employed by parents. This teaching procedure was subsequently adapted for use by preschool teachers with 4- to 5-year-old children (Lonigan & Whitehurst, 1998; Whitehurst et al., 1994, 1999; Zevenbergen, Whitehurst, & Zevenbergen, 2003). Dialogic reading is designed to encourage active participation by the child during shared reading. The parent (or preschool teacher or other adult reader) is taught to prompt the child for verbal answers relevant to the story or text. The parent is also encouraged to provide specific kinds of feedback about the child's response. The prompts and the feedback should be adjusted to reflect the child's level of language functioning and the child's familiarity with the story.

Children can learn a lot of language and literacy skills when sharing books with an adult: new words, more mature grammar, more accurate or precise speech articulation, phonological awareness, letter-sound associations and word recognition, typical story structures, and predicting and inferencing skills. Children cannot learn this diversity of skills all at once during the same shared reading event, however. Parents should be supported to choose a specific goal for each book. The goals should be matched to the child's speech and language learning needs. Prompts should be planned to challenge the child while being appropriate for the child's interests and potential for success. Here we will provide definitions of the prompts and feedback that adults should use along with examples in Table 6–3. The examples will demonstrate the use of the prompts to encourage the learning of new vocabulary and the use of a target phoneme [ɹ] in relation to the corresponding letters "R" and "r" along with some word recognition skills.

The kinds of prompts that parents might use are described using the CROWD acronym: completion, recall, open-ended, wh-questions, and distancing. Completion prompts are similar to a

Table 6–3. Definitions of Dialogic Reading Techniques with Examples Using the PEER Sequence

Technique	Definition	Vocabulary Example	Phoneme Example
Prompt	Elicit a response from the child.		
Completion		This is the story of Little Red Riding . . .	This is the story of Little Red Riding Hood. Rrred starts with the "rrr" sound. "rrr" goes with the letter . . .
Recall		Do you remember where she is going with her basket?	Do you remember which one is the word "red"?
Open-ended		What do you think she should put in the basket for Grandma?	How did the girl get her name?
Wh-questions		In this picture, where is Little Red Riding Hood?	What is this letter here?
Distancing		Do you remember when you went for a hike in the woods with Grandpa? Tell me about that.	Look, here is a word that we saw yesterday . . . at the market . . . Do you know what it says?
Evaluate	Provide feedback to indicate whether the response was correct or not.	Sort of a hat, but it is called a hood because it's attached to her cape.	No, it says "red." It's on the Red Rooster sign. It says "red."
Expand	Add information to the child's response.	Forest, yes, or in this book they call it the woods.	Yes, that's the letter "R" in the word "Red."
	Or get more information.	Who lives in the woods?	What is the word?
Repeat	Ask the child to repeat the correct response	What is the other word for forest? Say "woods."	What is this word? Say "red."
	or the new information.	Tell me, "Grandma lives in the woods."	Red, that's right, let's read Little Red Riding Hood.

time delay prompt: the adult produces a rhyme or phrase that reoccurs in the story, with a pause inserted to cue the end of the phrase or the next phrase that should occur. **Recall prompts** are a direct request to retell parts of the story, either as just read or as read on a prior day. When the adult reader expects a long answer (beyond yes/no or a single word), **open-ended prompts** are used ("Tell me what is happening here"). **Wh-questions** are the familiar "what" or "who" questions that may be easy to answer, but also the more complex "when" and "why" questions. **Distancing prompts** encourage children to link story content to their own experience.

The adult reader is also taught to evaluate the child's response to each prompt and provide informative feedback. If the child's answer is not correct, the adult can provide the correct answer and ask the child to repeat it. If the child's answer is correct, the adult can ask for more information and ask the child to repeat the expanded reply. The whole sequence of events follows **PEER**: prompt, evaluate, expand, repeat. The PEER sequence should be used sparingly during a single reading session, perhaps once every three pages or so. The prompts can become more complex as the story is repeated. This style of reading is used most often with younger children. Additional demonstrations, showing how to apply these techniques with younger and older children, are presented in Rvachew and Brosseau-Lapré (2018).

Meta-analyses have shown that dialogic reading is effective to enhance children's vocabulary development (Bus, Van Ijzendoorn, & Pellegrini, 1995; Mol, Bus, & De Jong, 2009; Reese & Cox, 1999). Mol et al. (2008) concluded that dialogic reading was most effective for toddlers and preschool-age children. Older children with

higher-level language skills may benefit from a different style of shared reading (Hindman, Connor, Jewkes, & Morrison, 2008; Reese & Cox, 1999). For example, the "performance style" of reading involves discussions of the story before reading to preview new vocabulary and to help the children connect important concepts to their own experience. After reading the book dramatically and without interruptions, further discussion ensures that the children have understood the story (Dickinson & Tabors, 2001); this style has been shown to be beneficial to language development in kindergarten-age children.

Practice 6–4

In pairs, and given the speech sounds that your pair targeted in Practice 6–3, choose a children's book that will provide a child with the opportunity to hear and produce words that contain that target sound. Create dialogic reading prompts using the CROWD acronym, that would be appropriate to implement when reading the book to a child with delayed speech and language skills. You might attach the prompts to the book using sticky notes. Practice reading the book to each other, with the designated adult reader using the PEER sequence to elicit responses from the listener and provide feedback as appropriate. Your prompts should focus on vocabulary or sound-symbol knowledge or phonological awareness but not a mix of all three.

Several studies have involved teaching the parents of children with language impairments to use dialogic reading techniques with their children (Dale, Crain-Thoreson, Notari-Synverson, & Cole, 1996; Kaderavek & Justice, 2002). Rvachew and Brosseau-Lapré (2015) combined dialogic reading with speech therapy as an intervention for French-speaking children with phonological delay. In a 12-week randomized control trial, children received individual speech therapy and group phonological awareness therapy, while their parents were taught to implement a dialogic reading intervention at home. We concluded that the dialogic reading intervention was most effective when combined with an input-oriented approach to speech therapy. We speculate that the input-oriented approach to therapy taught the children to listen carefully to speech input and improved their phonological processing abilities. This 6-week intervention component prepared the children to successfully participate in the dialogic reading component that followed. As a consequence, the parents who experienced this combination of intervention components achieved more success and were more satisfied with the home reading program.

Box 6–3. Dialogic Reading: Key Points

- Shared reading is an ideal context for providing high-quality language input.
- While sharing a book, the adult reader prompts the child to talk about the story.
- After eliciting a response, the adult evaluates or expands the response.
- The adult may ask the child to repeat the correct response.
- Dialogic reading enhances vocabulary skills.
- Dialogic reading may also improve phonological awareness and emergent literacy.

Chapter 6 Study Questions

The first column of this table lists intervention techniques that were discussed in this chapter. The second column shows descriptions of intervention techniques. Match the techniques to their descriptions by putting the number of the technique into the box next to the appropriate description.

Technique		Description
1 completion prompt	_____	child identifies well-produced exemplars of the target and mispronunciations of the target
2 error detection	_____	slow speech with exaggerated pitch contours
3 question prompts	_____	improves vocabulary and emergent literacy skills
4 focused stimulation	_____	helps the child link story content to his/her own experience

Technique		Description
5 expansion	_____	is an acronym for prompt, expand, evaluate, repeat
6 telegraphic speech	_____	should be adjusted to reflect the child's level of perceptual knowledge and/or language functioning
7 recast	_____	simplified, ungrammatical models of speech/language
8 distancing prompt	_____	pause to prompt the child to complete a well-known phrase
9 isolation	_____	repeat what the child says but with extra information
10 imitation	_____	repeat what the child says but correctly
11 auditory bombardment	_____	child and SLP shift gaze between play materials and each other's faces
12 dialogic reading	_____	running commentary about what the child is doing
13 ear training techniques	_____	used in the context of structured play activities to strengthen acoustic-phonetic representations of words
14 joint attention	_____	direct request to retell parts of the story
15 motherese	_____	a response that is used when the child has produced the target correctly
16 identification	_____	label, demonstrate, and describe the target phoneme
17 PEER	_____	present many good exemplars of the target phoneme, with amplification
18 parallel talk	_____	help the child develop an internalized auditory model of the phoneme
19 recall prompts	_____	SLP presents a variety of speech sounds in different contexts and the child signals when the target sound is produced

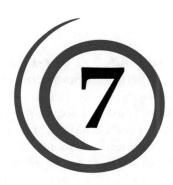

Output-Oriented Approaches

Learning Objectives

- Describe the primary goal of output-oriented approaches to phonology intervention.
- Identify the characteristics of children who are most likely to benefit from vocal play as a therapeutic procedure.
- List and describe six techniques for encouraging vocal play in young children.
- Describe the characteristics of children who will benefit from a sensorimotor approach to intervention.
- Provide a rationale for practicing nonsense syllable drills as implemented in the context of the sensorimotor approach.
- Define the "challenge point."

- Identify strategies for altering practice components to maintain practice at the optimum challenge point when the child's performance is too high versus too low.
- Distinguish "knowledge of performance" and "knowledge of results" feedback.
- Describe the characteristics of children who will benefit from traditional articulation therapy.
- Describe five types of procedures for establishing correct articulation of a new phoneme.
- List the steps in a traditional articulation therapy program as recommended by Van Riper.
- List 13 strategies for promoting transfer and maintenance of learning.

In the previous chapter, input-oriented procedures were described, which have the primary goal of strengthening children's acoustic-phonetic representations for words. These procedures facilitate speech accuracy by providing the child with clear targets for speech production. Although most children with a speech sound disorder (SSD) will benefit from an input-oriented intervention procedure, those interventions are not usually sufficient by themselves. Children, whether exhibiting a normal or a slow trajectory of phonological development, require years of practice to achieve adultlike speech accuracy and precision. In this chapter, procedures that target knowledge of **articulatory-phonetic representations** will be described.

7.1 RATIONALE FOR THE OUTPUT-ORIENTED APPROACH

Output-oriented procedures date back to the origins of the profession of speech-language pathology, reflecting the traditional view that speech errors have an articulatory basis (e.g., Morley, 1957). As discussed in Chapter 4, a child might have a disorder affecting the muscles so that precise control of the articulators is impossible, as in the case of dysarthria. A child might have difficulty with voluntary control of the multiple articulator movements required to produce specific speech sounds or reliably sequence those speech sounds, as in childhood apraxia of speech (CAS). A child might have mislearned the articulatory gestures associated with a particular phoneme, as in the case of persistent speech errors. Or a child might have structural anomalies that make it difficult to produce certain speech sounds without distortion. In all of these cases, an intervention approach that focuses on the learning of articulatory gestures will be required.

The treatment procedures in this chapter are organized to reflect key challenges as they emerge over the course of normal speech development. During the earliest stage of speech production development, the infant must explore the vocal system to expand the vowel space and discover the full range of resonance, phonation, and articulatory possibilities. Subsequently the infant must gain voluntary control of the vocal system to produce reduplicated and variegated strings of syllables in babble and first words. During the preschool period the child must add more complex speech sounds and syllable shapes and increase accuracy of production. Over the late school-age period the child must increase precision even while coping with changing articulatory structure and advanced linguistic complexity. The child with an SSD may need the assistance of an SLP to meet one or more of these challenges.

Over the years a great many approaches to remediation of speech errors have been described that in some cases include unique procedures and in others are made up of overlapping bundles of conventional procedures. A comprehensive review of many of these approaches is provided by Gordon-Brannan and Weiss (2006) and will not be repeated here. Rather, the focus will be on specific evidence-based procedures, organized by child needs at certain developmental junctions. These procedures can be combined concurrently or sequentially to create an individualized approach to meet the unique needs of each child with an SSD.

7.2 VOCAL PLAY

The SLP may be called on to treat children at the earliest stages of speech development. Children who have SSDs secondary to conditions that can be identified at birth may demonstrate marked delays in speech development at a very early age. Most commonly these secondary speech and language delays will be associated with craniofacial anomalies, genetic syndromes that involve multiple developmental delays, hearing impairment, or very low birth weight. Children with primary speech delay may also have markedly restricted repertoires of speech sounds, perhaps producing only [ə] or [ɡə] when vocalizing, even at ages as late as 3 or 4 years. Children with severe delays may also be unable to imitate new speech sounds, either due to their young age or secondary to cognitive delays or because of a deficit in speech motor control. The most *inappropriate* course of action would be to wait for the child to mature, delaying intervention until the child achieves readiness for a treatment program that relies on imitation procedures to teach new speech sounds. Rather, the goal of the speech therapy program should be to increase the child's repertoire of vocal behaviors. A number of techniques can be employed to encourage the toddler or child to engage in vocal play.

The SLP should plan child-directed play activities that encourage the child to freely explore the possibilities of the vocal system. The SLP should help the child to experience the full range of sensory and social effects that occur when different vocalizations are produced. In this case, the SLP should have a range of experiences in mind, but specific targets are not systematically provided or reinforced. The SLP must create a safe and positive environment for this exploration to occur because the child may have experienced disappointment or discouragement in the past if attempts to produce a particular word failed or screeching noises

were deemed to be socially unacceptable. At this stage of the therapy program, all vocalizations and especially a variety of vocalizations must be encouraged and celebrated.

Dethorne, Johnson, Walder, and Mahurin-Smith (2009) reviewed evidence for six techniques to encourage vocal play in young children who are not readily imitating speech sounds, specifically: (1) provide access to augmentative or alternative communication; (2) minimize pressure to speak; (3) imitate the child; (4) use an infant-directed speaking register (exaggerated pitch contours and slowed rate); (5) augment sensory and social feedback; and (6) avoid emphasis on nonspeech articulator movements. These techniques will be discussed briefly in turn.

When the child has a very limited vocal repertoire it is essential to introduce another means of communication. **Augmentative and alternative communication (AAC)** systems vary widely and include informal manual gestures, formal sign languages, picture boards, and digital devices. Issues related to the choice and implementation of AAC systems with these young children are beyond the scope of this book, and the reader is urged to consider other sources (Beukelman & Mirenda, 2013; Johnston, Reichle, & Evans, 2004; Lund, Quach, Weissling, McKelvey, & Dietz, 2017). However, it is clear that parallel introduction of an AAC system will complement and facilitate the emergence of spoken language (Romski et al., 2010).

Furthermore, while encouraging vocal play, it is essential to **minimize pressure to speak** as a means of communication. Parents, teachers, and other individuals who interact with the child must be counseled to accept all the means of communication that the child is using. It is essential to not expect or demand communicative use of vocal communication. The purpose of this phase of the intervention is to help the child freely explore the vocal system. No one should insist that the child try to control the vocal system for intentional communication just yet.

During the vocal play session, an important technique will be to imitate the child. Initially the child may be silent while playing with the toys provided. The SLP must play with the child, enthusiastically imitating the actions that the child uses while playing. Wait patiently for the child to produce any vocal noise and then imitate it immediately, whatever it is. Single subject research has shown that this technique results in significant increases in vocalizations and the number of different phonemes produced by nonverbal toddlers (Gill, Mehta, Fredenburg, & Bartlett, 2011).

When talking during the speech therapy session, an infant-directed speaking style will capture the child's attention: this means talking slowly with exaggerated pitch and loudness changes. This style should be used when talking to the child, modeling speech, or imitating the child's vocalizations. Talking should be playful and integrated with the toy play. Always follow the child's lead. For example, if the child pushes the snowplow and makes a small grunting noise, the SLP can imitate the grunt but vary the length, producing short and long grunts to match short and long pushes. Over time, the grunt might be expanded to include highly variable ambulance sirens, low-pitch truck horns, and high-pitch train whistles. Begin with sounds that are in the child's repertoire and encourage small variations in duration, resonance, voice quality, airflow, and places of closure in the vocal tract.

Practice 7–1

Recall that during the expansion stage of early vocal development, the infant explores many parameters of speech production, such as ingressive versus egressive air flow, oral versus nasal resonance, loud versus quiet sound production, high- versus low-pitch changes, open versus closed vocal tract, full versus partial closure, round versus spread lip gestures, and lip versus tongue movements. In pairs, pick a parameter and design a play routine that might encourage vocal productions that encourage vocal play with that parameter.

The fifth technique is to enhance sensory feedback, that is, find ways to help the child notice the sensory consequences of speech motor movements. Natural opportunities for sensory stimulation commonly occur in vocal play routines. For example, toddlers and parents often make "raspberry" sounds or prolonged "wawawa" vocalizations during face washing. Babies produce many sounds with hands or objects in their mouths. When playing with older children, the SLP's or caregiver's hands can be shaped into different kinds of wind instruments to create a pretend marching band. These kinds of prolonged or repeated sounds are important because they help the child to pair internal touch and movement feedback with the auditory consequences of speech sound articulation. With imagination, prolonged sound making can be encouraged in many pretend play routines.

The sixth technique is to avoid practicing nonspeech articulatory movements. Although vocal play is not focused on the meaningful use of speech, the vocalizations nonetheless occur in a functional context. Vocal play specifically involves learning the relationships between motor movements and their acoustic and sensory consequences. Movements are not practiced without sound. Sounds are not practiced in isolation from the playful context.

Box 7–1. Vocal Play: Key Points

- The vocal play procedure helps the child discover the links between articulatory movements and the associated sensory consequences.
- Vocal play should be implemented with a child who has a very limited repertoire of vocalizations and/or limited imitation abilities.
- An augmentative or alternative communication system must be provided during this period so that the child is under no pressure to use speech for communication.
- The SLP provides an unstructured free play environment and imitates the child's actions and vocalizations while encouraging expansion to a broader variety of vocalizations.

7.3 FUNDAMENTALS OF THE SENSORIMOTOR APPROACH

Recall from Chapter 2 that an important milestone in speech development is the emergence of babble—the production of repeated syllables, either reduplicated or variegated. Babbling provides the infant with a store of motor plans for basic syllables that later act as templates for the selection and production of early words. Some children with SSDs do not achieve babbling at the expected age—especially those who lack reliable access to sensory feedback, such as infants who are hearing impaired or infants with CAS. For these children, a sensorimotor treatment approach focuses on nonsense syllable drills with the goal of enhancing the child's awareness of sensory feedback associated with the production of the syllables: auditory sensations as the sound is transmitted through the air, tactile sensations as articulators come into contact with each other, movement sensations in the joints and muscles as the syllable is produced. The goal of heightening sensory awareness is shared with vocal play therapy techniques. However, there is an important difference at this stage of therapy and that is that the SLP and the child have a specific speech goal during each vocal production. On each practice trial the SLP will present an audiovisual model of a syllable or string of syllables for repetition and the child will attempt to reproduce those syllables. The child should initially be encouraged to monitor the sensory feedback and use that information to achieve the targeted movement goal. Subsequently, with high-intensity practice the child will acquire well-tuned motor plans for a repertoire of basic syllables that can be used to form words. One specific sensorimotor speech therapy program will be outlined here and some others that involve practice with nonsense syllables will be mentioned. Subsequently, in this section, the principles of motor learning will be discussed as a guide to the therapeutic techniques that should be employed while helping children acquire motor plans for the production of a basic repertoire of syllables.

7.3.1 Nonsense Syllable Drills

An important feature of sensorimotor approaches to speech therapy is the focus on nonsense syllable drills. There are three aspects of these drills that must be carefully explained to parents or other caregivers and communication disorders assistants so that they understand the nature of the program when they are helping to implement it. First, there is no practice of isolated phonemes (excepting vowels which can form a syllable by themselves). There is one program for the treatment of CAS that does include practice with some consonants in isolation (Nuffield Centre Dyspraxia Programme; Williams, 2009; Williams & Stephens, 2010). Typically, this is not advised, however, because it is known that children with motor speech disorders and especially CAS have difficulty with co-articulation of adjacent segments within syllables. Furthermore, most theories of linguistic organization suggest that there is a mental store of syllable-sized motor plans for speech production (Levelt, Roelofs, & Meyer, 1999).

The second unique aspect of these drills is that the syllables that are practiced are not meaningful; that is, they are nonsense syllables. Nonsense syllable drills are very common in the treatment of CAS because it is believed that they focus attention on the motor planning task that is the target of the intervention. Furthermore, nonsense syllable practice should reduce the cognitive load and avoid interference from misarticulated real words. For example, if the child has been pronouncing "Mummy" /mʌmi/ → [mʌji], it may be difficult to prevent this misarticulation during speech practice; it is better to practice [mimi], [mimʌ], [maʊmi] until the syllable [mi] has achieved **automaticity** in

a variety of contexts before introducing practice on the real word "Mummy." The ability to practice a core set of syllables automatically—that is, correctly without undue effort and conscious attention—is the goal of this intervention. The use of nonsense word stimuli in speech therapy for children has a long history and there is some research evidence for good generalization to real words (Gierut, Morrisette, & Ziemer, 2010; Sacks, Flipsen, & Neils-Strunjas, 2013; Strand & Skinder, 1999).

A final advantage of nonsense syllable material is that the practice syllables can be constructed specifically for each individual child. The nonsense syllables will usually be composed of segments that the child knows how to say unless the child has an extremely limited repertoire. It is expected that the child should be able to imitate each modeled utterance completely correctly. This means that the therapy sessions will not have the purpose of teaching the child to produce new sounds and family members may be puzzled by this aspect of the intervention. Consider the example posed above: if the child can say "Mummy" /mʌmi/ → [mʌji] approximately correct but cannot say his own name at all, "Sam" /sæm/ → [dʌ], the family may think that it is wiser to teach a new sound, /s/, than to practice a phoneme that is in the child's repertoire. Therefore, it will be necessary to explain that the goal of the intervention is to help the child achieve automatic and precise control of movement patterns rather than to produce new speech sounds specifically. In fact, a related feature of a sensorimotor intervention is that complexity is added to the speech practice material very gradually and the child is expected to achieve a high level of accuracy at each step of the program before passing to the next step. The nonsense syllables are also selected and ordered to balance repetition with variability so that the child achieves **dynamic stability**: this means that the child can produce the syllables in diverse phonetic contexts, in response to different environmental stimuli and for varied pragmatic goals.

A sequence of nonsense syllable drills that is very appropriate for young children with CAS was first recommended by Ling (1976) for children with severe hearing impairment. The sequence of practice targets is shown in Table 7–1. This program begins with the production and sequencing of vowels for those children with the most restricted phonetic repertoires. Next, a variety of CV syllables involving labial

consonants are mastered before introducing VCV and CVCV disyllables (that is, two syllable combinations). Although the VCV form is introduced before the CVCV form, many children find the VCV form to be more difficult because it is hard for them to combine an open syllable (V) with a closed syllable (CV). Notice that reduplicated forms (such as [bibi]) are practiced before variegated syllables (such as [bobi] or [baibu]). The most complex practice materials vary the consonant and the vowel within each item, as in [waʊfi]. The program ends with three syllable strings in which the stress pattern is systematically manipulated. The labial consonants are a good starting point because these targets provide visual feedback as well as

Table 7–1. *Modified Sequence of Practice Targets Adapted from Ling (1976)*

Level 1	**Corner vowels and vowel sequences (diphthongs)**
a.	V: [i], [u], [æ], [ɑ]
b.	Vv: [ei], [ou], [ɑi], [au], [oi]
Level 2	**Labial consonants in increasingly complex syllable sequences**
a.	CV, CVv: C = [w], [m], [b], [f], e.g., [wi], [wu], [wæ], [wɑ] . . .
b.	CVCV, CVvCVv: e.g., [bibi], [bubu], [baibai], [baubau] . . .
c.	V(v)CV(v): e.g., [awa], [iwi], [ouwou], [eiwei] . . .
d.	CV(v)$_1$CV(v)$_2$: e.g., [mimu], [mami], [mumai], [moimau] . . .
e.	C$_1$V(v)$_1$C$_2$V(v)$_2$: e.g., [fimu], [woubi], [bafai], [mæwau] . . .
f.	C$_1$V(v)$_1$C$_2$V(v)$_2$: vary intensity, pitch, stress patterns
Level 3	**Coronal consonants in increasingly complex syllable sequences**
a-e.	Repeat sequence of syllables as for Level 2 but C = [j], [n], [d], [s], and [l]

Note. Ling (1976) includes additional levels for remaining places of articulation and, finally, voicing contrasts; usually the child has attained sufficient control and a large enough repertoire of phones and syllable shapes in spontaneous speech at this point that the SLP can proceed to a sensorimotor approach that includes more complex syllable types or to a phonological approach after Level 3.

other sensory information. The sequence of practice items has a semi-random, semi-blocked practice schedule. Randomness is inherent in the number of consonants that are practiced, so that the target is changing from trial to trial; however, all the labial consonant targets are practiced in the first block (that is, Level 1). After the items composed of labial consonants are mastered, the program is repeated with a set of consonants produced with the tongue tip or blade. These coronal consonants also contrast the range of manner classes found in English. There are other levels in Ling's program, but after the labial and coronal levels are complete, the child will likely be ready to progress to more complex syllable structures. In some cases it may even be appropriate to switch to one of the phonological approaches described in Chapter 8 to ensure generalization to meaningful speech and maintenance in longer or linguistically complex utterances.

Although the treatment procedure recommended by Ling (1976) was first suggested many decades ago, the theoretical concepts that motivated the approach remain current, with a focus on the importance of feedforward and feedback control on the acquisition of speech motor control (for further discussion, see descriptions of the DIVA model [Directions Into Velocities of Articulators] and its application to speech therapy in Rvachew & Brosseau-Lapré, 2018). More recent approaches continue to use these same techniques with some modifications. For example, the Rapid Syllable Transition Treatment (ReST) is based on a similar procedure and has been shown to be effective in a randomized controlled trial (Murray,

McCabe, & Ballard, 2015; see also http://sydney.edu.au/health-sciences/rest/). Children are taught to produce three-syllable nonsense words with systematic variations in stress patterns while maintaining accurate consonant and vowel production and smooth transitions between syllables. The nonsense words are made up of four consonants, three long vowels, and schwa. The consonants and vowels are selected individually for each child by the SLP. The consonants are selected to be stimulable and different from each other—representing multiple manner classes and both voicing categories. In many respects the program is very similar to the teaching sequence recommended by Ling except that it starts at a higher level of difficulty.

Another program that employs nonsense syllable drills is the McDonald sensorimotor approach (for details of the teaching sequence, see Rvachew & Brosseau-Lapré, 2018). Similar to the ReST program, the SLP chooses the consonant and vowel content of the nonsense syllables individually for each child, selecting any consonants that the child produces correctly at least 50% of the time (that is, at the level of customary production). The nonsense syllable drills begin with disyllables, progress to three-syllable strings, and conclude with abutting consonant sequences (such as CVCCVC). As with all the sensorimotor approaches, there is an emphasis on systematic variation of consonants and vowels as well as stress patterns within items. Shine (1989) describes the complete approach in detail, which eventually incorporates teaching new phonemes that are not in the child's repertoire.

Practice 7–2

Imagine that you have decided to implement a sensorimotor approach with a 30-month-old boy, using the teaching sequence shown in Table 7–1. The child's complete productive vocabulary consists of "Mummy" /mʌmi/ → [mʌji] , [mʌ]; "Daddy" /dædi/ → [dʌji], [dʌ], [dʌdi]; "Sam" /sæm/ → [dʌ]; "Fred" /fɹɛd/ → [fː], [fəf]; "cookie" /kʊki/ → [dədə], [gəgə]; "milk" /mɪlk/ → [mʌ], [gʌ]; and "ball" /bɑl/ → [bʌ] (with within-word variability as shown). Sam has good nonverbal imitation skills but has difficulty with accurate verbal imitation. Write a script to explain to Sam's parents your choice of treatment approach. Enact a role play with a partner: taking turns with the parent and SLP roles, describe the treatment and explain the rationale.

7.3.2 Sensorimotor Therapy Procedures

It is assumed that at least some aspects of speech acquisition are similar to the learning of any other motor task, be it learning to tie shoelaces or ride a bike or play hockey. Given this assumption, the principles of motor learning should apply equally to all these contexts. Motor learning has been studied most often in artificial laboratory tasks (Wulf, Schmidt, & Deubel, 1993) or in sports (Guadagnoli, Holcomb, & Davis, 2002). Increasingly, the principles of motor learning are being applied to the acquisition of speech motor control (for a review of the principles and associated research, see Maas et al., 2008).

These principles will be outlined here within the context of the **challenge point framework**, which is based on the idea that the learner must receive just the right amount of information while practicing in order to learn a new skill (Guadagnoli & Lee, 2004).

An important concept in motor learning is the distinction between practice performance and learning. **Practice performance** is measured as the percentage of correct practice trials during a therapy or practice session. **Learning** is measured as (1) generalization to untrained speech material, and (2) maintenance of the new skill over a period of time, especially if practice or therapy has been discontinued. For example, the child might practice the syllables [fifi], [fufu], [fʌfʌ], and [fefe] in therapy on Monday, Wednesday, and Friday, achieving 95% correct performance on practice trials. During the weekend, the child's mother observes that the child continues to say "Fred" /fɹɛd/ → [wəf], "face" /fes/ → [səs], "fork" /fɔɹk/ → [gəg], and "feet" /fit/ → [də]. This means that the child has not yet learned the /f/ phoneme in the onset position: even though practice performance is high, generalization to meaningful speech in the home environment has not occurred. Another child achieves 100% correct practice performance for nonsense words like [ˈsæmˌkɪʃ] in therapy, and her father reports that she has started to pronounce "popcorn," "peacock," and "copycat" correctly. After the break for the winter holiday, the child is again saying [pɑptɔɹn], [pitɑt], and [tɑpitæt]. This return to [t] for /k/ substitutions in natural speaking situations shows that the child has not yet learned the /k/ phoneme: although practice performance is high, the child cannot maintain performance with real words, even during short breaks from therapy.

Differentiating between practice performance and learning is important because the conditions of practice that result in the best practice performance may not optimize learning. The principles of motor learning must be adjusted for each learner in real time to ensure that the learner is practicing at the challenge point—that is, receiving the appropriate amount of information to facilitate learning from practice. If the task is too easy or the SLP is providing too much support, the child will not be receiving useful information during practice to support learning. If the task is too hard or the SLP provides insufficient support, the child will not be able to process the information well enough to support learning. There are no general rules that will work for every child or even for any child at all phases of the learning process. The SLP must be alert to the child's performance and information needs and flexible in the application of the principles of motor learning at all times. Table 7–2 presents strategies for modifying the conditions of practice to help the child obtain optimum practice performance and maintain performance at the challenge point even as target complexity is gradually increasing.

The first step in determining the child's practice and information needs is to begin each session with a prepractice or warm-up period. The pace of intervention during prepractice will be slow. The purpose of this part of the therapy session is to identify the session targets for the child and determine the support that the child will require to achieve success. Some planned targets may even be altered or discarded if the child is not able to achieve the intended goals even with plenty of instruction. The identification procedures are the same as those described in Chapter 6 except the targets

will be syllables or syllable sequences instead of individual phonemes. Again, the auditory, articulatory, visual, and sensory characteristics of the targets should be modeled and described. If, for example, you are introducing Level 2b of the sequence shown in Table 7–1, you will want to be sure that the child can identify productions that involve "closed lips" compared with "round lips," and "one part" compared with "two parts." Auditory bombardment is also valuable in the prepractice session to ensure that the child has good knowledge of the targets. If the child understands the necessary concepts, error detection and self-monitoring tasks may also be included during prepractice. Sometimes the child's performance levels will not be consistent within steps of the Ling teaching sequence: for example, the child might be capable of producing reduplicated disyllables involving [m,b,w] but not [f]; in this case the SLP can decide to practice only monosyllabic items with [f] (i.e., single syllables such as [fi], [fu]) while continuing with the other disyllabic items (i.e., two-syllable items such as [bibi], [mumu]). Notice, however, that the random practice schedule is maintained: the SLP should not decide to switch to a blocked practice schedule in which only [f] items are practiced and the other labial targets are omitted from practice. The context for the session's practice activities can be determined by observing the child's performance during prepractice as well. If the child struggles to achieve the session goals, the practice activity should be a very simple drill-based activity without many distractions. However, the child might have practiced hard at home during the week and achieved a high degree of automaticity; in this case a more complex practice context that challenges the child to maintain accuracy while attending to

Table 7–2. *Strategies for Modifying the Conditions of Practice to Obtain Performance at the Challenge Point*

Practice Performance Is Too High	Practice Performance Is Too Low
Practice component: Intensity	
Increase treatment intensity to induce fatigue, i.e., increase dose or session duration.	Reduce treatment intensity to alleviate fatigue, i.e., reduce dose, shorten session, or take a break.
Practice component: Nominal task difficulty	
Increase task complexity, e.g., stops → fricatives; monosyllables → disyllables; disyllables → trisyllables; trochaic → iambic; singletons → clusters.	Decrease task complexity, e.g., fricatives → stops; disyllables → monosyllables; trisyllables → disyllables; iambic → trochaic; clusters → singletons.
Practice component: Complexity of context	
Increase context complexity, e.g., embed nonsense syllables in a functionally meaningful context and activity; or, practice the syllables in the context of a competing task (cutting out pictures, playing hopscotch, etc.).	Decrease context complexity, e.g., decrease all distractions in the environment; or reduce task to a simple stimulus-response-feedback routine; and ensure that feedback is simple and fast and does not distract from the task.
Practice component: Practice schedule and variability	
Increase variability of stimulus items from trial to trial (variable practice), e.g., ['fifi], ['bubu], [ba'ba], ['maemae], [wa'wa] . . .	Increase predictability of items from trial to trial (constant practice), e.g., ['bibi], ['bubu], ['baba] . . . ['mimi], ['mumu], ['mama] . . .
Practice component: Stimulus presentation	
Move down the integral stimulation hierarchy (see Table 7–3).	Move up the integral stimulation hierarchy (see Table 7–3).
Cue access to internalized representation of the target, obtaining spontaneous productions of the target form.	Provide a model of the target form with maximum multimodal information about its characteristics.
Practice component: Knowledge of performance	
Intermittently ask child for explicit evaluation of own performance.	Frequently provide explicit information about movement parameters during or after correct and incorrect responses.
Practice component: Knowledge of results	
Provide summative information about response accuracy after sets of responses.	Provide information about response accuracy immediately on each trial.

a secondary task would be advisable. Finally, the child's overall state should be observed and taken into account when planning the intensity of the practice portion of the treatment session.

Typically the **practice** part of the session should involve high-intensity practice, which means at least 50 and preferably 100 practice trials (Murray, McCabe, & Ballard, 2014; Williams, 2012). An efficient and focused SLP can lead a child through those practice trials in 10 to 20 minutes. It is best if the child completes many short sessions of intense practice (**distributed practice**) rather than attempting to cram a week's worth of practice trials into one long speech therapy session (**massed practice**). Furthermore, children with CAS require more frequent treatment sessions to obtain a measurable functional outcome (Campbell, 1999; Namasivayam et al., 2015). Therefore, it will be necessary to engage family members and school personnel in order to increase the number of practice sessions each week. Two to three sessions weekly with a professional, augmented by at least daily practice at home, are advisable for children with severe speech disorders.

Variability of practice can be modified in response to the child's practice performance. If the child is struggling to maintain accuracy, **constant practice** with repetition of items will help the child achieve fluid accuracy for each individual item; subsequently, **variable practice** should be introduced as soon as possible. It is convenient to work in five-trial blocks because it is easy to count groups of trials with your fingers. Returning to the example of practicing at Level 2b of the sequence shown in Table 7–1, the child might achieve four or five correct responses out of five attempts when imitating [bibi], [bubu], [boʊboʊ], [baibai],

[baʊbaʊ], as well as [mimi], [mumu], [moʊmoʊ], [maimai], [maʊmaʊ]. Therefore, it would be appropriate to switch from constant to variable practice by interleaving these items: [bibi], [mumu], [baibai], [baʊbaʊ], [moʊmoʊ]. On the other hand, the child would be performing well below challenge point if only one of the following items was imitated correctly: [fifi], [fufu], [foʊfoʊ], [faifai], [faʊfaʊ]. In this situation it would be necessary to practice each individual item with repetition: [fifi], [fifi], [fifi], [fifi], [fifi].

When the child is performing below challenge point (that is, less than four out of five correct responses) there are other adjustments that the SLP can make. Task difficulty can be reduced so that, for example, the child is returned to monosyllabic items as previously mentioned: [fi], [fu], [foʊ], [fai], [faʊ]. This is not the preferred option, however, because it is likely that the child's performance will return to a level of performance that is above challenge point. A better option is to provide more support to the child when stimulating the disyllabic models. The level of support that is provided when stimulating the child to produce the target item can be varied along the **integral stimulation hierarchy**. The integral stimulation hierarchy is an ordered series of prompts that the SLP can choose from in order to stimulate a response from the child (Gildersleeve-Neumann, 2007; Strand & Debertine, 2000). The purpose of the prompt is to define the target that the child is expected to achieve, either by providing a model for imitation or by prompting the child to access her/his own internal representation of the target. The prompt may also help the child select or construct a motor plan for achieving the target. As the child's performance improves, the SLP should provide less support by selecting prompts that are lower on the hierarchy. The integral stimulation hierarchy is shown in Table 7–3.

What should the SLP do if the child cannot achieve success during coproduction or while imitating the practice stimuli (that is, at Levels 1 or 2 of the integral stimulation hierarchy)? Theoretically this problem should not arise if the intervention is implemented according to the appropriate sequence: first, employ the vocal play procedure to ensure that the child has a detailed internal model of the full range of sensory and social effects that occur when different vocalizations are produced; second, practice speech movements in a slow progression from vowels through CV syllables and so on with small advances in complexity. However, specific difficulties may arise such as an inability to produce the complex articulatory gesture required for [f] or the uncommon combination of gestures required for the diphthong [oi]. Some popular approaches to the treatment of CAS include tactile and/or gestural prompts at the highest level of the integral stimulation hierarchy. Therefore, if the child is unable to produce the practice material, the SLP might prompt the child to produce the sequence of sounds by guiding the articulators and providing sensory information about targets

Table 7–3. *Integral Stimulation Hierarchy with Examples for Nonsense Syllable Stimulus*

Level	Prompts	Example
1	Imitative prompt Coproduction	SLP: Watch me and listen. Let's say [fufu]. SLP & Child together: [fufu].
2	Imitative prompt Mimed prompt	SLP: Watch me and listen. Let's say [fufu]. SLP: Mimes [fufu] while child says [fufu].
3	Imitative prompt Repetition prompt (with or without delay)	SLP: Watch me and listen. When I raise my finger, say [fufu]. (Raises one finger, immediately or with one- to three-second delay) Child: [fufu] SLP: (raises next finger) Child: [fufu] SLP: (raises next finger) Child: [fufu]
4	Graphic cue Coproduction	SLP: This is Little Rabbit [fufu]. When the rabbit hops, we're going to say the rabbit's name together, ready? Little Rabbit . . . SLP & Child together: [fufu]
5	Graphic cue (or other cue for spontaneous production such as printed text or a question)	SLP: Look at this picture. Who is this? It's Little Rabbit . . . Child: [fufu]

for articulatory movements. Usually this kind of prompting and feedback is provided via the SLP's own hands, placed on the child's face to stabilize the jaw and shape movements of the lips. PROMPT is a program that relies extensively on this kind of cueing (Dale & Hayden, 2013). Dynamic Temporal and Tactile Cueing (Strand & Skinder, 1999) incorporates tactile and gestural cueing as needed. These approaches require extensive training in the use of the prompts for effective application. It is essential when using these types of prompts and cues to fade their use as quickly as possible so that the child does not become dependent upon this kind of external information to select and implement motor plans. Furthermore, it is important when implementing tactile cueing to be aware that the sensory cues provided by the SLP might interfere with the child's efforts to process self-produced sensory feedback while speaking.

After the child attempts each stimulus item, internal and external feedback serve to strengthen the child's motor plan and contribute to learning. The type of feedback, timing of feedback, and schedule of feedback all play a role in facilitating learning. During the prepractice portion of the session, **knowledge of performance feedback** should be provided. This kind of feedback provides information about the quality of the articulatory movements and is best obtained via the child's own senses. The simplest kind of knowledge of performance feedback is obtained by children monitoring their own movements in the mirror and listening to their own speech while producing the target items. Children's awareness of articulatory movements may be enhanced by introducing cold ice or objects, sweet or spicy foods, or vibration into the oral cavity just before an articulatory attempt. Although these techniques are not sup-

ported by high-level research evidence, there are some case studies suggesting that they may be effective in certain cases (e.g., see use of electric toothbrush for oral stimulation in Lundeborg & McAllister, 2007). Furthermore, it has been demonstrated that some children with SSDs have reduced access to sensory feedback (Fucci, 1972; Fucci, Petrosino, Underwood, & Kendal, 1992; Hetrick & Sommers, 1988; McNutt, 1977; Sommers, Cox, & West, 1972). Access to feedback about articulatory performance may also be provided by real-time electropalatography or ultrasound technology. Finally, the SLP may enhance the child's awareness of performance feedback by commenting on the child's movements after the articulatory attempt has been completed: for example, "You rounded your lips when you said 'wa.' Good job!" or "Remember to make your lips round." This kind of verbal comment is in some respects more about the result of the movement than the performance of the movement but may remind the child to focus on certain aspects of the required articulatory gesture when attempting it on the next practice trial. All of these forms of external knowledge of performance feedback should be restricted to the prepractice portion of the treatment session as much as possible. This kind of feedback may help the child to successfully acquire a new movement pattern. Excessive focus of attention on the movement goal during practice may hinder the child's acquisition of automaticity and dynamic stability.

During high-intensity practice, the focus should be on **knowledge of results**: did the child produce an accurate or at least acceptable sounding version of the target? **Direct** knowledge of results feedback can be provided after each trial, informing the child about the correctness of each response. Unless the child is really struggling to achieve correct responses, however, it is best to provide **summative** knowledge of results feedback: this means that the SLP tells the child which of five responses were correct after each group of five trials. Summative feedback gives the child a chance to monitor intrinsic feedback and judge his/her own responses before receiving confirmation from the SLP. Even if providing direct feedback after each trial, the SLP can delay that feedback by one, two, or three seconds so that the child has an opportunity to process intrinsic feedback without interference from the SLP (Strand & Skinder, 1999). Overall, learning is optimized when the child can practice complex targets with a minimum of external feedback.

Velleman and Strand (1994) suggest a lesson plan outline for the implementation of a sensorimotor approach with young children with CAS. Each treatment session has four components: Warm-ups, Practicing the Scales, Practicing the Song, and Changing the Song. The Warm-up portion is the prepractice portion of the session as described above, intended to identify the target and provide the child with all the information required to achieve success in the production of the planned target items. Practicing the Scales is the high-intensity practice portion of the section, involving drill practice or drill-play activities to achieve 50 to 100 attempts to produce the target items. Practicing the Song provides the child with the opportunity to transfer one or more of the skills learned in the practice part of the session to meaningful words. Finally, Changing the Song involves using the new skills in a meaningful context and may foreshadow upcoming targets. A lesson plan is shown in Demonstration 7–1 along with two lines of the accompanying session notes. In this case, the imagined therapy client is "Sam" from the previous section, who has passed successfully through vocal play to begin Level 1 of the Ling program shown in Table 7–1.

Practice 7–3

Working in small groups, pretend that Sam is progressing through the practice sequence shown in Table 7–1. Design a lesson plan as demonstrated in Demonstration 7–1, one plan for each group, at a different level of the practice sequence.

Box 7–2. Sensorimotor Therapy Approach: Key Points

- Sensorimotor therapy helps the child to acquire well-tuned motor plans for a repertoire of basic syllables that can be used to form words.
- Typically, sensorimotor approaches focus on a graded sequence of nonsense syllable targets that are composed of stimulable consonants in increasingly complex syllable contexts.
- During high-intensity practice, the SLP should provide just enough stimulation to obtain a successful practice attempt and the appropriate amount of feedback to maintain practice performance at the challenge point.
- A useful structure for a sensorimotor lesson plan includes four parts: Warm-up (prepractice), Practicing the Scales (nonsense syllable drills), Practicing the Song (real word practice), and Changing the Song (practice in a meaningful context).

Demonstration 7–1

Lesson Plan to Practice Vowels with Hypothetical Toddler

1. Warm-ups (prepractice)

Instructional objective #1: Identify the visual symbol that is associated with each diphthong.

Activity #1: Attach with ticky tack 2 of 5 pictures to large mirror, below face level (e.g., "bandaid," "eye"); sitting side by side in front of mirror, produce the diphthongs [aʊ] and [ɑɪ] one at a time, slowly. Sam is to point to the picture that matches the sound. Discuss the lip movements that go with each diphthong. Discontinue after 7 consecutive responses or 2 minutes.

Instructional objective #2: Child imitates each diphthong correctly 3 times (constant practice schedule) while sitting side by side in front of mirror. Use knowledge of performance feedback. Provide mimed prompt or coproduction if necessary.

2. Practicing the scales (Ling sequence, Level 1b, see Table 7–1)

Instructional objective: Produce the diphthongs [aʊ], [ɑɪ], [eɪ], [oʊ], [oɪ]. Aim for 50 practice trials in groups of 5 trials with variable practice. Adjust integral stimulation hierarchy and schedule of knowledge of results feedback as necessary to maintain practice at challenge point.

Activity: Sam can put animal in barn after each group of 5 trials.

Record Keeping Sheet for Practice Trials (partial example)

Target	Accuracy	ISH	Feedback
aʊ ɑɪ oʊ eɪ oɪ	1̶ 2 3̶ 4 5̶ 2/5	imitation	Summative KR
aʊ ɑɪ oʊ eɪ oɪ	1 2 3 4 5̶ 4/5	coproduction	Summative KR

Demonstration 7–1 continues on next page.

214

3. Practicing the song

Instructional objective: Use the words "ow" and "eye" correctly in a meaningful context.

Activity 1: Hang 5 monkeys on a plastic tree. Sam shakes the tree until the monkeys fall off. Each monkey says… "ow" when it falls off the tree. After Sam says "ow" he can put a miniature bandaid on the monkey.

Activity 2: After Sam says "eye" he can put an "eye" sticker on paper cut-outs of dogs.

4. Changing the song

Instructional objective: Sing "ee ai ee ai oh" and attempt "woof, woof" as part of the song.

Activity: Encourage Sam to sing along to Old MacDonald. Each verse is repeated with "dog". Put a dog cut-out in his homework book with a paper clip to take home for further practice.

SOAP Notes for Session

S: Mum reports that Sam didn't want to practice at home because 'aw' and 'oy' was hard. I focused on diphthongs today and he enjoyed the activities and persisted even with difficult items. O: Sam practiced 60 trials during drill and achieved 80% accuracy at imitative level but struggled with delayed imitation. A: Session end probe: V = 100%, VV = 90% and CV = 50% in direct imitation with most difficulty observed for /f/; therefore, P: assign V and VV items for homework; begin next session by revising Ling 16 VV item and then progress to Level 2a with CV only.

7.4 TRADITIONAL ARTICULATION THERAPY

In the previous section, sensorimotor therapy procedures were directed at stabilizing movement patterns for the production of syllables composed of speech sounds that were in the child's phonetic repertoire. In this section, traditional articulation therapy procedures will be described. These procedures are employed with the goals of introducing new sounds into the child's repertoire and achieving mastery-level production of these new sounds in spontaneous speech. The traditional speech therapy program that is used to teach new speech sounds, developed by Van Riper (1978), is also sensorimotor in character because the focus is on integrating sensory feedback from multiple sources during production of the articulatory gestures to achieve dynamic stability for accurate production of the auditory target. However, this intervention focuses on one speech sound at a time, taking a vertical goal attack strategy. The children who are best suited to this approach have persistent speech errors, typically distortion errors on late developing phonemes such as sibilants or rhotics. Occasionally a child will demonstrate age-appropriate production of all phonemes except /k,g,ŋ/. In any case, there will be a few phonemes that are absent from the child's phonetic repertoire that require remediation. If the child presents with a broad range of error patterns, the phonological treatment procedures that are presented in Chapter 8 will be more appropriate. The steps that are followed in a traditional articulation therapy program are listed in Table 7–4 and will be described in the sections to follow.

Table 7–4. *Steps in Traditional Articulation Therapy*

Ear Training[a]	Identification
	Isolation
	Stimulation
	Error Detection
	Self-Monitoring
Establishment	Stimulability procedures
Stabilization[b]	Syllables: e.g., /sV, /Vs/, /VsV/, /sVC/, /CVs/, /cCVC/, and /CVs/
	Words: prevocalic target postvocalic target
	Phrases, patterned sentences
	Complex words
	Sentences
Transfer and Maintenance	Conversation

[a]Ear training procedures are described in Chapter 6.

[b]Stabilization steps are practiced first with imitative models and then spontaneous productions are elicited, in separate substeps of the program.

7.4.1 Ear Training

A crucial first step in articulation therapy is **ear training** using the four techniques described in Chapter 6 (see Table 6–2). These activities can be conducted during the first session that introduces a new phoneme target. Error detection tasks may be repeated briefly at the beginning of subsequent sessions. The example activities for implementation of these techniques given in Chapter 6 are for younger children, but clients with persistent speech errors may be older school-age children who will require modifications to take into account their interests as well as their higher level of cognitive and linguistic abilities. When working with older children, complex sentence level material can be prepared for misarticulation judgments. Often children with persistent errors will be receiving treatment in groups. The group of children receiving treatment to remediate dental distortion of /s,z/ could jointly prepare and record sentence-level material around a topic of interest, recruiting friends and family members to augment the recordings of misarticulated speech from among their group. Each session could begin with practice identifying the correct and incorrect productions of the target phoneme in the recorded sentences.

Error detection activities, in which the children identify errors in other's speech, should lead into **self-monitoring**, in which the children learn to identify correct and incorrect tokens of the target phoneme in their own speech while they are talking. Self-monitoring activities should begin with single words and proceed to progressively longer utterances. Van Riper (1978) recommended teaching self-monitoring in the second speech therapy session, directly after the ear training session, rather than waiting until the end of treatment when the child is in the maintenance phase. Sometimes the SLP delays self-monitoring until very late in the treatment program, which unnecessarily prolongs the stabilization phase and delays transfer of learning to the extra-clinic setting (Koegel, Koegel, & Ingham, 1986).

7.4.2 Establishment

Traditional articulation therapy is typically applied to **unstimulable** speech sound targets—that is, sounds that the child cannot say correctly, even when provided with an imitative model. When a child is not stimulable for a given speech sound, that child may simply lack the requisite "how-to" knowledge of the appropriate configuration of articulatory gestures; alternatively, the child may have specific underlying problems with the planning, programming, or execution of the requisite movements. In either case there are a variety of strategies that the SLP can bring to the task of helping the child achieve a correct production and then establish consistency in the execution of that production in syllables before proceeding to the sound stabilization phase of articulation therapy. The techniques to be covered here, in order, are: (1) stimulation, (2) contextual facilitation, (3) phonetic placement, (4) successive approximation, and (5) visual feedback. These techniques are defined with examples in Table 7–5. Specific guidance for applying these techniques to establish all the consonants and vowels in English can be found in Secord, Boyce, Donahue, Fox, and Shine (2007).

Stimulation can be applied while seated face-to-face with the child or while seated side-by-side at a large mirror. The child must be able to see the SLP's face without putting the neck in an uncomfortable position. The child must also be seated comfortably with adequate support for trunk and feet. As with the sensorimotor approach, most phonemes are presented for imitation in the context of a syllable, that is, stops, glides, and liquids. Nasals and fricatives can be presented in isolation but should be put in a syllable

Table 7–5. *Techniques to Establish a New Speech Sound*

Definition	Example
Stimulation	
Provide verbal instructions and an audiovisual model for imitation, with knowledge of performance feedback after the child's attempt.	Watch me. I am going to say "aaah" and while I do that I am going to lift my tongue up and down, fast, with a kind of flipping motion. When my tongue flips up and down we'll hear a singing sound. Watch me, and then it will be your turn, here we go: "aaalaaalaaalaaalaaa."
Contextual facilitation	
Practice the target sound in a syllable with another sound that shares similar articulatory gestures.	Watch. When I say [uː], my tongue is back and my lips are round. When I say [ʃː], my tongue is back and my lips are round. When I say [uʃː], my tongue is back and my lips are round, all the way through. Watch me again and then it's your turn, [uʃː].
Phonetic placement	
Physical manipulation of the child's articulators to move them into the correct location and configuration for accurate production of the target sound.	First I'm going to hold your chin here. Then I am going to put this tongue blade into your mouth, just a little bit, to hold down the front of your tongue here. Now I'm holding the front of your tongue down. Lift the back of your tongue and say [kː].
Successive approximation	
Shaping a new articulatory configuration by moving the child from a known articulatory configuration in a series of small steps toward the target sound.	First, say [tʰ]. Good, let's make lots, like this, [tʰ], [tʰ], [tʰ]. Excellent, now really fast [tʰ tʰ tʰ]. Now if we go really really fast it sounds like this [tststststs]. Can you hear the little whistle sound coming in? Let's make it a little longer: [tststsssss].
Visual feedback	
Use technology such as ultrasound or spectrographic feedback to provide information about tongue placement or results of articulation.	Watch, when I say [ʌ], we see three bumps (pointing to formant peaks on the real-time spectrograph), far apart. When I say [ʌɚ], the second bump and the third bump moved close together. Now, you try it. We'll watch your bumps on the app.

context as soon as possible. Stimulation consists of providing the child with an auditory and visual model of the target phoneme. Verbal instructions may also be added as necessary. The child is then asked to imitate the model and knowledge of performance feedback is provided after each attempt. The prompts suggested with respect to the integral stimulation hierarchy shown in Table 7–3 are stimulation techniques. Very often the child will be successful with just a little bit of added verbal instruction and careful attention to the SLP's model. The key to this approach may be to direct the child's attention to the articulatory movements rather than the speech sound target itself. Older children are usually aware that they "cannot say the [target] sound" and might be too discouraged to try. The child might be willing to imitate specific articulatory gestures, however, especially if some new configurations are suggested. Recall the concept of motor equivalence: if past unsuccessful attempts at [s] have involved the "tongue tip up" position, the version with the tongue tip down behind the lower incisors can be tried. Alternative articulatory gestures can be found to achieve or approximate most speech sound targets.

If the child is not successful after a few attempts, **contextual facilitation** techniques may help: this means modeling the target sound in the context of another sound that positions the articulators for producing the target more easily. Often, a facilitating context can be discovered by applying your knowledge of articulatory phonetics. For example, the vowel [u] involves pulling the tongue back somewhat and rounding the lips, articulatory gestures that overlap with [ʃ]; therefore it might help to target the sibilant in the syllable [uʃ] (Stokes & Griffiths, 2010). Con-

textual facilitation is a key procedure in the implementation of the **paired stimuli** technique for establishing new phonemes. With this technique, the child is asked to imitate a word or syllable in which the child can say the target and immediately after a new word or syllable, in rapid succession. This technique is intended to promote generalization of production from the facilitative context to other contexts in which the child misarticulates the phoneme. For example, the child might typically substitute [s] for /ʃ/, except in the word "wash," which is consistently produced /wɑʃ/ → [wɑʃ]. The child's difficulties with this phoneme may be particularly acute in the word onset position. The paired stimuli technique would involve asking the child to say the words, in order, "wash," "she," "wash," "show," "wash," "shy," "wash," "shoe"; it is expected that with repetition of this series, correct production of [ʃ] will emerge in the word onset position. Alternatively, a series of words with [ʃ] in the coda position could be interleaved with "wash" as in "wash," "bush," "wash," "fish," "wash," "mash," "wash," "hash."

The SLP may need to resort to **phonetic placement**, which involves physical manipulation of the child's articulators to move them into the correct location and configuration for accurate production of the target sound. Phonetic placement is usually combined with verbal instruction about articulatory placement. Phonetic placement may also include amplified sensory feedback about the position of the articulators (for example, cinnamon flavor on the alveolar ridge to provide a target for tongue tip placement). A large number of tools and products have been applied in the process, ranging from everyday objects such as pencils (Shriberg, 1980) to dental tools such as flavored sponges (toothettes) to specially created tongue placement devices such as the Speech Buddies (http://www.speechbuddy.com). Regarding the specific techniques that can be used for each speech sound, Secord et al. (2007) is the best resource over and above the guidance of experienced SLPs. Some general rules apply to the application of phonetic placement techniques, however. First, it is essential to consider safety at all times. Never place a choking hazard in a young child's mouth. Always ensure that the child is seated in a stable position, and stabilize the child's chin with one hand while placing any object in the child's oral cavity with the other. Be sure that the child is not allergic to any food items that you might use during phonetic placement (in general, ensure that the child and the parent agree to the placement of any objects or food items in the child's mouth).

Second, phonetic placement should only be used in the context of practicing speech sounds. For example, Table 7–5 suggests holding the front of the tongue down to elicit [k]: importantly, the child is attempting to produce a speech sound during this activity, even though it is a slightly distorted and prolonged version of [k:]. At no time will the SLP hold down the front of the tongue and require the child to practice silent tongue body movements.

Third, the phonetic placement technique should be **faded out** as quickly as possible to encourage independent production of the speech sound. After a few successful attempts with the tongue blade in the mouth, an independent production should be elicited: the SLP might elicit a sequence of [k] sounds, alternating the use of the tongue blade with independent imitative productions. Then a series of

imitated [k] productions can be elicited with the tongue blade close to but not in the child's mouth. Finally, and hopefully after only a few minutes of practice with the tongue blade in sight, it can be dispensed with altogether. The SLP should help the child proceed to syllable-level productions with no specific placement cues as quickly as possible.

Practice 7–4

In pairs, role-play the use of phonetic placement techniques to establish a frequently misarticulated consonant. One student takes the role of the SLP and the other takes the role of the child who is not stimulable for the selected consonant phoneme. The pair must research appropriate phonetic placement techniques seeking published sources and expert advice and obtain all necessary tools. In addition, bilingual students may wish to teach a foreign speech sound to their monolingual peers.

A useful adjunct to phonetic placement may be **successive approximation** or shaping to move the child from a known articulatory configuration to the new configuration in a sequence of small steps. Suggestions for shaping are also provided in Secord et al. (2007). Successful application of shaping procedures requires a careful task analysis, in other words, good knowledge of the articulatory-phonetic characteristics of the target sound and the similar phone that is currently in the child's repertoire. Subsequently, a series of intermediate gestures from the known phone to the new phone can be taught in sequential order. Shaping from [t] to [s] by teaching the child to insert excessive aspiration after the [t] is very common. As another example, Shriberg (1975) provided detailed instructions for moving the child from sustained production of the liquid [l] to vocalic [ɚ]. The original source should be consulted for a complete description of the protocol, but essentially the technique involves gradually moving the retroflex tongue tip back from the [l] position toward the [ɚ] position. Once having obtained a decent-sounding [ɚ] from the child through successive approximation, a related technique called **chaining** can be used to work the phone into syllables and words in varied syllable positions and contexts, for example: (1) prevocalic—[ɚ], [ɚɹɛ], [ɹɛ], [ɹɛd], [ɹid]; (2) postvocalic—[ɚ], [iɚ], [hiɚ], [hɛɚ], [pɛɚ]; and (3) intervocalic—[ɚ], [ɚɹi], [hɚɹi], [hɛɹi], [tʃɛɹi].

Often children with persistent speech errors are relearning a new configuration of articulatory gestures for which they have overlearned a distorted production, and for which the required gestures are invisible. Therefore it is impossible for them to see what is wrong with their own articulatory configuration and how to change it. This problem is particularly acute in the case of [ɹ] because three gestures are required (lip rounding, a bunched or retroflex tongue shape that creates a constriction in the palatal region of the oral cavity, and retraction of the tongue root in the pharynx, as illustrated in Figure 1–4. The pharyngeal constriction cannot be seen and is a movement that is especially hard to teach. Spectrographic feedback provides **visual feedback** about the result of these gestures because when they are implemented correctly the second and third formants will move closer together on the spectrogram

(McAllister Byun, 2017; Shuster, Ruscello, & Toth, 1995). Ultrasound feedback will provide information about the shape and location of the tongue in the oral cavity (Bernhardt, Gick, Bacsfalvi, & Adler-Bock, 2005; Preston et al., 2014). These technologies are often referred to as **biofeedback**, which is intended to bring an unconscious process to overt awareness so that it can be consciously manipulated. Biofeedback is appropriate during the establishment phase because it helps the child become aware of overlearned and maladaptive articulatory gestures in order to establish new articulatory gestures through conscious effort. After the new configuration of articulatory gestures has been established, however, the child will have the opposite goal: now the child must practice the new sound until it can be produced automatically—that is, consistently, effortlessly, without conscious control. Therefore, it is important to fade out the visual feedback as quickly as possible and not carry over biofeedback techniques to the stabilization phase of therapy.

7.4.3 Stabilization of New Phonemes

After the new phoneme is established in isolation or a simple syllable, therapy shifts to the goal of stabilizing production in utterances of increasing length and complexity. A vertical goal attack strategy is used to encourage high-intensity practice of the target in syllables, words, phrases, and sentences, as outlined in Table 7–4. The child is expected to demonstrate automatic production at a high level of accuracy at each level of complexity before the next level is introduced. Within each level of complexity the SLP will usually begin with imitated productions and then proceed to spontaneous productions of the desired target structures. Principles of motor learning should be employed during practice sessions, being sure to maintain performance at the challenge point using the techniques listed in Table 7–2. Compared with the stimulation phase, the SLP will be shifting to less frequent feedback, focusing on knowledge of results rather than performance. Knowledge of performance feedback should not be required on a regular basis, perhaps only for a minute or two in prepractice activities as each new level is introduced.

Notice that the traditional procedure is to systematically work through all possible word positions early in the program. For example, if the target phoneme were /s/: (1) syllables, in order /sV/, /Vs/, /VsV/, /sVC/, /CVs/; (2) words, prevocalic position, such as "soap," "sun"; (3) words, postvocalic position such as "mouse," "lace"; (4) words, intervocalic position such as "racing," "messy"; (5) phrases or patterned sentences such as "I like/don't like sardines/ice cream/salmon/sausage/lettuce/seaweed"; (6) complex words such as "necessary," "possible"; and (7) sentences such as "I bought three bars of soap at the pharmacy today" and "I like to eat ice cream sundaes with chocolate sauce." Some SLPs might even work the cluster contexts into this sequence, including /sCVC/ and /CVCs/ syllables at the first level and introducing s-cluster words just prior to the patterned sentences level. Furthermore, at each level, many different words presenting a broad range of phonetic contexts are practiced. These procedures are consistent with the principle of variable practice and therefore conducive to generalization of learning from the practice context to speaking in the extra-clinic environment.

The practice context at all of the levels shown in Table 7–4 can be drill or drill-play. **Drill practice** involves simple rapid practice of the target behavior with knowledge of results feedback provided at the desired schedule. The reinforcement could be direct one-to-one (after each trial), random (for example, on 20% of trials, randomly selected), or summative (at the end of a block of trials, indicate the total score). Reinforcement might be tangible (real items that the child values such as stickers or treats) or social (such as verbal praise). The reinforcement system must be designed with the child's personality, interests, and skill level taken into account. Elaborate systems for commenting on and rewarding the child's performance slow down the activity and may actually reduce the child's motivation to engage in drill practice. Research indicates that tangible rewards undermine intrinsic motivation to participate in an activity when they are provided simply for engaging in an activity that is already intrinsically rewarding; under these conditions the child perceives the reward system to be controlling and the reward undermines perceived autonomy (Cameron, Pierce, Basko, & Gear, 2005). On the other hand, tangible reinforcers can be motivating when they are provided to reward achievement of a specific goal. When rewards provide information about improved levels of practice performance, the reward system serves to enhance the child's perceived competence. Therefore it is important to design the reinforcement system to provide knowledge of results information, rather than control behavior. A common reinforcement system that is used with drill practice is a **token** economy: tokens are provided for correct responses and the tokens are exchanged for an activity or an object that the child desires. As in computer games, the level of practice performance that is required to earn a token can be increased as the child's skill level improves over the course of the therapy program. The exchange system must be negotiated with the child and possibly the child's family. A portion of a hypothetical drill practice session is shown in the left-hand column of Demonstration 7–2. Notice in this example that the child and the therapist are scoring the child's productions so that self-monitoring is encouraged. Summative knowledge of results feedback is provided after each block of five trials. Knowledge of performance feedback can be provided if necessary and the pair can discuss disagreements about the correctness of each item. The difficulty level of the task and the required performance level to earn tokens can be adjusted in response to the child's practice performance after each activity or session.

A second hypothetical example is shown in the right-hand column of Demonstration 7–2, in this case illustrating the characteristics of drill-play. A **drill-play** activity is designed to elicit a large number of practice trials in a relatively authentic context in which the reinforcement for accurately produced target items is built into the game. In the example shown, the SLP and child are playing battleships. The game has been modified slightly to require both child and adult to produce a full sentence that is loaded with /ɹ/ sounds in order to confirm a hit or a miss. There are plenty of opportunities to produce the target phoneme in casual conversation during the course of the game. Neither tangible rewards for correct articulations nor specific feedback about misarticulations occurs. Rather, naturalistic consequences are built into the game play.

The examples of drill and drill-play activities shown in Demonstration 7–2 each lend themselves to easy assignment of homework. The list of words practiced as a drill activity is meant to be sent home for continued drill practice. If the child achieves a high level of practice during the speech therapy session, task difficulty can be increased for home practice: perhaps the parent could give a clue about each word and the child could supply the answer without reading it (e.g., "a type of bird"—[ɹabɪn]); alternatively, the child could make a sentence with each word (e.g., "a [ɹabɪn] eats worms"). The SLP should try the higher-level task in therapy first, however, to ensure that the child will achieve a high level of success with the assigned activity at home. Furthermore, homework is most valuable when the parent understands both the goal and the structure of the activity. The drill-play activity can also be sent home as additional game cards can be supplied to the family along with printed rules for game play. The parent or other family members who play the game must be able to detect correct and incorrect pronunciations of the "r" sound in the child's speech, however, and this is not always the case. It has been shown that home practice yields the best results when mothers are trained to carry out the home program and when mothers have good auditory discrimination skills (Sommers, 1962). Traditional articulation therapy has been shown to be effective compared with no therapy in randomized control trials (Sommers et al., 1961), but the effectiveness of this approach is correlated with the amount of home practice (Günther & Hautvast, 2010).

Demonstration 7–2

Comparison of Drill and Drill-Play Activities

A. Spontaneous single word /ɹ,ɝ/ drill activity

SLP: I have pasted some "ɹ" words into your homework book. They are listed in rows, I want you to read each row slowly. After each word, you and I will mark whether you said the word correctly, like this: ✓✗

Child: What about the tokens?

SLP: After each row, we'll count the check marks. If you say 4 or 5 words correct you get 5 tokens. If you get less than 4 checkmarks, no tokens. I have to agree with your checkmarks, don't make a check unless you say the word correctly!

Child: OK, then I get my new computer game.

SLP: When you have a 1000 tokens. So far you have 565. Today you could get maybe 80 to 100 more, we'll see, so you're getting there. Start the first line.

B. Spontaneous sentences /ɹ,ɝ/ drill-play activity

SLP: We each take one of these battleship cards. It's a secret, don't show me! Each card has a destroyer, a frigate, and an aircraft carrier marked off. We are going to bomb each other's oceans by calling instructions to the fighter pilots like this: Fire on grid target A3, or whichever space you want. If you say all the "ɹ" sounds correct, I will say "hit" or "miss." If you mispronounce any "ɹ" sounds, I will say "abort, abort" and there will be no bombing, you get that? OK, and you have to listen to me carefully, because I might mispronounce the "ɹ" sounds on my turn. You start.

Child: [fɑɹɚ ɔn ɡɹɪd tɑɝɡɪt B5].

SLP: That's a hit! OK, my turn.

[fɑɹɚ ɔn ɡɹɪd tɑʊʊɡɪt D7].

Listen: [ɡɹɪd tɑʊʊɡɪt D7].

Demonstration 7–2 continues on next page.

A. Spontaneous single word /ɹ,ɝ/ drill activity continued

Child:	[bɛɝ] [ɹɑbɪn] [kwaʊn] [ɹɑɪs] [tʃɛɹi]
	Look, I have four!
SLP:	No, sorry, I have only 3, bear, robin, rice. We both have crown wrong but I don't agree cherry is correct. Try the next one.
	Remember, when you see the letter "r" you have to move your tongue back.
Child:	[stɔɝ] [bɹaʊn] [ʌn] [ɹɑfəl] [pɛɹɪt]
	Now I have four!
SLP:	Totally, you get 5 tokens. You are having a bit of trouble with "r" in the middle. Try those words like parrot a bit slower and remember to bring your tongue back, ok?
Child:	OK, I wanna get five good on the next one.
SLP:	I think you will. Just remember to be extra careful when the "r" is in the middle of the word.

B. Spontaneous sentences /ɹ,ɝ/ drill-play activity continued

Child:	[ʌbɔɝt] [ʌbɔɝt]
SLP:	Abort! No fire. OK, your turn again.
Child:	[fɑɪɝ ɔn gɹɪd tɑɝgɪt B foʊɹ].
SLP:	Abort, abort!
Child:	Oh! I was sure I had a hit.
SLP:	Maybe, but the fighter pilot couldn't understand you. It's my turn now.
	[fɑɪɝ ɔn gɹɪd tɑɝgɪt D7].
Child:	Miss, that's a miss, haha.
	Now, [fɑɪɝ ɔn gɹɪd tɑɝgɪt B foɝ].
SLP:	Another hit.
Child:	Yay, I bet it's a destroyer.
SLP:	[fɑɪɝ ɔn gɹɪd tɑɝgɪt G9].
Child:	G9! You finally got a hit.

7.4.4 Transfer and Maintenance

The final stage of phonological development is characterized by a long period of gradual refinement that is marked by two progressive changes toward adult-like speaking ability: (1) increased consistency with which certain phonemes are produced, resulting in improved accuracy across phonetic contexts and speaking environments, and (2) increased stability in the achievement of speech motor goals, resulting in improved precision. Increased accuracy may occur rapidly or gradually. In some cases, a child will show rapid diffusion of a new phoneme throughout the lexicon followed by relatively sudden mastery of correct production, when the speech therapy program has barely progressed through the syllable level of formal practice (e.g., see Powell & McReynolds, 1969). More often, however, SLPs have reported that achieving transfer of correct production from practice sessions to spontaneous speech in the extraclinic environment is a difficult challenge that is not met for many children with persistent speech errors. Acquiring age-appropriate levels of precision may also be a particular problem for children with SSD: all children must adapt continuously to changing articulatory structure and expectations for increasing linguistic complexity. A child with an SSD might show fluctuating levels of precision in the production of speech sounds while adapting to these challenges. Therefore, it is necessary to design the speech therapy program to promote transfer of learning and follow-up with the child after discharge from formal therapy to ensure that learned skills are maintained over time.

Although Table 7–4 implies that transfer and maintenance occur during a separate phase of the traditional articulation therapy program, it is best to use procedures during the stabilization phase that will facilitate transfer of learning all along. Some strategies to promote generalization, transfer, and maintenance of learning are shown in Table 7–6. **Generalization** of learning is achieved when the child correctly produces the target in words or word positions that were not practiced in the clinic. **Transfer** of learning occurs when the child transfers (or carries over) correct production of the sound from practice sessions to spontaneous speech in the extraclinic environment (in other words, stimulus generalization as defined in Chapter 5). **Maintenance** is observed as sustained accuracy in the production of the target phoneme after formal treatment is discontinued.

Practice 7–5

Discuss with a partner a time when you learned a skill but could not or had difficulty transferring the skill to a new context. How might you have modified your practice to promote transfer? Discuss with a partner a skill that you learned or knowledge that you acquired but subsequently lost. How could you modify your practice to maintain the skill or retain the knowledge longer?

The most important strategy is to ensure that the child has an excellent acoustic-phonetic representation of the target phoneme. Good knowledge of the target will allow the child to generalize that knowledge, first through lexical diffusion (changing the underlying representations of all the words that share the target

Table 7–6. *Tips to Promote Generalization, Transfer, and Maintenance*

1.	Ensure that the child has a good acoustic-phonetic representation for the target.
1a.	Use ear training procedures (see Chapter 6).
1b.	Provide auditory models of the target during the establishment phase.
2.	Use a phonological approach to therapy when appropriate (see Chapter 8).
3.	Apply principles of motor learning during the establishment and stabilization phases.
3a.	Maintain performance level during practice at the "challenge point" (see Table 7–2).
3b.	Do not "overpractice." Practice with variable stimuli at multiple levels in a single session.
3c.	Provide knowledge of performance feedback during a prepractice "warm-up."
3d.	Provide intermittent, summative, or delayed feedback of results during the practice activity.
4.	Plan for stimulus generalization.
4a.	Reduce difference between treatment and natural environment.
4b.	Plan activities that provide naturalistic reinforcement for correct use of target.
4c.	Include family members and school personnel in the treatment program.
5.	Empower the child to take responsibility for carryover.
5a.	Teach the child to self-monitor early in the treatment program (after "ear training").
5b.	Reinforce spontaneous self-corrections when they occur.
5c.	Prescribe brief but regular periods of self-monitoring in the extraclinic environment.

phoneme), then through self-monitoring (using feedback to strengthen the motor plan for the production of words containing that speech sound). Without this internal knowledge, the child is dependent on the SLP to provide feedback about accuracy of production. When the SLP is not present, accuracy will decline. A related strategy is to provide less and less external feedback during practice sessions so that the child learns to rely on self-produced feedback. Ensuring that the child practices in the extraclinic environment is also critical to transfer and maintenance: the child must take responsibility for transferring learning to these other environments. A simple and powerful way to do this is to ask the child to keep a record of correct productions, as produced in narrative or conversation-style speech, in different extraclinic environments (Koegel et al., 1986).

Box 7–3. Traditional Speech Therapy Approach: Key Points

- Van Riper's traditional approach to speech therapy is a sensorimotor approach applied to a single phoneme using a vertical goal attack strategy.
- The phases of the traditional approach to speech therapy are ear training, establishment, stabilization, and transfer/maintenance.
- Techniques for establishing a new phoneme include stimulation, contextual facilitation, phonetic placement, successive approximation, and visual feedback.
- Stabilization involves high-intensity practice of variable stimuli at progressively greater levels of complexity from syllables through sentences.
- The key to transfer and maintenance is to empower the child to take responsibility for carry over of accurate speech to the extraclinic environment.

Chapter 7 Study Questions

Respond to the following multiple choice questions by choosing the one best answer to each question.

1. You have assessed a child aged 30 months who is able to produce only the sounds [ə] and [gə]. The child has a mild intellectual delay and a receptive language age of 20 months and will not attempt to imitate speech sounds. You should recommend that:
   a. an early intervention worker at his child care center teach him to imitate before speech therapy is initiated.
   b. the SLP begin the Ling program at Level 1a (vowels).
   c. the SLP and the family engage the child in vocal play to increase his vocal repertoire.
   d. phonetic placement be used to establish some consonants in his repertoire.

2. When introducing an AAC system for a child with limited oral communication abilities, it is important that the family understand that:
   a. an AAC system will complement and facilitate the emergence of spoken language.
   b. a decision has been made that the child will never be capable of spoken language.
   c. the child will need extra encouragement to use speech as a means of communication.
   d. the parents must insist that the child use speech and the AAC system simultaneously.

3. Which of the following is the most important vocal play technique for increasing vocalizations in a preverbal child?
   a. Enhance sensory feedback.
   b. Practice nonspeech oral movements.
   c. Use an infant-directed speaking register when presenting models for imitation.
   d. Imitate the child's actions and vocalizations during play.

4. Which of the following are justifications for the focus on nonsense syllable drills in sensorimotor approaches to speech therapy?
   a. Nonsense syllables focus attention on the speech motor planning task that is the target of the sensorimotor intervention.
   b. Nonsense syllables can be constructed specifically to meet the needs of each individual child, in relation to the child's limited phonetic repertoire.
   c. Research shows that practice with nonsense syllables will generalize to real words.
   d. All of the above.

5. When practicing nonsense syllables, it is important to balance repetition with variability so that the child achieves dynamic stability, which means that:
   a. the child generalizes from taught sounds to new sounds not practiced in therapy.
   b. the child is ready to practice in meaningful speech.
   c. the child can produce the syllables in varied phonetic contexts.
   d. only variegated syllable strings are practiced in therapy.

6. The unique aspect of the ReST program, a sensorimotor program for treating CAS, is that it:
   a. focuses on prosody, with systematic variations in stress patterns over three-syllable nonsense words.
   b. includes practice with complex abutting consonant strings (e.g., CVCCVC).
   c. begins with the practice of isolated sounds before combining them into syllables.
   d. practices consonants at one place of articulation at a time.

7. The challenge point framework is based on the idea that:
   a. the learner must practice at least 100 practice trials in order to be challenged enough.
   b. the learner must receive the right amount of information while practicing to learn a new skill.
   c. better practice performance during therapy leads to better learning outside the clinic.
   d. practicing hard tasks is more challenging and leads to better learning.

8. Which of the following was NOT mentioned as a purpose of the prepractice portion of the sensorimotor speech therapy session?
   a. Identify the session's speech targets for the child.
   b. Warm up the speech muscles in preparation for high-intensity practice.
   c. Teach the child to monitor for and self-correct errors.
   d. Determine the challenging level of practice for each speech target.

9. When the child's practice performance is too high, which of the following lists contains three strategies for moving the child's practice performance back toward the challenge point?
   a. Increase intensity, reduce stimulation, provide less frequent feedback.
   b. Increase variability of stimulus items, move up the integral stimulation hierarchy, provide knowledge of performance feedback.
   c. Increase complexity of context, increase predictability, increase stimulation.
   d. Reduce intensity, reduce stimulation, reduce frequency of feedback.

10. When the child's practice performance is too low, which of the following lists contains three strategies for moving the child's practice performance back toward the challenge point?
    a. Reduce intensity, increase predictability, provide less frequent knowledge of results feedback.
    b. Reduce nominal task difficulty, reduce complexity of context, reduce feedback.
    c. Reduce complexity of context, move up the integral stimulation hierarchy, provide direct knowledge of performance feedback.
    d. Reduce nominal task difficulty, reduce variability of practice schedule, reduce stimulation.

11. The first step in Van Riper's traditional articulation therapy program is:
    a. ear training.
    b. establishment.
    c. self-monitoring.
    d. phonetic placement.

12. Which of the following is the correct definition of phonetic placement as a technique for establishing a new speech sound in the child's repertoire?
    a. Providing the child with an auditory and visual model of the target phoneme for imitation.
    b. Modeling the target sound in the context of another sound that positions the articulators for producing the target more easily.
    c. Physically manipulating the child's articulators to move them into the correct location and configuration.
    d. Bringing an unconscious process to overt awareness so that it can be consciously manipulated.

13. Which of the following is the traditional sequence of practice targets for stabilizing a new phoneme?
    a. Prevocalic position, syllables-words-phrases-sentences; then repeat for postvocalic position and repeat again for intervocalic position.
    b. Prevocalic position, syllables-words-phrases-sentences; stop and wait to see if generalization occurs to other word positions.
    c. Words, all positions mixed; phrases, all positions mixed; sentences, all positions mixed
    d. Syllables, CV, VC, VCV, CVC; words, prevocalic-postvocalic-intervocalic; phrases, all word positions; sentences, all word positions.

14. Which of the following is the most important strategy for ensuring that the child achieves transfer and maintenance of a new speech sound?
    a. Provide lots of knowledge of results feedback about accuracy of production.
    b. Involve the family in therapy, asking them to keep a record of the child's correct productions at home.
    c. Provide a homework book so that the child practices in the extraclinic environment.
    d. Ensure that the child has an excellent acoustic-phonetic representation of the target phoneme.

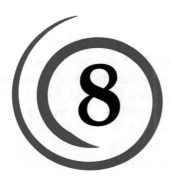

Phonological Approaches

Learning Objectives

- Describe two unique characteristics of phonological approaches to intervention.
- Describe the characteristics of children who might benefit from the core vocabulary approach.
- Identify the goal of the core vocabulary approach and describe the two procedures that are used to achieve this goal.
- Given a specific treatment goal, create a lesson plan for a single session that is consistent with the cycles phonological remediation approach.
- Given an intermediate treatment goal, identify minimal pair words that could be used for targeting the goal.
- Describe the four steps required to implement the method of meaningful minimal pairs.
- Explain why it is essential to ensure that children with speech sound disorders (SSDs) have adequate metaphonological awareness skills.
- Distinguish three contexts in which the speech-language pathologist (SLP) may intervene to improve a child's metaphonological knowledge.
- Plan activities to teach awareness of syllables, onsets, rimes, phonemes, and features.

Thus far treatment approaches that address phonetic knowledge have been presented. Chapter 6 covered treatment procedures that strengthen the child's knowledge of the acoustic-phonetic properties of words and phonemes. Chapter 7 covered treatment procedures that strengthen the child's knowledge of the articulatory characteristics of syllables and speech sounds. In this final chapter, procedures to strengthen the child's phonological knowledge of words, syllables, and phonemes will be presented. The procedures are presented in developmental order. In early phonological development the toddler organizes phonological knowledge at the level of word templates, increasing the number of templates so as to maintain lexical contrast. Eventually the child's vocabulary outgrows the number of available templates, and knowledge of individual phonemes emerges. Gradually the child develops an adultlike organization of underlying phonological representations for prosodic structures and segmental features. Finally, as the child's vocabulary continues to grow, metalinguistic access to phonological structure emerges and the child demonstrates explicit phonological awareness of syllables, onsets, rimes, and individual phonemes, facilitating the acquisition of reading.

8.1 RATIONALE FOR A PHONOLOGICAL APPROACH

For any given child it is likely that the SLP will need to select and order different treatment procedures to meet the child's needs as they change with developmental time. In other words, no one treatment approach will meet all the child's needs at all times. However, all children need to have adultlike knowledge at all levels of representation—that is, acoustic-phonetic, articulatory-phonetic, and phonological—in order to achieve intelligible and age-appropriate speech sound accuracy. By definition, children with a primary SSD will require an intervention that attends to underlying knowledge of the phonological system of their language at some point in their developmental trajectory. In fact, even those children with secondary SSDs will benefit from a phonological approach at certain developmental junctures (Pamplona, Ysunza, &

Espinoza, 1999). Furthermore, phonological approaches to intervention are typically more efficient than the traditional approach to articulation therapy when the child has many speech sound errors (Klein, 1996).

The efficiency of phonological interventions is grounded in the phonological approach to generalization. The phonological approach is very different from the sensorimotor approach to generalization that was introduced in Chapter 7. When using a sensorimotor approach it is necessary to practice target sounds in many different phonetic contexts, and therefore, the more practice words targeted in therapy sessions the better. Encouraging speech practice in a variety of environmental settings alongside teaching the child to self-monitor are also important strategies to ensure that the child transfers learning from the clinic to extraclinic settings. When implementing a phonological approach, however, reorganizing the child's phonological knowledge is expected to accomplish generalization and transfer with relative ease because phonological patterns are targeted rather than specific speech sounds. For example, if a child produces fricatives in the coda position but substitutes stops for fricatives in the onset position, this pattern appears to be **rule governed**. Practice with a small number of words with a fricative in the onset might change the rule, resulting in rapid emergence of all the fricatives in the syllable onset position. Therefore, there would be no need to teach all the fricatives and no need to practice them before all possible vowels to achieve generalization to untaught words.

A critical aspect of the phonological treatment program is the selection and ordering of treatment goals. Treatment goals are selected and ordered to maximize the possibility of generalization from treated targets to untreated targets, taking the structure of the underlying phonological hierarchy into account. Shared features between potential treatment targets provide information about possible patterns of generalization. Many studies have shown that generalization within and across natural classes of phonemes can occur without specific attention to a "transfer" phase of therapy (Costello & Bosler, 1976; Elbert, Dinnsen, & Powell, 1984; Elbert, Dinnsen, Swartzlander, & Chin, 1990; Elbert & McReynolds, 1985; McReynolds & Bennett, 1972). For example, teaching a child to produce /tʃ/ may facilitate the emergence of several other phonemes, specifically /dʒ/, /ʃ/, /ʒ/, because all of these phonemes share the feature Coronal:[−anterior].

Generalization across word positions can also be predicted (Forrest, Dinnsen, & Elbert, 1997; Forrest, Elbert, & Dinnsen, 2000). If the child has a common error pattern across all word positions, it is possible to treat the error pattern in only one word position and expect generalization to the other word positions: therefore, if the child stops fricatives in onsets and codas, the SLP could choose to treat /f/ in the onset and might observe generalization to /f/ and /s/ in the coda (that is, generalization to another fricative and to another word position is expected in this case). However, when the error pattern is not shared across word positions, there is not likely to be generalization: therefore, if the child stops fricatives in the coda but glides fricatives in the onset, treating /f/ in the coda might generalize to /s/ in the coda, but gliding of fricatives in the onset will remain unless this error is targeted specifically. Nonetheless, these expected patterns of generalization mean that the SLP does not need to treat each phoneme

to mastery, one after another, using a vertical goal attack strategy, as would be the case if the traditional approach to articulation therapy were employed. Rather, a few strategically selected phonemes can be treated using either a horizontal or cycles goal attack strategy. When the child has achieved 40% to 60% accuracy, a short break from therapy can be implemented. Monitoring of the child's progress is likely to reveal spontaneous progress toward mastery of the treatment goals because the child's knowledge of new phonological features will result in change across the lexicon.

Another unique aspect of phonological interventions is the use of procedures to heighten the child's awareness of the functional significance of phonological structure. It is natural that young children's speech utterances are inconsistent, inaccurate, and hard to understand. Most adults will go to some trouble to understand the message that the young child is trying to communicate and adapt to the child's inability to produce accurate speech. When the child's phonological knowledge lags behind age expectations, it may be necessary to make a special effort to communicate the linguistic impact of inconsistent or inaccurate speech to the child. This means that speech therapy will involve meaningful activities so that the child is motivated to speak more clearly to communicate intended messages accurately. Therefore there should be no activities that involve imitation of nonsense syllables or words with no meaning component, as was common in the sensorimotor procedures described in Chapter 7. There might be prepractice activities designed to heighten the child's explicit knowledge of phonological structures (e.g., features, onsets, rimes, syllables); however, during practice, meaningful consequences should naturally occur in response to correct or incorrect pronunciations. In other words, the child should have opportunities to use target words for the purpose of communicating meaning; when misarticulations of the target words result in a communication breakdown, this is a powerful intervention procedure that is intentionally employed in phonological approaches.

Practice 8–1

Assume that you are selecting treatment targets for a child aged 3;6 whose preferred word shapes are CV, CVC, and CVCVC with the following consonant repertoire: [p,b,m,t,d,n,w,j] (onset position); [t,d,n,k,g,s] (coda position). Choose two treatment goals that are most likely to maximize reorganization of the child's phonological system in the shortest period of time. Describe each goal in terms of the target segment (phoneme) and identify the syllable position and word shape into which it will be inserted for practice.

Box 8–1. Phonological Approach: Key Points

- The efficiency of phonological interventions is grounded in the phonological approach to generalization.
- Treatment targets are selected to promote generalization from taught to untaught items, based on similarities in features.
- Phonological interventions use procedures to heighten the child's awareness of the functional significance of phonological structure.

8.2 WORD-BASED PHONOLOGY: CORE VOCABULARY APPROACH

Very young children at the earliest stages of phonological development organize their phonological systems in the lexicon at the level of whole-word units. These whole-word units, called templates, need only be distinct enough to support comprehension in context. Therefore if a child has a four-word vocabulary, [dus] might be understood as "juice" in the kitchen and "shoes" when getting dressed for the park, whereas [ba] is understood to be "ball" in the park and "book" at bedtime. If the child adds "bye," it can be adapted to the [ba] template, differentiated by the simultaneous gesture. The addition of the word "banana" may require the acquisition of a new template, [nænæ]. The words produced with this limited number of templates can be understood even if the child's productions of the words are highly inconsistent so that the child might be pointing at the refrigerator and saying [dus], [duʃ], [dɪs], [diʃ], [dus̠], and the mother will understand the toddler's demand every time. As the vocabulary grows, however, the challenge of understanding the child's speech will grow. Typically, vocabulary growth will force a reorganization of lexical representations to include phoneme-level specificity as well as improved phonological planning skills so that the child is more consistent in the production of words. Sometimes, however, a child with a significant phonological planning deficit will continue to demonstrate a high level of within-word inconsistency even as the vocabulary grows. These children will have the characteristics of **inconsistent phonological disorder** when tested with the *Diagnostic Evaluation of Articulation and Phonology*

(Dodd, Zhu, Crosbie, Holm, & Ozanne, 2006): specifically, greater than 40% inconsistency on the word inconsistency test alongside atypical error types, not easily identified as natural phonological processes. Therefore an intervention that targets phonological patterns will be ineffective. Rather, the appropriate approach will target the inconsistency itself: this approach is called the core vocabulary approach.

The **core vocabulary approach** is designed to stabilize consistent production of a core set of functional vocabulary items (Crosbie, Holm, & Dodd, 2005; Dodd & Bradford, 2000). This approach has two critical procedures, the first being the selection of the core vocabulary words for practice, and the second being a unique procedure for stabilizing consistent production of those words.

A pool of core vocabulary items is constructed by the child's family, choosing words that are functionally important in the child's environment but produced inconsistently by the child. It is recommended that there be 50 words to start with and then the SLP chooses five words from the pool to practice first. The SLP works with the child to establish a "best pronunciation" for each of the five practice words. The best pronunciation may not be completely accurate but should be reasonably close or acceptable, as in, for example, "grandma" /ɡɹænma / → [gwæma]. After an acceptable target is established for each word, the goal is consistent production of this best pronunciation in clinic and extraclinic environments.

Although Dodd and colleagues do not take phonological factors into account in the selection of the words, it is possible to select the practice words from the list in order to deliberately expand the child's repertoire of preferred word templates in an orderly fashion. The templates that are currently in use by the child can be iden-

tified by conducting a multilinear analysis of the child's speech. Even though the child will not be using natural phonological processes (as the child has inconsistent and atypical errors by virtue of the diagnosis), there are often templates that can be identified by looking for certain preferred combinations of word shapes and features by syllable position. Case Study 8–1 presents some assessment data from a child who presents with a severe inconsistent phonological disorder, as indicated by 86% inconsistency on the Word Inconsistency Assessment. Percentage of Consonants Correct on the Diagnostic Evaluation of **Articulation** and Phonology (DEAP) assessment was only 61% despite a relatively complete phonetic repertoire in the onset and coda positions (/ð/ and /θ/ being the only absent phones). He also presented with severe difficulties in phonological memory as measured by the Syllable Repetition Task, with no corresponding evidence of transcoding difficulties, confirming the conclusion that the underlying problem is with phonological planning rather than motor planning (for more information about this child and interpretation of these test results, see Rvachew & Matthews, 2017b). Although his errors on the Phonology Assessment and in spontaneous speech could not be described as natural phonological processes, there was some predictability in his speech production nonetheless, as indicated by the quick nonlinear analysis shown in Part D of the case study (the procedures for multilinear analysis are described in detail in Rvachew & Brosseau-Lapré, 2018; a brief analysis is provided here by describing the child's strengths and needs at different levels of the phonological hierarchy when scanning his productions on the DEAP). Generally, he was able to produce simple one-syllable words correctly, such as "boy" /bɔɪ/ → [bɔɪ] and "van" /væn/ → [væn].

Case Study 8–1

Selected Assessment Data from a Candidate for Core Vocabulary Intervention

A. Case Description

This male child (TASC21), aged 5;5, participated in a treatment study in which interventions targeting phonological planning versus motor planning were compared for children with inconsistent speech errors. He and his family were bilingual (English and Arabic). His nonverbal intelligence was in the low average range and he was reported to have some difficulties with fine motor skills. He was diagnosed with primary speech and language delay. Single and multisyllable repetition rates were slow for age.

B. Prekindergarten Assessment at Age 59 Months

PPVT-III	SS = 69
MLU	1.41
DEAP Articulation	0.4 percentile
DEAP Phonology	3rd percentile
Word Inconsistency	85%
SRT memory	$z = -4.29$
SRT transcoding	$z = 0.28$

Notes. PPVT = Peabody Picture Vocabulary Test (Dunn & Dunn, 1997); MLU = Mean Length of Utterance (in morphemes); Diagnostic Evaluation of Articulation and Phonology; SRT = Syllable Repetition Task. Tests are described in Chapter 3.

C. Selected Word Productions from DEAP Phonology Assessment

pig	/pɪg/→[bɪk]	elephant	/ɛləfʌnt/→[ʊfʌnt]
knife	/naɪf/→[maɪs]	swing	/swɪŋ/→[swɪm]
crab	/kræb/→[kræts]	giraffe	/dʒəˌɹæf/→[ɹæf]
snake	/sneɪk/→[seɪk]	basket	/bæskɪt/→[pekes]
fishing	/fɪʃɪŋ/→[fɪdʒɪŋ]	square	/skwɛɚ/→[kus]
spider	/spaɪdə/→[paɪsə]	strawberry	/stɹɑbɛɹi/→[tupə]
umbrella	/ʌmbɹɛlʌ/→[gəˌɹɛlʌ]	web	/wɛb/→[bɛd]

Selected Assessment Data from a Candidate for Core Vocabulary Intervention

D. Quick Multilinear Analysis

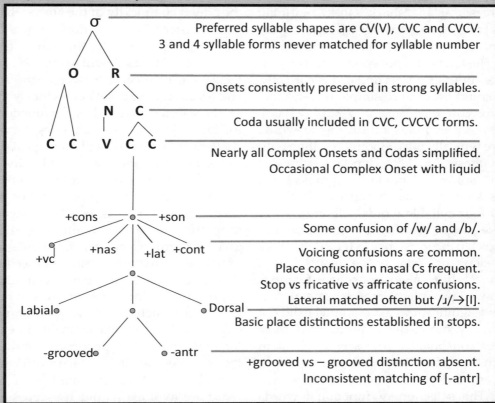

Preferred syllable shapes are CV(V), CVC and CVCV.
3 and 4 syllable forms never matched for syllable number

Onsets consistently preserved in strong syllables.

Coda usually included in CVC, CVCVC forms.

Nearly all Complex Onsets and Codas simplified.
Occasional Complex Onset with liquid

Some confusion of /w/ and /b/.

Voicing confusions are common.
Place confusion in nasal Cs frequent.
Stop vs fricative vs affricate confusions.
Lateral matched often but /ɹ/→[l].

Basic place distinctions established in stops.

+grooved vs – grooved distinction absent.
Inconsistent matching of [-antr]

E. Suggested Treatment Goals

1. Improve consistency of production of functional words, reducing occurrence of phonemic and semantic paraphasias.

2. Limit initial word set to one and two syllable words.

3. Expand repertoire of basic syllables to include CCVC.

4. Increase use of two-syllable words, especially with word internal CC sequences (CVCCV, CVC.CVC structures).

5. Reduce confusion between sonorants and obstruents.

6. Reduce confusion between fricatives and affricates.

7. Reduce place confusion within nasal class.

8. First five words: Batman, ride, Mindy, snack, Chase

When the word contained later developing phonemes or complex syllable structure, errors and inconsistency would increase, as in "shark"/ʃɑɪk/ → [ʃats], [ʃak] and "crab"/kræb/ → [kræts]. Apart from occasional correct production of a liquid cluster, he did not spontaneously produce complex onsets and codas correctly. He could pronounce simple two-syllable words correctly, "yucky" /jʌki/ → [jʌki], but more complex multisyllable words were typically mispronounced, often with metathesis: "basket" /bæskɪt/ → [pekes] and "spider" /spaɪdɚ/ → [paʊsɚ]. He was unable to match syllables in three- and four-syllable words. All attempts at these longer words were imitative and subject to inconsistency in the attempts, as in "elephant" /ɛləfʌnt/ → [ʊfʌnt], [ɛlfəs], [gonæs]. In terms of consonant features, knowledge of place among the nasal class was a significant weakness, and he did not have any knowledge of [–grooved]. Most other consonant errors seemed to stem from the difficulties he was having selecting and ordering segments within words.

The selection of functional words for practice can take his phonological knowledge into account. It might be best to choose five target words for this child that he will be able to approximate, which means a limit of one- to two-syllable target words for the first practice set. Increasing the complexity of single-syllable words and constructing two-syllable words from basic syllables might help him to achieve success in the early days of the treatment program. Therefore, if names of favorite action heroes are part of the 50-word pool, "Batman" might be a better starting point than "Spiderman." Words that contain s-clusters would be an excellent choice but preferably in single-syllable environments, such as in the word "snack."

The dog's name Mindy provides another opportunity to reinforce labial versus coronal place within the nasal class with the added complexity of the ambisyllabic nasal cluster. The verb "ride" targets the [ɹ]-[l] confusion. Finally the name of his best friend, "Chase," will serve nicely to tackle the confusion between affricates and fricatives. The point here is that words can be selected so that they are functional for the child while also targeting current challenges in the child's phonological system at an achievable level of difficulty.

After the practice words have been selected and the best pronunciation for each target word has been established (hopefully an accurate pronunciation, given careful selection), the words are practiced in treatment using a procedure that is unique to the core vocabulary approach. The intervention procedure is designed to help the child gain knowledge of the individual segments in each target word and independently construct the phonological plan for each word when producing it. Imitative models of the word are avoided as much as possible. Typically children with inconsistent phonological disorder will achieve much better success in imitation than in spontaneous speech. It is imperative that the child practice producing the words without a prior imitative model: therefore, other strategies to cue selection and ordering of the appropriate segments are provided to support the child's efforts. The techniques that are used to accomplish this goal are illustrated in Demonstration 8–1.

As with any treatment approach the first step is to identify the target for the child, which in this case is an entire word, "snack." Segmentation is the next technique, used to teach the child the individual sounds in the target word. Each

Core Vocabulary Approach: Teaching Procedure

A. Identify the target word

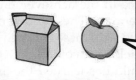

> This is a picture of a *snack*. Do you ever have apples and milk for snack? Today you will learn to say the word "snack." The word "snack" has four sounds in it. We are going to practice each sound, one at a time.

B. Segment the word and cue articulation of each sound in the word

> We're going to watch ourselves in the mirror and practice the sounds. The first sound is the snake sound like this: "ssss," you try it. Good, now the nose sound, like this: "nnnn." And this sound we make with the mouth open, "aaaa." Good. The last sound, I make with my tongue going up at the back, fast and hard, like this: "k."

s n a ck

C. Chain the sounds back together

s n a <u>ck</u>

s n <u>ack</u>

s <u>nack</u>

<u>snack</u>

> Now, we are going to put the sounds back together to make the word, remember this sound, make it with the back of your tongue. Perfect. Next, the open mouth sound (underline "a" slowly and into the "k" to encourage joining the sounds together"). Good you put these two sounds together. Do it again, a little faster. Now, start with the nose sound. Again. And again. Now, the snake sound... keep going. You got it. That's snack.

D. Drill-play to practice word without imitative models

> Let's play memory. Try to find the same snack on two cards. OK, apple slices, you eat them for…
> Oops, you forgot the snake sound. Let's look at the cue cards to practice the word….

sound in the word is practiced individually using **cued articulation** techniques. It can be helpful to practice the sounds in the word while sitting side-by-side at a large mirror. Cue cards that represent each sound can be attached to the mirror one at a time and practiced with verbal instruction and phonetic placement if required. Imitative models can be used at this step if required. The visual symbols on the cue cards can be any cue that is helpful to the child. When the children are school age, letters are advised, taking care to note the relationship between sounds and letters. The word "snack" has more letters than sounds and this is reflected in the way that the cues are placed on the cards. If the word was "snake," some additional cues would help to link letters to pronunciation, such as "s—n—ā—k¢." Pictograms can be added to the cue cards to represent articulatory gestures or sound characteristics, such as, for example, a snake to the "s" card or a nose to the "n" card. It is also possible to add or substitute finger spelling cues for the cards, but a static visual representation can be very helpful to children who have severe difficulties with phonological memory. Touch cues or manual prompts (in which the SLP puts her hands on the child's face to stimulate a muscle movement or indicate an articulatory target) are often used because these can be a powerful means of producing accurate production during therapy sessions. Excellent practice performance with these cues may make it difficult to achieve good generalization to the extra-clinic environment, however. The touch cues provide too much information about the target and interfere with the child's processing of feedback during speech production. Therefore, the touch cues are

not consistent with the goal of teaching children to independently construct their own phonological plan and monitor their own performance in the achievement of the planned utterance. These touch cues should be avoided with these children just as imitative models are avoided.

After the child has learned the association between each visual cue and each sound in the target word, **chaining** is used to teach the child to put the sounds back together to form the complete word. Usually it works best to start with backward chaining (that is, start with the last sound in the word) and then move to forward chaining. Some trial and error may be required to identify the best technique for a given word and child. When teaching multisyllabic words, the SLP may need to teach the child each syllable first, and then chain the syllables together. During the chaining step, the child should be encouraged to use the cue cards to remember the sounds and say them in the correct order. The SLP can underline the sounds, move the cards together, or use a sliding finger to get across the idea of joining them together smoothly. Imitative models should be avoided here but imitating the child can be used as positive reinforcement: when the child says "sssss—nack," the SLP can answer with, "That's right, when you put the snake sound on you get the word 'snack.' Let's practice the word again, a little faster this time. I'm going to move the snake sound closer. You try, the word is . . . "

When the child is able to chain the sounds together to produce the word spontaneously it is time for some drill practice. For example, the child could play memory with the SLP, turning over pairs of cards to find two that show the same snack food. After the child turns each card, the SLP produces a cue for spontaneous production, as in "Apples, you can eat them for . . ." If the child says "snack" using the pre-established best production (perhaps [ṣnæk] is acceptable), game play continues. If the child's production is unacceptable (such as [nakṣ]), game play is momentarily suspended while the cue cards are used to correct the production.

Finally, important actors in the child's environment are taught to cue the words in the home and school environment. The child's parents, grandmother, and kindergarten teacher will need to know the practice words for the week, the acceptable productions and some appropriate cues to use for stimulating use of those words in natural communication exchanges. The practice contexts and the cues to use in those contexts should be negotiated with care to ensure that they are feasible and that family members and school personnel know how to implement elicitation strategies that avoid the provision of imitative models. The cues and contexts should provide the child with opportunities to experience the natural consequences of consistent and intelligible production of the target words. If the child achieves consistent use of those practice words during the week, a new set of five practice words can be started during the next therapy session. If not, continued practice in therapy, perhaps increasing to phrase-level stimuli, can be implemented.

Experimental and nonexperimental studies have compared the core vocabulary approach with standard phonological approaches that target phonological contrasts (Crosbie et al., 2005; Dodd & Bradford, 2000). These studies demonstrate that the core vocabulary approach can be effective with children who have inconsistent phonological disorder, whereas phonological contrast therapy is better suited to children who have phonological delay. Although not directly tested, the pattern of results among the children in these studies suggests that the core vocabulary approach is best suited to children who have inconsistent speech errors despite a large phonetic inventory. Some children are inconsistent but have very limited phonetic inventories and may benefit from a sensorimotor approach prior to the implementation of any phonological approach to speech therapy.

Box 8–2. Core Vocabulary Approach: Key Points

- The Core Vocabulary Approach is intended for children with Inconsistent Phonological Disorder.
- Treatment targets are selected from a list of functional words provided by the client's family.
- When teaching target words, consistency is the goal rather than accuracy.
- The primary teaching techniques are segmentation, chaining, and production practice using visual cues for the phonemes in the word so that the child is forced to create her/his own phonological plan for production of the word without hearing an imitative model.
- An important aspect of the approach is providing opportunities for the child to use target words in authentic contexts at home and school.

8.3 PHONOLOGICAL PATTERNS: CYCLES REMEDIATION APPROACH

Most preschool-aged children with an SSD can be expected to have delayed phonological development, characterized by phonological error patterns that are commonly observed in younger children (Broomfield & Dodd, 2004; Dodd et al., 2017). Collectively these children are likely to have difficulties with phonological processing as measured by tests of speech perception and implicit phonological awareness (Rvachew, Ohberg, Grawburg, & Heyding, 2003) and oral motor skills as measured by diadochokinetic rates (Bradford & Dodd, 1996). Interestingly, deficits in underlying phonological knowledge do not seem to be the primary difficulty unless the child also has delayed receptive vocabulary skills (Munson, Edwards, & Beckman, 2005a, 2005b). In any case, a prudent approach to the treatment of these children's speech error patterns is to address the children's phonological knowledge at multiple levels of representation. The cycles approach (Hodson & Paden, 1983) is a commonly used and effective intervention that targets acoustic-phonetic, articulatory-phonetic, and phonological levels of representation. This comprehensive and developmental approach is characterized by a unique procedure for selecting and targeting treatment goals followed by the implementation of a structured combination of commonly used treatment procedures.

Each child's treatment program is organized within a series of cycles. Hodson (2007) defines a cycle as a period of time during which all of the selected target patterns for a given child are presented. Cycle duration is individualized for each child because it is determined by the number of pattern deficiencies that are identified for that child as potential intermediate targets and the number of stimulable phonemes that are available as potential specific targets. Specific guidelines for the selection and ordering of patterns are provided in Table 8–1 (as summarized from Hodson, 1989; Hodson & Paden, 1983). Generally, this approach would be used with a child that has unintelligible speech and a large number of predictable error patterns. Therefore a child could receive treatment for a broad range of intermediate goals in the first cycle, such as, for example, final consonant deletion, velar fronting, /s/-cluster simplification, and liquid gliding. Each phoneme within a target pattern receives 60 minutes of treatment per cycle and each pattern is targeted for 2 or more hours per cycle. Given that the child is expected to receive 60 minutes of intervention per week, specific goals might target one per week in order as follows: word final /m/, word initial /g/, /sp/ clusters, word initial /l/, word final /d/, word final /k/, /st/ clusters, and word initial /ɹ/. However, the exact specific goals and their order cannot be decided at the beginning of the cycle because only stimulable phonemes can be targeted with this approach: the SLP is expected to probe for potential stimulable targets repeatedly as the intervention progresses because the child's skill levels will change over time. Recycling of a target pattern (intermediate goal) is discontinued when generalization to conversation occurs, typically after two or three cycles. When the child generalizes all the initial goals to conversation, a treatment rest could be implemented; alternatively, new intermediate goals could be selected from the secondary target list if,

Table 8–1. *Cycles Remediation Approach:Target Patterns in Preferred Order of Selection*

Pattern	Target
	Primary Targets
Word structures (omissions)	Stops, nasals, and glides in CV syllables
	Compound words and 2- to 3-word phrases
	CVC (word-final consonants)
	VCV (within-word consonants)
Anterior-posterior contrasts	Fronting of velars, and/or
	Backing of alveolar or labial consonants
/s/ clusters	Stimulable word-initial clusters
	Stimulable word-final clusters
Liquids	Word-initial /l/ or /ɹ/ at the end of each cycle
	Secondary Targets
Palatals	/j, ʃ, tʃ, dʒ, ɝ, ɚ/
Other consonant sequences	Word-internal sequences
	Glide clusters
Singleton stridents	/s/ or /f/
Voicing contrasts	
Assimilations	
Any remaining idiosyncratic patterns	

Note. Summarized from Hodson (2007), Hodson and Paden (1983), and Hodson (1989).

for example, fronting of palatals and glide clusters remain as class deficiencies in the child's speech.

Regarding intervention procedures, each treatment session targets a single specific goal following a standard sequence of activities and using the same procedures each time. A mix of input-oriented, output-oriented, and phonological procedures are employed to enhance and integrate the child's knowledge across all types of phonological knowledge. Specifically, auditory bombardment is an important procedure that is applied twice during each treatment session and during home practice because Hodson (2011) claims that children learn speech "primarily by listening." A large part of each session is devoted to production practice so that the children can associate kinesthetic and auditory feedback during the acquisition of new phonological patterns.

However, this practice involves a small set of words carefully selected to maximize both phonetic context effects and phonological transfer. Importantly, these practice words are selected so that the child is stimulable for accurate production of the target phoneme. A high level of accurate production is expected during the practice session and during assigned homework activities. The standard outline for each session is shown in Table 8–2 with a justification and description of each intervention technique that is expected to be provided in order as shown.

The cycles approach has been shown to be effective in numerous studies (Almost & Rosenbaum, 1998; Montgomery & Bonderman, 1989; Pamplona et al., 1999; Rudolph & Wendt, 2014; Tyler, Edwards, & Saxman, 1987), including two randomized controlled trials. The studies also provide evidence that this intervention can be effective when provided to children individually as intended, or in small groups. The intervention takes a developmental, gradual approach, and therefore it is not surprising that in many cases, noticeable change is not observed until the second or third cycle (Rudolph & Wendt, 2014). One issue with this approach is that the assessment and target selection procedures tend to bias the SLP to focus on segment level goals while ignoring precursor word shape goals (this is not necessary because word structure goals are supposed to be selected first as indicated in Table 8–1). Nonetheless, children with severe delays and unintelligible speech may organize their phonology at the level of word length templates, in which case it is not appropriate to target phonological patterns that assume knowledge of natural classes of phonemes; rather, a multilinear analysis of the child's speech error patterns should be conducted and inconsistency should be considered to determine if the core vocabulary approach might be more effective. Other children with unintelligible speech have such limited repertoires of phones and syllables that a sensorimotor approach as described in Chapter 7 might be a more appropriate starting point. Some children do appear to be clear candidates for the cycles remediation approach because their error patterns are consistently characteristic of natural phonological processes; however, the child has very few stimulable phones available as specific goals. In these cases, the effectiveness of the cycles remediation approach can be enhanced by ensuring perceptual knowledge and stimulability of a small set of phonemes, using ear training and phonetic placement techniques, prior to the onset of the first cycle (Rvachew, Rafaat, & Martin, 1999).

Practice 8–2

Assume that you are targeting velar fronting as the intermediate goal and word-initial /k/ as the specific goal on the first day of the first cycle given a male child aged 3;9. Write a lesson plan following the outline for the Cycles Remediation Approach shown in Table 8–2. For each activity, indicate the objective; the procedure you will use; a description of the activity, materials, and the stimuli; the response the child is expected to make on each trial; and the feedback you will provide for correct and incorrect responses. Provide a detailed description of the homework assignment.

Table 8–2. *Cycles Remediation Approach: Session Outline and Treatment Procedures*

Procedure	Identification
Justification	Congruent with gradual acquisition trajectory of normal development, a new phoneme is targeted each week. Therefore, it is especially important that the child and caregiver or paraprofessional who will carry out homework knows what the target is for the session.
Description	SLP identifies the target for the child by briefly demonstrating the auditory, visual, articulatory, and tactile-kinesthetic properties of the sound.
Procedure	Auditory bombardment
Justification	Hodson includes this activity because children learn speech "primarily by listening." The ear training activity is intended to strengthen the child's acoustic-phonetic representation for the phoneme.
Description	SLP presents words to the child with amplification, taking care to not distort the target sound through overemphasis. Prerecorded words containing the target may be presented (with amplification, over headphones) as a substitute. Many words are presented, not just those that will be used for production practice during the session.
Procedure	Stimulation
Justification	It is important to establish accurate production of the target words, prior to practice. This activity helps the child associate the auditory target with kinesthetic and auditory feedback while speaking.
Description	Provide models of five carefully selected target words, with amplification, for imitation. Chaining and phonetic placement may be provided if necessary, but the words should be stimulable; therefore, these additional establishment techniques should not be required.
Procedure	Production practice
Justification	Helps establish new kinesthetic images ("integrative rehearsal").
Description	Drill-play activities (typically two) are used to provide practice with the five words that have been selected for practice. Adjust task difficulty and complexity as required to optimal challenge point (i.e., increase utterance length as performance improves).
Procedure	Auditory bombardment (repeat as above)
Procedure	Identify stimulable words for next session.
Justification	Children should be optimally challenged but also successful from the beginning of treatment.
Description	Probe stimulability of words containing the target for the next session.
Procedure	Assign homework, including auditory bombardment, production practice, and phonological awareness activity.
Justification	Children and families must be active participants in the intervention. All levels of representation must be integrated.

Box 8–3. Cycles Remediation Approach: Key Points

- The cycles approach targets patterns of error produced by children with moderate or severely delayed phonology.
- A cycle is a period of time during which all of the selected target patterns for a given child are presented.
- Cycle duration is individualized for each child based on the number of targets that are selected.
- Cycles are repeated until generalization for all target patterns is observed.
- Each pattern is targeted for 2 or more hours per cycle; within a pattern, each specific speech sound is targeted for 60 minutes; only stimulable phonemes are targeted.
- A standard lesson plan is implemented for each phoneme, including procedures such as auditory bombardment and drill-play activities for production practice.

8.4 MEANINGFUL MINIMAL PAIRS PROCEDURE

The method of meaningful minimal pairs is a uniquely phonological approach that targets the child's underlying knowledge of a distinctive feature contrast (Blache & Parsons, 1980). Therefore it is meant for children who lack phonological knowledge of specific phoneme contrasts within a natural class of phonemes defined by a distinctive feature. These might be chil-

dren who simplify contrasts in a manner similar to younger children with normally developing speech. For example, children with speech delay who front velars, /k,g/ → [t,d], and palatals, /ʃ,ʒ/ → [s,z], will benefit from this approach. Dodd and Bradford (2000) suggest that children with consistent atypical phonological disorder will especially benefit from this intervention—for example, a child who substitutes glides for ambisyllabic voiced consonants, "bigger" /bɪgɚ/ → [bɪjɚ] and "puddle" /pʌdl̩/ → [pʌjo]. In addition to the presence of predictable phonemic contrast errors, the child should have articulatory and perceptual knowledge of the sounds involved in the phonemic contrasts before implementing this procedure.

The method of meaningful minimal pairs is a conceptual approach to phonological intervention that has the goal of changing the child's production of an entire sound class (Weiner, 1981). The procedure has two key components: (1) teaching the child a pair of words that differ by a single phoneme, i.e., a minimal pair; and (2) arranging the environment so that the child experiences a communication breakdown if both words are produced as a homophone—meaning that the two words sound the same when they mean something different, thus motivating a change in production to avoid confusion. Phonological generalization is expected in other word pairs and phonemes that differ by the feature of interest. For example, "peak" /pik/ versus "beak" /bik/ are a minimal pair because they differ by one phoneme; specifically, the words share the same rime /ik/ but the onset consonant is different, /p/ versus /b/. If a child is prone to prevocalic voicing, these two words that mean something different will be produced as homophones, "peak"→ [bik] and "beak"→ [bik]. When the child is playing a game in which a climber goes on each "peak," confusion will arise if he says [bik] when asked where the climber goes (the climber will look pretty silly on the bird's beak!). The key to the intervention lies with the SLP's response to these homophones; when the child says [bik], the SLP must respond as if she heard the word "beak" even if she knows the child meant something else. Over time the child will learn that these words must be pronounced differently in order to communicate clear messages, "peak" /pik/ → [pik] versus "beak" /bik/ → [bik]. Notice that in this case, allophonic variation is an important part of the child's knowledge of this contrast: the child might have a **covert contrast** in which "peak" /pik/ → [pik] is heard by the listener to be the word "beak" /bik/ because the voice-onset time is too short and there is no aspiration when the child says word-initial /p/. Therefore, even if the child has underlying knowledge of the /p/ versus /b/ contrast, he must learn to produce it with enough phonetic distinction, /p/ → [pʰ] versus /b/ → [b], for listeners to perceive it. After learning a small number of minimal pairs that contrast these phonemes, correct production of the feature contrast [−voice] versus [+voice] should generalize to all consonants in the onset position of syllables, or at least to all the stop consonants.

Application of the method begins with a thorough linguistic analysis of the child's phonological system and the selection of a feature contrast as the therapy target. Most features of interest will impact a large number of phoneme pairs (for example, voicing impacts all the stops and fricatives). Therefore the SLP must decide which phoneme pairs to target and the order for introducing those specific phoneme contrast goals. Blache and Parsons

(1980) suggested tackling the affected phoneme pairs in developmental order. If the error pattern affects more than one word position, begin in word-initial position and then proceed to word-final if spontaneous generalization across word positions does not occur. Finally, in the treatment planning stage, select three to five word pairs that differ only by the feature of interest. The word pairs must be produced as homophones by the child. Some speech error patterns do not lend themselves well to remediation with the minimal pairs technique because the child's error does not create an easily pronounceable homophone. For example, if the child distorts the /ɹ/ phoneme so that "rake" /ɹek/ → [ɹek], it could be more confusing than helpful to practice the words "rake" and "wake."

It may be difficult to think of minimal-pair words that a young child will know and that are easy to manipulate in therapy (in the form of small toys or picture cards). In this case, it is acceptable to make up nonsense words, but the nonsense words must be linked to an object so that the word has meaning even if it is made up. For example, the target word pair could be "thief" /θif/ and "zief" /zif/ in which the first word is a picture of a robber and the second is a space alien. As another example, "rasp" /ɹæsp/ and "rast" /ɹæst/ could be contrasted by pairing the first word with an actual rasp and the second with an unusual object such as a chinoise-style strainer. The point is that the contrasting word must mimic the child's error production for the target word.

When teaching meaningful minimal pairs, proceed through the sequence of four steps listed in Table 8–3 with the corresponding instructions. First, it is necessary to ensure that the child knows the words and recognizes the pictures (or

Table 8–3. *Steps in the Meaningful Minimal Pairs Procedures*

	Step	Instructions (for example pair *peak/beak*)
1	Tests for concepts	(Show the child the pictures representing the concepts "peak" and "beak.") "This one is peak. This one is beak. Which one is the top of the mountain? That's right, a mountain climber wants to get to the peak at the very top of the mountain, here is the peak. Which one is the bird's beak? Yes, here is the bird's beak. The bird can crack hard nuts with its beak."
2	Test for discrimination	(Sit beside or behind the child. Show the child the picture of the "peak" and "beak" side by side on the table.) "Touch peak. Touch beak." (Move pictures around, rearrange in random order between trials.) "Touch beak. Touch peak." (Repeat with random ordering of pictures and trials until child achieves 7 consecutive correct response pairs.)
3	Production practice	(Place five pictures of "peak" and 4 pictures of "beak" in a haphazard arrangement on the table.) "Now it is your turn to be the teacher. Your job is to get me to pick up all the pictures on the table. When I have all the cards picked up, the climber can go one step up the path toward the peak of the mountain, OK? Start now, tell me what to pick up first."
4	Generalization	Repeat steps 1 to 3 as needed with new word pairs and phonemes until generalization has been achieved across the sound class at the word level. Then use traditional procedures to promote generalization to untrained words and to sentence-level material and conversational speech as needed.

objects) that have been chosen to represent the word pairs; the child's understanding that the words have different meanings is an essential aspect of the intervention. The second step ensures that the child has good perceptual knowledge of the phonemic contrast. It is important to sit beside or behind the child when asking him or her to point to the cards when you name them during this step. The child must be able to identify the words from the sounds in the word, without using visual cues from the SLP's face. Blache and Parsons (1980) point out that seven consecutive correct responses (to both members of the word pair) indicate above chance level responding. When the child achieves this level of performance, proceed to production practice by reversing roles. Now it is the child's turn to talk: the child tells the SLP which cards to pick up or otherwise manipulate. It will be obvious by following the child's eye gaze which item is the intended target even if the child misarticulates the intended word. However, it is essential to the procedure that the SLP pick up the item that is indicated by the child's speech. If the child says "Pick up *beak*" when he meant "Pick up *peak*," the SLP must pick up the *beak* card. If there are no more *beak* cards on the table, the SLP can provide informative feedback, such as: "I think you want me to pick up the *peak* card but I keep hearing *beak*; when I hear the buzzing sound at the beginning, that means the bird's beak; when I hear the puff of air, [pʰik], I will pick up the mountain peak." After two incorrect attempts, it is acceptable to offer additional verbal instructions or even phonetic placement in addition to the model, to help the child achieve the intended articulation. The point is to ensure that the child learns the two categories by producing linguistically and functionally different responses in relation to the two items and experiencing different functional outcomes. This sequence of three steps should take no more than ten minutes to complete.

The meaningful minimal pairs procedure is quite different from the more artificial imitative learning scenario where the child produces a nonfunctional response and receives feedback about the accuracy of the response. The game can be modified to involve more active participation by the child, but the essential procedure must remain the same. For example, a mountain peak could be drawn on one page of his homework book and a toucan with a large beak on the other. The child draws a sticker out of a bag and indicates whether the climber or nut sticker goes on the "peak" or the "beak" (however, the parrot spits the climber stickers out, back into the bag). After the child has learned the first pair, the SLP probes for generalization to other word pairs that contrast /p/-/b/ (i.e., "pea" versus "bee" and "pole" versus "bowl"). If the child is now producing these words correctly, a new phoneme contrast for the feature voice should be taught (e.g., "coat" versus "goat").

Baker (2010) conducted an extensive review of the scientific literature on the method of meaningful minimal pairs therapy and found 42 studies covering multiple levels of evidence, including nonexperimental studies, quasi-experiments, single-subject experiments, and two randomized controlled trials. Taken together, these studies demonstrate that the procedure is effective and efficient. The procedure may be implemented by itself or as part of a more comprehensive phonological approach to therapy such as Metaphon (Dean & Howell, 1986) or Parents and Children Together (Bowen & Cupples, 2006). In some cases children are taught words that differ by one phoneme, but the feature contrast is not minimal; this means that the word pairs can contrast phonemes that differ by many features (e.g., "cane" versus "chain"), as in the multiple opposition approach (Williams, 2010) and the maximal opposition approach (Barlow & Gierut, 2002).

The method of meaningful minimal pairs is best suited to children who have delayed phonological development, ideally of mild or moderate severity, as indicated by a few consistent patterns of phonological error in their speech. The child should be stimulable for the phoneme pairs that are targeted in therapy. There should be parent involvement in the therapy and a structured home practice component. Many studies have shown that generalization can occur after practice with between three and five word pairs and it may not be necessary to practice beyond the word level to achieve carry-over to conversation (Elbert et al., 1990; Elbert, Powell, & Swartzlander, 1991). In fact, if learning and carry-over have not occurred after five word pairs and 500 practice trials, the approach is not appropriate for the client. A thorough reevaluation of the child's needs should be conducted in order to identify a more appropriate choice of approach.

Practice 8–3

Think of three minimal word pairs that could be used to target the following distinctive feature contrasts when providing intervention to a 4- or 5-year-old child (see Table 1–5 for feature definitions):

[Coronal] versus [Dorsal] (alveolar vs. velar consonants);

[+consonantal][+continuant] versus [+consonantal][−continuant], (stops vs. fricatives);

[Coronal][+anterior] versus [Coronal][−anterior], (alveolar vs. post-alveolar fricatives);

Coda versus No Coda (syllables with vs. without a final consonant);

[Sonorant] versus [Sonorant][Consonantal], (/w/ vs. /ɹ/ or /l/).

If the child reduces /s/ clusters, what problem might arise if you attempt to resolve this problem using a pair such as "spot" versus "pot"?

Box 8–4. Meaningful Minimal Pairs: Key Points

- The method of **meaningful minimal pairs** is a uniquely phonological approach that targets the child's underlying knowledge of a distinctive feature contrast.
- A minimal pair consists of two words that differ by one phoneme.
- The method of meaningful minimal

pairs involves arranging the environment so that the child experiences a communication breakdown if both words are produced as a homophone.

- Usually children generalize their knowledge of the target contrast after learning three to five minimal pairs.

8.5 METAPHONOLOGICAL KNOWLEDGE

Metalinguistic awareness is a specific form of metacognition—knowing about knowing—that involves explicit awareness of linguistic structure rather than understanding meaning. For example, a toddler may understand that [bɹɪŋjə-stʌfi] means to get her favorite toy and take it in the car while not being aware that the phrase consists of three words; it may be months before she realizes that [gɛt] can be substituted for [bɹɪŋ] without changing

the meaning and many years before she learns that [bɹɪŋ] is a verb and [stʌfi] is a noun. **Metaphonological knowledge** pertains to phonological structure at all levels of the phonological hierarchy—specifically, words, syllables, onsets and rimes, phonemes, and features. Children with SSDs often have poor awareness of these structures, regardless of diagnosis, meaning that children with articulation disorder, phonological delay, consistent atypical and inconsistent phonological disorder, and childhood apraxia of speech should all be assessed for phonological awareness skills prior to and after school entry. These problems with metaphonological awareness put children at risk for difficulties with the acquisition of literacy (Anthony et al., 2011; Bird, Bishop, & Freeman, 1995; Nathan, Stackhouse, Goulandris, & Snowling, 2004a, 2004b). This is because a crucial reading skill is **decoding**, which means the ability to sound out printed words and link the spoken sounds to lexical and semantic representations. Decoding requires knowledge of the correspondence between letters and phonemes (e.g., "p"→[p], "a"→[æ]) and between combinations of letters such as **digraphs** and phonemes (that is, pairs of letters such as "ck"→[k], "sh"→[ʃ]). Knowledge of sound-letter correspondences is also known as the **alphabetic principle.** However, children cannot use their knowledge of the alphabetic principle to decode words if they do not have explicit knowledge of the phonemes that make up words. In other words, the child cannot easily learn to decode words such as "mushroom" if the child is not aware that spoken words are made up of syllables and syllables are made up of individual speech sounds. According to the "simple view of reading," the child's reading comprehension skills are determined jointly by decoding skills and oral language comprehension (Gough & Tunmer, 1986). Many children with an SSD have adequate language comprehension skills, but their decoding skills are likely to fall behind expectations (Rvachew, 2007) because phonological processing deficits are so common in this population (Rvachew & Grawburg, 2006). Therefore it is essential to assess and, when necessary, intervene to ensure that children with SSDs have age-appropriate phonological awareness abilities in order to prevent delays in the acquisition of literacy.

Practice 8–4

How many phonemes are in each of these words when you say them out loud? Laughter; spaghetti; division; fox; passion; telecommunications; treacle; post-script; grandma; wreath; messed; character; eight; poacher; slowed; sleight; maximum; computer; choir; easy; telephone.

Try to diagram the syllable structure of some of these words at the syllable, foot, onset-rime, and skeletal tiers of the phonological hierarchy.

There are three ways to address the phonological awareness skills of children with SSDs. In some approaches the activities are integrated into speech therapy sessions in which the primary goal is to reorganize the child's phonological system in order to improve speech intelligibility and accuracy; in this case, advances in phonological awareness skills are a fortunate side effect. However, given the frequent correspondence of reading and speech difficulties, these children are prime candidates for programs that target emergent literacy skills as a means to prevent reading disability. In the school environment, preventative programs are often implemented in the context of a "response to intervention" program. In this case, the SLP may work with kindergarten teachers to ensure that all children receive evidence-based instruction targeting phonological awareness and emergent literacy. The SLP should also implement a screening program to identify children who require additional small group or individualized support when they are not meeting the goals expected from the classroom program. Finally, SLPs are increasingly involved in the treatment of dyslexia and may intervene directly to improve children's decoding and spelling skills. The application of treatment procedures to improve metaphonology in each of these three contexts is discussed briefly in this chapter.

8.5.1 Speech Therapy Procedures That Promote Phonological Awareness

Many procedures for enhancing a child's metaphonological knowledge are easily integrated into a typical speech therapy session whether using an input-oriented, output-oriented, or phonological approach. In fact, metaphonology intervention can and should be introduced prior to school entry, when children with speech impairments are as young as 3 years old (Gillon, 2005) and many studies have demonstrated excellent results for 4- to 6-year-old children with SSD. These studies suggest that integrating speech therapy and phonological awareness intervention leads to significantly improved speech intelligibility and age-appropriate phonological awareness prior to school entry, which is a critical point for the prevention of literacy delays (Bernhardt & Major, 2005; Gillon, 2000; Hesketh, Adams, Nightingale, & Hall, 2000; Nathan et al., 2004; Rvachew & Brosseau-Lapré, 2015).

Young children can be taught awareness of words, syllables, rimes, onsets, phonemes, and features. Typically, larger units such as syllables and rimes are easier to learn than smaller units such as phonemes and may be the starting point when working with the youngest children. When teaching children to manipu-

late word onsets and phonemes within words, they should be encouraged to associate sounds with letters. Most teaching activities that are used with preschoolers will involve matching words that share the same unit or feature. Some preschool-aged children can also be taught to segment words into smaller units or blend smaller units into words, when provided with visual cues and sufficient coaching. The units that are the focus of intervention should be matched to the speech production goal. Some examples of potential phonological awareness activities are shown in Table 8–4.

The first activity is designed to raise the child's awareness of word-internal weak syllables that are presumably deleted in the child's speech. The activity is a variation on matching in which cards are sorted into two toy trains (with open cars), one with two cars and the other with three. In this activity the pictures are named by the SLP and the cards do not have printed text on them so that the child's judgment about the number of syllables is based solely on the sound of the word. The SLP should take care to produce the words with normal prosody. This sorting activity can be modified so that the child must sort words to match particular three-syllable prosodic patterns: "potato" could go in the train with a short-long-short car sequence, whereas "telephone" would go in the train with a long-short-long train sequence. These sorting activities would provide the child with listening experience and explicit vocabulary for talking about syllable number and stress characteristics. This new vocabulary and awareness will support self-monitoring when practicing production of words such as "elephant," "telephone," and "pelican."

The second activity would be a useful precursor to production practice with a

Table 8–4. Examples of Phonological Awareness Activities

Specific Speech Goal	Phonological Awareness Goal	Therapy Activity
Weak syllable deletion: 3 syllable word with word internal weak syllable.	Sort 3 syllable and 2 syllable words.	Child selects pictures from a card deck representing 2 and 3 syllable words (earwig, talon; elephant, telephone). SLP names the picture. Child puts it in the 2 or 3 car train.
Cluster reduction: single syllable words with /s/ cluster onset.	Segment and blend "s" → /s/ with rest of word and match to corresponding picture card.	Magnet board is used to create matching sets of pictures and letter combinations for pairs of words, pot-spot, top-stop, etc.
Velar fronting: word final /k/	Matching words to the letters "k" and "t" based on last sound.	SLP writes the letters "k" and "t" on facing pages in the child's homework book. The child cuts out pictures (puck, pat, meat, lock, etc.) and glues them on the appropriate page.
[+consonantal] [+continuant]	Identify sounds as short or long.	SLP writes letters in the child's homework book, down the side of the page: t, s, f, p, sh, k, z, d, v, b. Pronounce each sound in isolation. Child draws short (–) or long (—) line next to each letter or digraph to indicate whether it sounds short or long.

child who reduces /s/ clusters. The activity involves segmenting the /s/ sound from the rest of the word as well as blending it with the rest of the word to discover that different words with new meanings result. For example, one word pair would require a picture of a top (spinning top), a stop (red signal light), two cards with the letters "top" written on them, one smaller card with "s" written on it, and a smaller card that is blank to indicate a silent onset. The SLP explains that joining "s" plus "top" makes a word that goes with the "stop" picture, whereas "silent card" plus "top" goes with the "top" picture. After three word pairs have been introduced, the child can recreate the words to match to each of the six pictures. This activity can be carried out with plain index cards affixed to a mirror with reusable adhesive, or blank puzzle pieces can be purchased to create any stimuli required. Preschool-aged children may find segmentation and blending of phonemes difficult but an introduction to the concept can be made with continuant sounds prior to school entry when plenty of practice is provided with the support of visual props.

The third activity is a good example of the intersection between phonological therapy and phonological awareness. When the specific goal is to suppress Velar Fronting as a phonological process, it is good therapeutic practice to heighten the child's awareness of the phonemic contrast between /k/ and /t/. Matching words to letters is an activity that is commonly used to promote awareness of phonemes in words, teach the alphabetic principle, and support knowledge of a phonemic contrast. Therefore, sorting words into categories based on the child's target sound in comparison to the child's error sound is especially powerful for targeting speech accuracy and phonological awareness at the same time. Note again that the target letters should be written down for matching but the stimulus pictures should not have written words on them. The child should not be matching printed "k" to printed "k." Rather, in this activity the child must learn to match heard [k] at the end of [pʌk] to the letter "k" when printed on the white board or mirror or in the child's homework book.

Finally, it is possible to teach the child awareness of distinctive features as targeted in the fourth example activity. This activity would be appropriate for a child who is substituting stops for fricatives. The child is expected to listen and learn that some sounds are short ([−continuant], whereas others are long [+continuant]. The activity can proceed to word length stimuli after the child learns the association when the speech sounds are presented in isolation. This is another activity that provides the child with some vocabulary and listening skills that will support self-monitoring and self-correction when production practice with fricative sounds begins. These kinds of metaphonological procedures are an integral part of the Metaphon program (Dean & Howell, 1986).

The phonological awareness activities suggested in Table 8-4 are easily administered to small groups of children. In fact, a meta-analysis indicated that small group instruction was more efficient and effective compared with individual or whole class instruction in phonological awareness (Ehri et al., 2001). Furthermore, phonological awareness instruction can be provided effectively by paraprofessionals and supplemented by computer instruction. Therefore, an efficient service delivery model for children with SSDs may be for small groups to receive phonological awareness sessions from a paraprofessional as a supplement to weekly individual speech therapy sessions from the SLP. One program that is well suited to this treatment model when the clients are 4-year-old children is Sound Foundations (Byrne & Fielding-Barnsley, 1991). This intervention is meant to be delivered over 12 weeks, with twice-weekly half-hour sessions. The program focused on seven consonants and two vowels: initial /s/, /ʃ/, /m/, /p/, /l/, /t/, /g/, final /s/, /m/, /p/, /t/, /l/, and the vowels /æ/ and /ɛ/ (notice that four of the consonants are frequently misarticulated by children with SSDs). The lessons are play-based but use matching and sorting activities similar to those described in Table 8–4. When delivered to children with average speech and language skills in preschool classrooms, the impact on nonword decoding abilities was apparent through fifth grade. Recently the intervention has been modified to include sensorimotor instruction of letter forms and dialogic reading to strengthen vocabulary skills and reading skills in children who were at risk for reading impairment (Hindson, Byrne, Fielding-Barnsley, Hine, & Shankweiler,

2005). Justice, Chow, Capellini, Flanigan, and Colton (2003) compared an explicit phoneme awareness intervention, similar to the Sound Foundations approach, with a shared reading/dialogic reading control condition. Growth in emergent literacy skills was significantly greater for children in the experimental intervention that taught phonological awareness explicitly.

Practice 8–5

Imagine you are treating a small group of four 9-year-old boys for persistent speech errors that include dental distortion of /s/, derhoticization of /ɪ/, and a tendency to misarticulate longer or more complex words (e.g., "computer" → [pʊɾɚ], "ambulance" → [æmələnz]). You ask a speech disorders assistant to complete a 12-week phonological awareness program with these boys to supplement your weekly speech therapy sessions. Design the first lesson plan for this program.

8.5.2 Structured Emergent Literacy Interventions

An important role for the school SLP is to join together with other school personnel to support teachers in the selection and implementation of evidence-based curricula to ensure acquisition of adequate literacy skills by all primary grade students. This task is crucial in schools that have a high proportion of students at risk for literacy delays due to social or biological risk factors. An essential characteristic of the most effective curricula is early implementation, during the pre-kindergarten year or even earlier if possible. When chil-

dren enter into reading instruction with poor phonological awareness skills, they develop inefficient "whole word" **orthographic representations**—that is, representations of printed words are memorized one at a time (Harm, McCandliss, & Seidenberg, 2003). Some children can develop quite large sight reading vocabularies but be unable to decode nonwords because they are unable to sound out words that they have not been taught. It is very difficult to change orthographic representations to reflect relationships between letters and subsyllabic units later in life, after these inefficient representations have been acquired. Consequently, the child struggles to make the transition from "learning to read" in the primary grades to "reading to learn" in the later grades when the child is expected to independently acquire new words such as "convergent" and "lithosphere" from printed texts. Therefore, the effectiveness of emergent literacy programs is highly dependent upon the time at which they are introduced; specifically, phonological awareness and the alphabetic principle must be introduced prior to the onset of formal reading instruction.

A second characteristic of the most effective curricula for at risk children is that they are comprehensive—using best practices to target vocabulary and other oral language skills, phonological awareness, alphabet knowledge, and other print concepts in a coordinated and explicit fashion (Piasta, 2016). Relatedly, the teachers who provide the program must receive sufficient training and ongoing support to implement the teaching procedures across this range of learning goals (Lennox, Garvis, & Westerveld, 2017; Wasik, Bond, & Hindman, 2006). Teachers' explicit knowledge of language and print structure varies widely but is directly related to their use of best practices and their students' literacy acquisition (Piasta, Connor, Fishman, & Morrison, 2009). Speech-language pathologists are well positioned to support teachers and other school personnel in the provision of evidence-based language and literacy curricula.

Some curricula that have been shown to be effective with preschool-aged children will be briefly described as examples but there are many others that meet the criteria of explicitly targeting both the oral language and code related precursors to literacy acquisition. Snow et al. (2014) taught an explicit framework to teachers and principals to promote vocabulary, grammar, narrative skills, phonological awareness, and working memory to children in preschool and first-grade classrooms. A cluster randomized trial was implemented to compare oral language and reading outcomes for over 600 children who received the intervention compared with control children who received the standard curriculum. The schools that received the intervention obtained significantly better outcomes for some aspects of oral language and for reading compared with the control schools. The findings were important because the program was provided to disadvantaged children over 18 months and resulted in grade level reading ability at follow-up.

The Teaching Emergent Literacy and Language (TELL) curriculum was found to be effective in a randomized controlled trial when implemented specifically with children who had speech, language, and other developmental delays (Wilcox, Gray, Guimond, & Lafferty, 2011). This curriculum consists of a structured series of curriculum components that were required to be implemented on a daily or weekly basis, targeting phonological awareness, print concepts, alphabet knowledge, vocabulary, writing, and

grammar. The curriculum was completely integrated into the kindergarten program, encompassing small group, large group, circle time, snack time, craft activities, and all other activities that typically occur throughout the entire school year. The teachers were taught to use supportive and explicit teaching practices while implementing the activities (such as using a slow rate of speech and pointing to important words while reading). Speech-language pathology services were also provided to children in the experimental classrooms as needed. Their randomized controlled trial showed that children who received the TELL curriculum achieved higher levels of oral language proficiency and were significantly more likely to reach benchmarks for phonological awareness in comparison to the children in control classrooms.

Another effective program that provides a comprehensive array of elements targeting oral language and preliteracy skills is PAVEd for Success (Phonological Awareness and Vocabulary Enhancement; Schwanenflugel et al., 2010). This large-scale quasi-experimental study investigated both the effectiveness and sustainability of the program in pre-kindergarten classrooms in low-income rural communities. Furthermore, the study was designed to investigate the effectiveness of the individual components of the program to reduce the risk of reading disability; ultimately the study showed that the intervention was most effective when teachers implemented all components, specifically: (a) teach a new letter each week; (b) provide interactive storybook reading daily, in small and large groups; (c) create a print rich classroom; (d) document short conversations with each child weekly, to promote personal narratives and complex vocabulary; (e) teach phonological awareness lessons three times weekly; (f) plan for explicit vocabulary teaching based on weekly themes and incorporated into the preschool routine. The researchers also found that ongoing expert support was important to help teachers implement the curriculum appropriately throughout the school year.

Taken together these studies suggest that a combined approach that targets emergent literacy and oral language skills is essential for children who have speech and language impairments and impoverished access to language input or who are English language learners. These studies also show that the SLP is a key player in the successful implementation of these classroom interventions. Ehren and Ehren (2001) discuss strategies for expanding the SLP role to include collaborations with teachers in the provision of literacy programs. Schuele and Boudreau (2008) provide excellent guidance for school SLPs who are implementing phonological awareness interventions, either directly or through school personnel.

8.5.3 Reading and Spelling Interventions

Even among children who are able to access speech therapy as preschoolers, a good proportion of children with an SSD are likely to struggle with literacy in school. The risk is especially high if the speech difficulties persist beyond the preschool period (Bird et al., 1995; Glogowska, Roulstone, Peters, & Enderby, 2006; Lewis & Freebairn, 1992; Lewis, Freebairn, Hansen, Iyengar, & Taylor, 2004; McNeill, Wolter, & Gillon, 2017; Nathan et al., 2004). The risk of reading impairment is even greater if there is a concomitant language disorder. Children with a history of SSD are likely to have difficulties with spelling regardless of whether there

is concomitant language delay. Children with childhood apraxia of speech are at particular risk and are very likely to require individual therapy during the school years for treatment of speech, language, and literacy problems. For those children who arrive in third grade with an identified reading or spelling disability, individual treatment, implemented by an SLP or paraprofessional working under the supervision of an SLP, is required. The intervention should be carefully designed to specifically target gaps in the child's repertoire of language and literacy skills.

Reading and spelling deficits usually arise from a core deficit in phonological processing. Older children will require continued attention to phonological awareness but combined with intensive phonics instruction. The inclusion of activities to enhance morphological awareness may also help. Randomized controlled trials suggest that a multisensory approach to the mapping of phonological and orthographic representations is effective (Joly-Pottuz, Mercier, Leynaud, & Habib, 2008; Porkorni, Worthington, & Jamison, 2004; Wise, Ring, & Olson, 1999). The Lindamood Phoneme Sequencing Program promotes phonological awareness in older children with reading impairments and this program appears to be especially well suited to children with severe and persistent speech impairments. This program explicitly teaches awareness of the articulatory gestures associated with phonemes as well as relationships between phonemes in terms of place and manner of articulation. This knowledge is then incorporated into analytical exercises that target letter-sound relationships, manipulation of sounds within words, and spelling-sound patterns. There is evidence that a focus on phoneme manipulation tasks can be helpful for children with apraxia of speech when the outcomes are speech accuracy and phonological awareness (Moriarty & Gillon, 2006).

Phonics instruction is a systematic approach to teaching children the alphabetic principle and the correspondence between spelling patterns and sounds. A phonics intervention that has been shown to be effective with 7- to 10-year-old children with poor reading skills is the Word Building program (Beck, 2018). This program has the goal of improving the quality of the child's orthographic and phonological representations by forcing the child to attend to each letter in the printed word. A series of progressively ordered lessons build words from the CVC through the CCCVCC word shapes, with separate units for different word families (e.g., short vowels, long vowels). The child forms words with letter cards: inserting, deleting, and exchanging cards according to instructions provided by a tutor. Each new word is read by the child with support as needed from the tutor. In a small sample randomized controlled trial, McCandliss, Beck, Sandak, and Perfetti (2003) found that children demonstrated statistically and clinically significant gains in phonological awareness, nonword decoding, real word reading, and reading comprehension, relative to a no-treatment control group, after 20 one-hour lessons provided during the summer break from school.

Children with speech and language impairments may also benefit from interventions to improve **morphological awareness**, that is, awareness of morphemes, the minimal units of meaning in words. Four types of morphemes are used to create words, with the root morpheme being the base form: **root morphemes** can be a word by itself ("dog," "teach," "happy"). Bound morphemes can be joined to a root morpheme to make a more complex word: **prefixes** change

meaning but not grammatical class, as in "unhappy"; **suffixes** change meaning and grammatical class as in "teacher"; and **inflections** provide information about grammatical categories such as number and verb tense, as in "dogs" or "teaching." Often when root and bound morphemes are combined, there are phonological consequences: for example, "divide" and "division" involve a different pronunciation of the second "i." Furthermore, root morphemes may be spelled differently when bound morphemes are added, as in the extra "n" in the word "funnier." Morphological awareness predicts future development of vocabulary, reading, and spelling skills (Sparks & Deacon, 2013; Wolter, Wood, & D'zatko, 2009). Some interventions are being developed to teach children the relationship between spelling patterns and the morphological structure of words. The effectiveness of these interventions in comparison to phonological awareness and phonics instruction is not yet clear, however, as the studies are yielding mixed results (Arnbak & Elbro, 2000; Wolter & Dilworth, 2013; Kirk & Gillon, 2009).

Spelling can be taught directly, using a variety of multisensory techniques to support the acquisition of difficult words; these techniques include visualizing words with eyes closed before writing them, tracing words before writing from memory, and pronouncing words and spelling out loud before writing or typing the component letters. This type of practice should focus on words that will be used in the child's writing, specifically targeting those words that the child cannot spell accurately. It is important that spelling instruction for clients with speech, language, and learning disorders is fully individualized to the child's specific needs. Children with spelling difficulties will need more practice per word and more concentrated periods of study to learn new words than children who do not have learning disabilities. Therefore, therapy time and concentrated practice time should not be used to overpractice words that have already been mastered. In addition to structured practice with common orthographic and morphological patterns, the child must integrate new words into authentic reading and writing activities with support. More information about spelling interventions for SLPs is provided by Masterson and Crede (1999), Masterson and Apel (2010), and Scott (2000).

Box 8–5. Metaphonological Knowledge: Key Points

- Metaphonological knowledge involves explicit awareness of phonological units such as syllables, onsets, rimes, phonemes, and features.
- Phonological awareness intervention can be integrated into speech therapy sessions, leading to excellent outcomes for speech accuracy and emergent literacy skills.
- SLPs can support teachers in the selection and implementation of evidence-based curricula to support oral language and literacy learning in preschool classrooms.
- High-quality early years curricula include structured activities to teach vocabulary, narrative skills, phonological awareness, alphabet knowledge, and print concepts.
- Older children with past or current histories of SSDs may require individualized interventions targeting phonological awareness, morphological awareness, phonics, and spelling to succeed at school.

8.6 CONCLUSION

The way in which treatment procedures across multiple levels of phonological representation are combined must be individualized for the needs of each child. Furthermore, it is important to understand that the child's needs will change over time as maturation and therapy change the child's skill levels and the environment presents new challenges. The SLP must reconsider the child's needs at regular intervals and combine treatment components to meet those individual needs, sequentially and concurrently. A young child with a severe inconsistent phonological disorder may benefit from the combination of focused stimulation, as described in Chapter 6, to strengthen perceptual knowledge of the target words, provided concurrently with the core vocabulary approach, described in this chapter, to improve consistency in the production of those same words. A child with childhood apraxia of speech (CAS) may require the sensorimotor approach described in Chapter 7 to acquire a repertoire of motor plans for basic syllables; subsequently it is likely that the child will develop a productive phonological system consisting of common phonological patterns that will benefit from the broad-based cycles approach to phonological intervention described in this chapter; at a later age it is likely that the same child will benefit from the traditional articulation therapy approach described in Chapter 7 to remediate persistent speech errors, provided concurrently with interventions to strengthen phonological awareness, phonics, and spelling knowledge, as described in this chapter.

Children with phonological delay in particular are known to have difficulties with phonological processing as discussed in Chapter 4. Therefore, these children benefit from a combination of intervention procedures that target knowledge of acoustic-phonetic and phonological representations. Rvachew and Brosseau-Lapré (2015) obtained good results with the combination of procedures listed in Table 8–5. The treatment program was effective because the combination of procedures carefully targets the difficulties common to children with phonological delay in a coherent manner. Specifically, individual sessions during the first six weeks of the program targeted the children's acoustic-phonetic representations, using focused stimulation, auditory bombardment, and error detection tasks. The children were also taught to identify speech production errors in their own speech. When the children began to produce words containing the target structures spontaneously during speech therapy sessions, minimal pairs contrast therapy was introduced. This treatment procedure strengthened the children's knowledge of the linguistic significance of the target contrast and provided opportunities for production practice. Parents observed the sessions and completed homework activities with their

Table 8–5. *Recommended Procedures for an Input-Oriented Approach to Phonological Intervention*

Service Delivery	Treatment Procedure	Information Sources
First six weeks		
Individual sessions, provided by SLP, once weekly for 6 weeks (usually 45 minutes or 15 minutes for each of 3 phonological targets) with parent observing and home practice.	Focused stimulation	Fey et al. (2003); Chapter 6
	Ear training	Van Riper (1978); Chapter 7
	Speech perception training (SAILS)	Rvachew & Brosseau Lapré (2015); Chapter 6
	Meaningful Minimal Contrast Therapy	Weiner (1981); Chapter 8
Second six weeks		
Parent administered program provided daily with 6 once weekly training sessions provided to small groups of parents.	Dialogic Reading Home Program	Whitehurst et al. (1988); Chapter 6
Administered by paraprofessionals or student SLPs, once weekly for 6 weeks, to small groups of children.	Phonological Awareness Groups (Sound Foundations)	Byrne & Fielding-Barnsley (1991); Chapter 8

Note. These are the procedures that were used in the Essai Clinique Randomisé sur les Interventions Phonologiques (Randomized Clinical Trial of Phonological Interventions; ECRIP trial) as described in Rvachew and Brosseau-Lapré (2015).

children. During the second six weeks the children received a small group phonological awareness intervention modeled on the Sound Foundations program, targeting awareness of syllables, onsets, and rimes. Concurrently, parents were taught to use dialogic reading techniques at home during shared storybook reading to teach new vocabulary and highlight phonological awareness. This study shows that it is possible to provide an intervention that meets children's multiple needs in an efficient manner because these treatment components can be delivered over a 12-week period by a combination of providers, including individual speech therapy provided by an SLP, group therapy provided by paraprofessionals, and a supported home program component. With creativity and an understanding of the foundations of speech pathology practice, the SLP can provide an efficient and evidence-based speech therapy program to every child with an SSD.

Chapter 8 Study Questions

Question 1. Answer the following short-answer questions regarding the core vocabulary approach:

a. This core vocabulary approach is meant for children with which diagnosis?

b. What are the criteria that are used to select targets when implementing this approach?

c. What is the level of processing targeted by the procedures used in this approach?

d. Describe four teaching procedures that are used during a speech therapy session when implementing this approach.

e. What is the primary purpose of these teaching procedures?

Question 2. Answer the following short-answer questions regarding the cycles remediation approach:

a. This cycles remediation approach is best suited to children with which diagnosis or diagnoses?

b. What are the criteria used to select target patterns (intermediate goals) and target words (specific goals) when implementing this approach?

c. What levels of representation are targeted by the procedures used in this approach?

d. What are the procedures used during each treatment session when implementing this approach?

e. What kind of homework exercises should be assigned each week when implementing this approach?

Question 3. Answer the following short-answer questions regarding the method of meaningful minimal pairs:

a. The method of meaningful minimal pairs is best suited to children with which diagnosis or diagnoses?

b. What are the criteria used to select target patterns (intermediate goals) and target words (specific goals) when implementing this approach?

c. What level of representation is targeted by the method of meaningful minimal pairs?

d. What are the procedures used during each treatment session when implementing the method of meaningful minimal pairs?

Question 4. Answer the following short-answer questions regarding phonological awareness interventions:

a. Phonological awareness interventions are best suited to children with which diagnosis or diagnoses?

b. What is the best age to integrate phonological awareness treatment procedures into speech therapy sessions?

c. Describe some procedures for improving awareness of syllables, onsets, and rimes.

REFERENCES

Adler, S. (1984). *Cultural language differences: Their educational and professional implications.* Springfield, IL: Charles C. Thomas.

Allen, M. M. (2013). Intervention efficacy and intensity for children with Speech Sound Disorder. *Journal of Speech, Language, and Hearing Research, 56*(3), 865–877.

Almost, D., & Rosenbaum, P. (1998). Effectiveness of speech intervention for phonological disorders: A randomized controlled trial. *Developmental Medicine and Child Neurology, 40,* 319–325.

Alwan, A., Narayanan, S., & Haker, K. (1997). Toward articulatory-acoustic models for liquid approximants based on MRI and EPG data. Part II. The rhotics. *Journal of the Acoustical Society of America, 101,* 1078–1089.

American Speech-Language-Hearing Association. (1996). *Inclusive practices for children and youths with communication disorders* [Technical Report]. Available from www.asha.org/policy

American Speech-Language-Hearing Association. (1997–2018a). *Central auditory processing disorder.* ASHA Practice Portal, http://www.asha.org/practice-portal/clinical-topics/central-auditory-processing-disorder/

American Speech-Language-Hearing Association. (1997–2018b). *Childhood hearing screening.* http://www.asha.org/practice-portal/professional-issues/childhood-hearing-screening/

American Speech-Language-Hearing Association. (2002). *Childhood apraxia of speech* [Technical Report]. Retrieved from http://www.asha.org/docs/html/TR2007-00278.html#r8

American Speech-Language-Hearing Association. (2009). *Prekindergarten NOMS Fact Sheet: Does treatment time affect SLP outcomes in preschoolers?* NOMS National Data Reports and Fact Sheets. Retrieved from http://www.asha.org/members/research/noms/noms_data.htm

American Speech-Language-Hearing Association. (2010a). *Cultural competence checklist—personal reflection.* Available from https://www.asha.org/uploadedFiles/Cultural-Competence-Checklist-Personal-Reflection.pdf

American Speech-Language-Hearing Association. (2010b). *Cultural competence checklist—policies and procedures.* Available from https://www.asha.org/uploadedFiles/Cultural-Competence-Checklist-Policies-Procedures.pdf

American Speech-Language-Hearing Association. (2010c). *Cultural competence checklist—service delivery.* Available from https://www.asha.org/uploadedFiles/Cultural-Competence-Checklist-Service-Delivery.pdf

American Speech-Language-Hearing Association. (2011). *National Outcome Measurement System (NOMS) for Pre-Kindergarten.* Rockville Pike, MD.

American Speech-Language-Hearing Association. (2013). *Speech-language pathology assistant scope of practice* [Scope of Practice]. Available from www.asha.org/policy

American Speech-Language-Hearing Association. (2017). *Issues in ethics: Cultural and linguistic competence.* Available from www.asha.org/Practice/ethics/Cultural-and-Linguistic-Competence/

American Speech-Language-Hearing Association. (2018). *Childhood fluency disorders.* ASHA Practice Portal. https://www.asha.org/Practice-Portal/Clinical-Topics/Childhood-Fluency-Disorders/

Anthony, J. L., Aghara, R., Dunkelberger, M., Anthony, T. I., Williams, J. M., & Zhang, Z. (2011). What factors place children with Speech Sound Disorders at risk for reading problems? *American Journal of Speech-Language Pathology, 20,* 146–160.

Arnbak, E., & Elbro, C. (2000). The effects of morphological awareness training on the reading and spelling skills of young dyslexics. *Scandinavian Journal of Educational Research, 44*(3), 229–251.

Baker, E. (2010). Minimal pair intervention. In A. L. Williams, S. McLeod, & R. J. McCauley (Eds.), *Interventions for speech sound disorders in children* (pp. 41–72). Baltimore, MD: Brookes.

Baker, E., Croot, K., McLeod, S., & Paul, R. (2001). Psycholinguistic models of speech development and their application to clinical practice. *Journal of Speech, Language, and Hearing Research, 44,* 685–702.

Baker, L., & Cantwell, D. P. (1982). Developmental, social and behavioral characteristics of speech and language disordered children. *Child Psychiatry and Human Development, 12,* 195–206.

Baker, L., & Cantwell, D. P. (1987). A prospective psychiatric follow-up of children with speech/language disorders. *Journal of the American Academy of Child and Adolescent Psychiatry, 26*(4), 546–553.

Ball, M. J., Müller, N., & Rutter, B. (2010). *Phonology for communication disorders.* New York, NY: Psychology Press.

Bankson, N., & Bernthal, J. E. (1990). *Bankson-Bernthal Test of Phonology.* Austin, TX: Pro-Ed.

Bankson, N., & Bernthal, J. (2004). Etiology/factors related to phonologic disorders. In J. E. Bernthal & N. W. Bankson (Eds.), *Articulation and phonological disorders* (pp. 139–200). Boston, MA: Allyn & Bacon.

Barlow, J. A., & Gierut, J. A. (2002). Minimal pair approaches to phonological remediation. *Seminars in Speech and Language, 23*(1), 57–67.

Barratt, J., Littlejohns, P., & Thompson, J. (1992). Trial of intensive compared with weekly speech therapy in preschool children. *Archives of Disease in Childhood, 67,* 106–108.

Beck, I. L. (2018). *Word building.* Retrieved from https://www.education.pitt.edu/Education alResources/Teachers/LEADERS/Teaching Strategies/WordBuilding.aspx

Beitchman, J. H., Nair, R., Clegg, M., Patel, P. G., Ferguson, B., Pressman, E., & Smith, A. (1986). Prevalence of speech and language disorders in 5-year-old kindergarten children in the Ottawa-Carleton region. *Journal of Speech and Hearing Disorders, 51,* 98–110.

Bennett, K. E., & Haggard, M. P. (1999). Behavior and cognitive outcomes from middle ear disease. *Archives of Disease in Childhood, 80,* 28–35.

Bernhardt, B., Gick, B., Bacsfalvi, P., & Adler-Bock, M. (2005). Ultrasound in speech therapy with adolescents and adults. *Clinical Linguistics & Phonetics, 19*(6/7), 605–617.

Bernhardt, B., & Major, E. M. (2005). Speech, language and literacy skills three years later: A follow-up study of early phonological and metaphonological intervention. *International Journal of Language and Communication Disorders, 40,* 1–27.

Bernhardt, B., & Stemberger, J. P. (1998). *Handbook of phonological development from the perspective of constraint-based phonology.* San Diego, CA: Academic Press.

Bernhardt, B., & Stemberger, J. P. (2000). *Workbook in nonlinear phonology for clinical application.* Austin, TX: Pro-Ed.

Bernhardt, B., & Stemberger, J. P. (2002). Intervocalic consonants in the speech of English-speaking Canadian children with phonological disorders. *Clinical Linguistics & Phonetics, 16,* 199–214.

Bernhardt, B., Stemberger, J. P., & Major, E. M. (2006). General and nonlinear phonological intervention perspectives for a child with resistent phonological impairment. *Advances in Speech-Language Pathology, 8,* 190–206.

Bernhardt, B. M., & Holdgrafer, G. (2001). Beyond the basics I: The need for strategic sampling for in-depth phonological analysis. *Language, Speech and Hearing Services in Schools, 32,* 18–27.

Beukelman, D. R., & Mirenda, P. (2013). *Augmentative and alternative communication: Supporting children and adults with complex communication needs* (4th ed.). Baltimore, MD: Brookes.

Bird, J., Bishop, D. V. M., & Freeman, N. H. (1995). Phonological awareness and literacy development in children with expressive phonological impairments. *Journal of Speech and Hearing Research, 38,* 446–462.

Bishop, D. V. M., Snowling, M. J., Thompson, P. A., Greenhalgh, T., & CATALISE-2 consortium. (2017). Phase 2 of CATALISE: A multinational and multidisciplinary Delphi consensus study of problems with language development: Terminology. *Journal of Child Psychology and Psychiatry, 58*(10), 1068–1080.

Blache, S. E., & Parsons, C. L. (1980). A linguistic approach to distinctive feature training. *Lan-*

guage, Speech and Hearing Services in Schools, *11,* 203–207.

Blakeley, R. W., & Brockman, J. H. (1995). Normal speech and hearing by age 5 as a goal for children with cleft palate: A demonstration project. *American Journal of Speech-Language Pathology, 4*(1), 25–32.

Bleile, K. (2002). Evaluating articulation and phonological disorders when the clock is running. *American Journal of Speech-Language Pathology, 11,* 243–249.

Blood, G. W., Ridenour, V. J. J., Qualls, C. D., & Hammer, C. S. (2003). Co-occuring disorders in children who stutter. *Journal of Communication Disorders, 36,* 427–448.

Bloom, K. (1988). Quality of adult vocalizations affects the quality of infant vocalizations. *Journal of Child Language, 15*(3), 469–480.

Bountress, N. G., Sever, J. C., & Williams, J. (1989). Relationship between two nontraditional procedures for assessing speech-sound discrimination. *Perceptual and Motor Skills, 69,* 499–503.

Bowen, C., & Cupples, L. (2006). PACT: Parents and children together in phonological therapy. *Advances in Speech Language Pathology, 8*(3), 282–292.

Bradford, A., & Dodd, B. (1996). Do all speech disordered children have motor deficits? *Clinical Linguistics & Phonetics, 10,* 77–101.

Broomfield, J., & Dodd, B. (2004). The nature of referred subtypes of primary speech disability. *Child Language and Teaching Therapy, 20*(2), 135–151.

Bus, A. G., Van Ijzendoorn, M. H., & Pellegrini, A. D. (1995). Joint book reading makes for success in learning to read: A meta-analysis on intergenerational transmission of literacy. *Review of Educational Research, 65,* 1–21.

Byrne, B., & Fielding-Barnsley, R. (1991). Evaluation of a program to teach phonemic awareness to young children. *Journal of Educational Psychology, 83*(4), 451–455.

Campbell, T. F. (1999). Functional treatment outcomes in young children with motor speech disorders. In A. Caruso & E. A. Strand (Eds.), *Clinical management of motor speech disorders in children* (pp. 385–395). New York, NY: Thieme Medical.

Campbell, T. F., Dollaghan, C. A., Rockette, H. E., Paradise, J. L., Feldman, H. M., Shriberg, L. D., . . . Kurs-Lasky, M. (2003). Risk factors for speech delay of unknown origin in 3-year-old children. *Child Development, 74,* 346–357.

Cantwell, D. P., & Baker, L. (1987). Prevalence and type of psychiatric disorder and developmental disorders in three speech and language groups. *Journal of Communication Disorders, 20*(2), 151–160.

Catts, H. W. (1993). The relationship between speech-language impairments and reading disabilities. *Journal of Speech and Hearing Research, 36,* 948–958.

Catts, H. W., Fey, M. E., Zhang, X., & Tomblin, J. B. (2001). Estimating the risk of future reading difficulties in kindergarten children: A research-based model and its clinical implementation. *Language, Speech, and Hearing Services in Schools, 32,* 38–50.

Cheour, M., Ceponiene, R., Lehtokoski, A., Luuk, A., Allik, J., Alho, K., & Näätänen, R. (1998). Development of language-specific phoneme representation in the infant brain. *Nature Neuroscience, 1,* 351–353.

Chiappe, P., Siegel, L. S., & Gottardo, A. (2002). Reading-related skills of kindergartners from diverse linguistic backgrounds. *Applied Psycholinguistics, 23*(01), 95–116.

Chomsky, N., & Halle, M. (1968). *The sound pattern of English.* New York, NY: Harper & Row.

Cirrin, F. M., Schooling, T. L., Nelson, N. W., Diehl, S. F., Flynn, P. F., Staskowski, M., . . . Adamczyk, D. F. (2010). Evidence-based systematic review: Effects of different service delivery models on communication outcomes for elementary school-age children. *Language, Speech and Hearing Services in Schools, 41*(3), 233–264.

Claessen, M., Heath, S. M., Fletcher, J., Hogben, J., & Leitão, S. (2009). Quality of phonological representations: A window into the lexicon. *International Journal of Language & Communication Disorders, 44*(2), 121–144.

Claessen, M., & Leitão, S. (2012). Phonological representations in children with SLI. *Child Language and Teaching and Therapy, 28,* 211–233.

Claessen, M., Leitão, S., & Barrett, N. (2010). Investigating children's ability to reflect on stored phonological representations: The Silent Deletion of Phonemes task. *Journal of Language & Communication Disorders, 45,* 411–423.

Coady, J. A., & Evans, J. L. (2008). Uses and interpretation of nonword repetition tasks in children with and without specific language impairments (SLI). *International Journal of Language & Communication Disorders, 43,* 1–40.

Colledge, E., Bishop, D. V. M., Koeppen-Schomerus, G., Price, T. S., Happe, F. G. E., Eley, T. C., . . . Plomin, R. (2002). The structure of language abilities at 4 years: A twin study. *Developmental Psychology, 38*(5), 749–757.

Conboy, B. T., Brooks, P., Meltzoff, A. N., & Kuhl, P. K. (2015). Social interaction in infants' learning of second-language phonetics: An exploration of brain-behavior relations. *Developmental Neuropsychology, 40*, 216–229.

Coplan, J., & Gleason, J. R. (1988). Unclear speech: Recognition and significance of unintelligible speech in preschool children. *Pediatrics, 82*, 447–452.

Costello, J., & Bosler, S. (1976). Generalization and articulation instruction. *Journal of Speech and Hearing Disorders, 41*(3), 359–373.

Crosbie, S., Holm, A., & Dodd, B. (2005). Intervention for children with severe speech disorder: A comparison of two approaches. *International Journal of Language and Communication Disorders, 40*(4), 467–491.

Dale, P. S., Crain-Thoreson, C., Notari-Synverson, A., & Cole, K. N. (1996). Parent-child book reading as an intervention technique for young children with language delays. *Topics in Early Childhool Special Education, 16*, 213–235.

Dale, P. S., & Hayden, D. A. (2013). Treating speech subsystems in childhood apraxia of speech with tactual input: The PROMPT approach. *American Journal of Speech-Language Pathology, 22*, 644–661.

Dawson, J. L., & Tattersall, P. J. (2001). *Structured Photographic Articulation Test* (2nd ed.). DeKalb, IL: Janelle.

Dean, E., & Howell, J. (1986). Developing linguistic awareness: A theoretically based approach to phonological disorders. *British Journal of Disorders of Communication, 31*, 223–238.

DeCasper, A. J., & Fifer, W. P. (1980). Of human bonding: newborns prefer their mothers' voices. *Science, 208*, 1174–1176.

Delattre, P., & Freeman, D. C. (1968). A dialect study of American r's by X-ray motion picture. *Linguistics, 44*, 29–68.

Dethorne, L. S., Johnson, C. J., Walder, L., & Mahurin-Smith, J. (2009). When "Simon Says" doesn't work: Alternatives to imitation for facilitating early speech development. *American Journal of Speech-Language Pathology, 18*, 133–145.

Diehl, R. L., Lotto, A. J., & Holt, L. L. (2004). Speech perception. *Annual Review of Psychology, 55*, 149–179.

Dodd, B. (1995). Procedures for classification of subgroups of speech disorder. In B. Dodd (Ed.), *The differential diagnoses and treatment of children with speech disorder* (pp. 49–64). San Diego, CA: Singular.

Dodd, B. (2011). Differentiating speech delay from disorder: Does it matter? *Topics in Language Disorders, 31*, 96–111.

Dodd, B. (2014). Differential diagnosis of pediatric speech sound disorder. *Current Developmental Disorders Reports, 1*(3), 189–196.

Dodd, B., & Bradford, A. (2000). A comparison of three therapy methods for children with different types of developmental disorder. *International Journal of Language and Communication Disorders, 35*(2), 189–209.

Dodd, B., & McIntosh, B. (2008). The input processing, cognitive linguistic and oro-motor skills of children with speech difficulty. *International Journal of Speech-Language Pathology, 10*, 169–178.

Dodd, B., Ttofari-Eecen, K., Brommeyer, K., Ng, K., Reilly, S., & Morgan, A. (2018). Delayed and disordered development of articulation and phonology between four and seven years. *Child Language Teaching and Therapy, 34*(2), 87–99.

Dodd, B., Zhu, H., Crosbie, S., Holm, A., & Ozanne, A. (2006). *Diagnostic Evaluation of Articulation and Phonology (DEAP)*. London, UK: Pearson Education.

Dollaghan, C. A., & Campbell, T. F. (1998). Nonword repetition and child language impairment. *Journal of Speech, Language, and Hearing Research, 41*, 1136–1146.

Dworkin, J. P. (1980). Characteristics of frontal lispers clustered according to severity. *Journal of Speech and Hearing Disorders, 55*, 37–44.

Dworkin, J. P., & Culatta, R. A. (1980). Tongue strength: Its relationship to tongue thrusting, open-bite, and articulatory proficiency. *Journal of Speech and Hearing Disorders, 45*(2), 277–282.

Ehren, B. J., & Ehren, T. C. (2001). New or expanded literacy roles for speech-language pathologists: Making it happen in the schools. *Seminars in Speech and Language, 22*, 233–243.

Ehri, L. C., Nunes, S. R., Willows, D. M., Schuster, B. V., Yaghoub-Zadeh, Z., & Shanahan, T. (2001). Phonemic awareness instruction helps children learn to read: Evidence from the national reading panel's meta-analysis. *Reading Research Quarterly, 36*(3), 250–287.

Eicher, J. D., Stein, C. M., Deng, F., Ciesla, A. A., Powers, N. R., Boada, R., . . . Gruen, J. R. (2015). The DYX2 locus and neurochemical signaling genes contribute to speech sound disorder and related neurocognitive domains. *Genes, Brain and Behavior, 14*(4), 377–385.

Eilers, R. E., & Oller, D. (1994). Infant vocalizations and the early diagnosis of severe hearing impairment. *Journal of Pediatrics, 124*(2), 199–203.

Eiserman, W. D., Weber, C., & McCoun, M. (1995). Parent and professional roles in early intervention: A longitudinal comparison of the effects of two intervention configurations. *Journal of Special Education, 28*, 20–44.

Eising, E., Carrion-Castillo, A., Vino, A., Strand, E. A., Jakielski, K. J., Scerri, T. S., . . . Fisher, S. E. (2018). A set of regulatory genes co-expressed in embryonic human brain is implicated in disrupted speech development. *Molecular Psychiatry*, 1–14. doi:10.1038/s41380-018-0020-x

Elbert, M., Dinnsen, D. A., & Powell, T. W. (1984). On the prediction of phonological generalization learning patterns. *Journal of Speech and Hearing Disorders, 49*, 309–317.

Elbert, M., Dinnsen, D. A., Swartzlander, P., & Chin, S. B. (1990). Generalization to conversational speech. *Journal of Speech and Hearing Disorders, 55*, 694–699.

Elbert, M., & McReynolds, L. V. (1985). The generalization hypothesis: Final consonant deletion. *Language and Speech, 28*, 281–294.

Elbert, M., Powell, T. W., & Swartzlander, P. (1991). Toward a technology of generalization: How many exemplars are sufficient? *Journal of Speech and Hearing Research, 34*, 81–87.

Ertmer, D. J., & Nathani Iyer, S. (2012). Prelinguistic vocalizations in infants and toddlers with hearing loss: Identifying and stimulating auditory-guided speech development. In M. Marschark & P. E. Spencer (Eds.), *Identifying and stimulating auditory-guided speech development*. Oxford Handbooks Online. Oxford University Press. Retrieved from http://www.oxfordhandbooks.com/view/10.1093/oxfordhb/9780195390032.001.0001/oxfordhb-9780195390032-e-024

Esling, J. (2015). iPA Phonetics (version 1.1) [Mobile application software]. Retrieved from http://itunes.apple.com

Fairbanks, G., & Bebout, B. (1950). A study of minor organic deviations in 'functional' disorders of articulation: 3. The tongue. *Journal of Speech and Hearing Disorders, 15*, 348–352.

Feldman, H. M., Dollaghan, C. A., Campbell, T. F., Colborn, D. K., Janosky, J., Kurs-Lasky, M., . . . Paradise, J. L. (2003). Parent-reported language skills in relation to otitis media during the first 3 years of life. *Journal of Speech, Language, and Hearing Research, 46*, 273–287.

Felsenfeld, S., Broen, P. A., & McGue, M. (1994). A 28-year follow-up of adults with a history of moderate phonological disorder: Educational and occupational results. *Journal of Speech and Hearing Research, 37*, 1341–1353.

Fey, M. E. (1992). Articulation and phonology: An addendum. *Language, Speech, and Hearing Services in Schools, 23*, 277–282.

Fey, M. E., Cleave, P. L., & Long, S. H. (1997). Two models of grammar facilitation in children with language impairments: Phase 2. *Journal of Speech, Language, and Hearing Research, 40*, 5–19.

Fey, M. E., Long, S. H., & Finestack, L. H. (2003). Ten principles of grammar facilitation for children with specific language impairments. *American Journal of Speech-Language Pathology, 12*(1), 3–15.

Fletcher, S. G. (1972). Time-by-count measurement of diadochokinetic syllable rate. *Journal of Speech and Hearing Research, 15*, 763–770.

Flipsen, J. P., & Ogiela, D. A. (2015). Psychometric characteristics of single-word tests of children's speech sound production. *Language, Speech, and Hearing Services in Schools*, 1–13.

Flowers, H., Girolametto, L., Weitzman, E., & Greenberg, J. (2007). Promoting early literacy skills: Effects of in-service education for early childhood educators. *Canadian Journal of Speech-Language Pathology and Audiology, 31*, 6–18.

Forrest, K., Dinnsen, D. A., & Elbert, M. (1997). Impact of substitution patterns on phonological learning by misarticulating children. *Clinical Linguistics & Phonetics, 11*, 63–76.

Forrest, K., Elbert, M., & Dinnsen, D. A. (2000). The effect of substitution patterns on phonological treatment outcomes. *Clinical Linguistics & Phonetics, 14*, 519–531.

Fox, A. V., & Dodd, B. (2001). Phonologically disordered German-speaking children. *American Journal of Speech-Language Pathology, 10*, 291–307.

Francis, D. J., Fletcher, J. M., Shaywitz, B. A., Shaywitz, S. E., & Rourke, B. P. (1996). Defining learning and language disabilities: Conceptual and psychometric issues with the use of IQ tests. *Language, Speech and Hearing Services in Schools, 27,* 132–143.

Fucci, D. (1972). Oral vibrotactile sensation: An evaluation of normal and defective speakers. *Journal of Speech and Hearing Research, 15,* 179–184.

Fucci, D., Petrosino, L., Underwood, G., & Kendal, C. (1992). Differences in lingual vibrotactile threshold shifts during magitude-estimation scaling between normal-speaking children and children with articulation problems. *Perceptual and Motor Skills, 75,* 495–504.

Fudala, J. B. (2000). *Arizona Articulation Proficiency Scale—Third Edition.* Los Angeles, CA: Western Psychological Services.

Gathercole, S., & Baddeley, A. (1996). *Children's Test of Nonword Repetition (CNRep).* London, UK: Psychological Corporation.

Gerken, L. (2009). *Language development.* San Diego, CA: Plural.

Gibbon, F. E. (1999). Undifferentiated lingual gestures in children with articulation/phonological disorders. *Journal of Speech, Language, and Hearing Research, 42,* 382–397.

Gick, B., Allen, B., Roewer-Després, F., & Stavness, I. (2017). Speaking tongues are actively braced. *Journal of Speech, Language, and Hearing Research, 60*(3), 494–506.

Gierut, J., Morrisette, M. L., & Ziemer, S. M. (2010). Nonwords and generalization in children with phonological disorders. *American Journal of Speech-Language Pathology, 19,* 167–177.

Gierut, J. A. (1986). On the assessment of productive phonological knowledge. *Journal of the National Student Speech-Language-Hearing Association, 14,* 83–100.

Gierut, J. A. (1998). Treatment efficacy: Functional phonological disorders in children. *Journal of Speech, Language, and Hearing Research, 41,* S85–S100.

Gierut, J. A., Morrisette, M. L., Hughes, M. T., & Rowlands, S. (2001). Phonological treatment efficacy and developmental norms. *Language, Speech, and Hearing Services in Schools, 27,* 215–230.

Gildersleeve-Neumann, C. E. (2007, November 6). Treatment for childhood apraxia of speech. *The ASHA Leader.* Retrieved from http://www.asha.org/Publications/leader/2007/071106/f071106a.htm

Gill, C., Mehta, J., Fredenburg, K., & Bartlett, K. (2011). Imitation therapy for non-verbal toddlers. *Child Language Teaching & Therapy, 27*(1), 97–108.

Gillon, G. T. (2000). The efficacy of phonological awareness intervention for children with spoken language impairment. *Language, Speech, and Hearing Services in Schools, 31,* 126–141.

Gillon, G. T. (2005). Facilitating phoneme awareness development in 3- and 4-year-old children with speech impairment. *Language, Speech, and Hearing Services in Schools, 36,* 308–324.

Girolametto, L., Pearce, P. S., & Weitzman, E. (1997). Effects of lexical intervention on the phonology of late talkers. *Journal of Speech, Language, and Hearing Research, 40*(2), 338–348.

Girolametto, L., Weitzman, E., & Greenberg, J. (2003). Training day care staff to facilitate children's language. *American Journal of Speech-Language Pathology, 12*(3), 299–311.

Glaspey, A. M., & MacLeod, A. A. N. (2010). A multi-dimensional approach to gradient change in phonological acquisition: A case study of disordered speech development. *Clinical Linguistics & Phonetics, 24*(4–5), 283–299.

Glaspey, A. M., & Stoel-Gammon, C. (2007). A dynamic approach to phonological assessment. *Advances in Speech Language Pathology, 9,* 286–296.

Glogowska, M., Roulstone, S., Enderby, P., & Peters, T. (2000). Randomised controlled trial of community based speech and language therapy in preschool children. *British Medical Journal, 321,* 923–928.

Glogowska, M., Roulstone, S., Peters, T. J., & Enderby, P. (2006). Early speech- and language-impaired children: Linguistic, literacy, and social outcomes. *Developmental Medicine and Child Neurology, 48,* 489–494.

Goldman, R., & Fristoe, M. (2015). *Goldman Fristoe Test of Articulation—Third Edition.* Minneapolis, MN: Pearson Assessments.

Goldstein, B. A. (2004). *Bilingual language development and disorders in Spanish-English speakers.* Baltimore, MD: Brookes.

Goldstein, B. A., Fabiano, L., & Washington, P. S. (2005). Phonological skills in predominantly English-speaking, predominantly Spanish-speaking, and Spanish-English bilingual children. *Language, Speech, and Hearing Services in Schools, 36,* 201–218.

Goldstein, H., Fabiano, L., & Iglesias, A. (2004). Spontaneous and imitated productions in Spanish-speaking children with phonological disorders. *Language, Speech, and Hearing Services in Schools, 35,* 5–15.

Goozée, J. V., Murdoch, B., Ozanne, A., Cheng, Y., Hill, A., & Gibbon, F. (2007). Lingual kinematics and coordination in speech-disordered children exhibiting differentiated versus undifferentiated lingual gestures. *International Journal of Language & Communication Disorders, 42,* 703–724.

Gordon-Brannan, M. (1994). Assessing intelligibility: Children's expressive phonologies. *Topics in Language Disorders, 14,* 17–25.

Gough, P. B., & Tunmer, W. E. (1986). Decoding, reading, and reading disability. *Remedial and Special Education, 7,* 6–10.

Graham, L. W., & House, A. S. (1971). Phonological oppositions in children: A perceptual study. *Journal of the Acoustical Society of America, 49*(2B), 559–566.

Graham, S. A., & Fisher, S. E. (2015). Understanding language from a genomic perspective. *Annual Review of Genetics, 49*(1), 131–160.

Gray, S. (2006). The relationship between phonological memory, receptive vocabulary, and fast mapping in young children with specific language impairment. *Journal of Speech, Language, and Hearing Research, 49,* 955–969.

Grunwell, P. (1981). *The nature of phonological disability in children.* London, UK: Academic Press.

Grunwell, P. (1987). *Clinical phonology* (2nd ed.). London, UK: Chapman Hall.

Grunwell, P. (1992). Processes of phonological change in developmental speech disorders. *Clinical Linguistics & Phonetics, 6,* 101–122.

Guadagnoli, M., Holcomb, W., & Davis, M. (2002). The efficacy of video feedback for learning the golf swing. *Journal of Sports Sciences, 20*(8), 615–622.

Guadagnoli, M. A., & Lee, T. D. (2004). Challenge point: A framework for conceptualizing the effects of various practice conditions in motor learning. *Journal of Motor Behavior, 36,* 212–224.

Günther, T., & Hautvast, S. (2010). Addition of contingency management to increase home practice in children with speech sound disorder. *International Journal of Language & Communication Disorders, 45,* 345–353.

Harm, M. W., McCandliss, B. D., & Seidenberg, M. S. (2003). Modeling the successes and failures of interventions for disabled readers. *Scientific Studies of Reading, 7*(2), 155–182.

Haskill, A. M., & Tyler, A. A. (2007). A comparison of linguistic profiles in subgroups of children with specific langauge impairment. *American Journal of Speech-Language Pathology, 16,* 209–221.

Hauner, K. K. Y., Shriberg, L. D., Kwiatkowski, J., & Allen, C. T. (2005). A subtype of speech delay associated with developmental psychosocial involvement. *Journal of Speech, Language, and Hearing Research, 48,* 635–650.

Hayden, D., & Square, P. (1999). *Verbal Motor Production Assessment for Children.* San Antonio, TX: Psychological Corporation.

Healy, T. J., & Madison, C. L. (1987). Articulation error migration: A comparison of single word and connected speech samples. *Journal of Communication Disorders, 20,* 129–136.

Hearnshaw, S., Baker, E., & Munro, N. (2018). The speech perception skills of children with and without speech sound disorder. *Journal of Communication Disorders, 71,* 61–71.

Hesketh, A., Adams, C., Nightingale, C., & Hall, R. (2000). Phonological awareness therapy and articulatory training approaches for children with phonological disorders: a comparative outcome study. *International Journal of Language and Communication Disorders, 35*(3), 337–354.

Hetrick, R. D., & Sommers, R. K. (1988). Unisensory and bisensory processing skills of children having misarticulations and normally speaking peers. *Journal of Speech and Hearing Research, 31,* 575–581.

Hillenbrand, J., Minifie, F. D., & Edwards, T. J. (1979). Tempo of spectrum change as a cue in speech-sound discrimination by infants. *Journal of Speech and Hearing Research, 22*(1), 147–165.

Hind, S. (2006). Survey of care pathway for auditory processing disorder. *Audiological Medicine, 4,* 12–24.

Hindson, B., Byrne, B., Fielding-Barnsley, R., Hine, D. W., & Shankweiler, D. (2005). Assessment and early instruction of preschool children at risk for reading disability. *Journal of Educational Psychology, 97*(4), 687–704.

Hodson, B. W. (1989). Phonological remediaton: A cycles approach. In N. A. Creaghead, P. W. Newman, & W. A. Secord (Eds.), *Assessment and remediation of articulatory and phonological disorders* (2nd ed.). New York, NY: Macmillan.

Hodson, B. W. (2004). *Hodson Assessment of Phonological Patterns—Third Edition.* Austin, TX: Pro-Ed.

Hodson, B. W. (2007). *Evaluating and enhancing children's phonological systems: Resarch and theory to practice*. Wichita, KS: Phonocomp.

Hodson, B. W. (2011). Enhancing phonological patterns of young children with highly un-intelligible speech. *The ASHA Leader, 16*, 16–19.

Hodson, B. W., & Paden, E. P. (1983). *Targeting intelligible speech: A phonological approach to remediation*. Boston, MA: College Hill.

Hodson, B. W., Sherz, J. A., & Strattman, K. H. (2002). Evaluating communicative abilities of a highly unintelligible preschooler. *American Journal of Speech-Language Pathology, 11*(3), 236–242.

Hoffman, P. R., Daniloff, R. G., Bengoa, D., & Schuckers, G. (1985). Misarticulating and normally articulating children's identification and discrimination of synthetic [r] and [w]. *Journal of Speech and Hearing Disorders, 50*, 46–53.

Hoffman, P. R., Stager, S., & Daniloff, R. G. (1983). Perception and production of misarticulated /r/. *Journal of Speech and Hearing Disorders, 48*(2), 210–215.

Höhle, B., Pauen, S., Hesse, V., & Weissenborn, J. (2014). Discrimination of rhythmic pattern at 4 months and language performance at 5 years: A longitudinal analysis of data from German-learning children. *Language Learning, 64*(s2), 141–164.

Holm, A., Crosbie, S., & Dodd, B. (2013). Treating inconsistent speech disorder. In B. Dodd (Ed.), *Differential diagnosis and treatment of children with speech disorders* (pp. 182–201). Hoboken, NJ: Wiley.

Holm, A., Dodd, B., Stow, C., & Pert, S. (1999). Identification and differential diagnosis of phonological disorder in bilingual children. *Language Testing, 16*(3), 271–292.

Holm, A., Farrier, F., & Dodd, B. (2007). Phonological awareness, reading accuracy and spelling ability of children with inconsistent phonological disorder. *International Journal of Language & Communication Disorders, 43*, 300–322.

Hurtado, N., Grüter, T., Marchman, V. A., & Fernald, A. (2014). Relative language exposure, processing efficiency and vocabulary in Spanish–English bilingual toddlers. *Bilingualism: Language and Cognition, 17*, 189–202.

Hustad, K. C. (2012). Speech intelligibility in children with speech disorders. *Perspectives on Language Learning and Education, 19*, 7–11.

Imada, T., Zhang, Y., Cheour, M., Taulu, S., Ahonen, A., & Kuhl, P. K. (2006). Infant speech perception activates Broca's area: A developmental magnetoencephalography study. *Neuroreport, 17*, 957–962.

Iuzzini, J., & Forrest, K. (2010). Evaluation of a combined treatment approach for childhood apraxia of speech. *Clinical Linguistics & Phonetics, 24*, 335–345.

Jacewicz, E., & Fox, R. A. (2014). The effects of indexical and phonetic variation on vowel perception in typically developing 9- to 12-year-old children. *Journal of Speech, Language, and Hearing Research*, 1–17.

Jacoby, G. P., Levin, L., Lee, L., Creaghead, N. A., & Kummer, A. W. (2002). The number of individual treatment units necessary to facilitate functional communication improvements in the speech and language of young children. *American Journal of Speech-Language Pathology, 11*, 370–390.

Joanisse, M. F., Manis, F. R., Keating, P., & Seidenberg, M. S. (2000). Language deficits in dyslexic children: Speech perception, phonology, and morphology. *Journal of Experimental Child Psychology, 77*, 30–60.

Johnson-Root, B. A. (2015). *Oral-facial evaluation for speech-language pathologists*. San Diego, CA: Plural.

Johnson, C. J., Beitchman, J. H., Escobar, M., Atkinson, L., Wilson, B., Brownlee, E. B., . . . Wang, M. (1999). Fourteen-year follow-up of children with and without speech/language impairments: Speech/language stability and outcomes. *Journal of Speech, Language, and Hearing Research, 42*, 744–760.

Johnston, S. S., Reichle, J., & Evans, J. (2004). Supporting augmentative and alternative communication use by beginning communicators with severe disabilities. *American Journal of Speech-Language Pathology, 13*(1), 20–30.

Joly-Pottuz, B., Mercier, M., Leynaud, A., & Habib, M. (2008). Combined auditory and articulatory training improves phonological deficit in children with dyslexia. *Neuropsychological Rehabilitation, 18*(4), 402–429.

Jusczyk, P. W., & Thompson, E. (1978). Perception of a phonetic contrast in multisyllabic utterances by 2-month-old infants. *Perception & Psychophysics, 23*(2), 105–109.

Justice, L. M. (2006). Evidence-based practice, response to intervention, and the prevention of reading difficulties. *Language, Speech and Hearing Services in Schools, 37*, 284–297.

Justice, L. M., Chow, S., Capellini, C., Flanigan, K., & Colton, S. (2003). Emergent literacy intervention for vulnerable preschoolers: Relative effects of two approaches. *American Journal of Speech-Language Pathology, 12,* 320–332.

Kaderavek, J. N., & Justice, L. M. (2002). Shared storybook reading as an intervention context: Practices and potential pitfalls. *American Journal of Speech–Language Pathology, 11,* 395–406.

Kehoe, M. (2013). *The development of prosody and prosodic structure.* New York, NY: Nova Science.

Kehoe, M. M., & Lleo, C. (2002). Intervocalic consonants in the acquisition of German: Onsets, codas or something else? *Clinical Linguistics & Phonetics, 16,* 169–182.

Keith, R. W. (2009). *Tests for auditory processing disorders for children (SCAN-3:C).* San Antonio, TX: Pearson.

Kenney, K. W., Prather, E. M., Mooney, M. A., & Jeruzal, N. C. (1984). Comparisons among three articulation sampling procedures with preschool children. *Journal of Speech and Hearing Research, 27,* 226–231.

Kent, R. D. (1997). *The speech sciences.* San Diego, CA: Singular.

Kent, R. D. (2004). The uniqueness of speech among motor systems. *Clinical Linguistics & Phonetics, 18,* 495–505.

Khan, L. M., & Lewis, N. P. (2015). *Khan-Lewis Phonological Analysis—Third Edition.* Circle Pines, MN: American Guidance Services.

Kirk, C., & Gillon, G. T. (2009). Integrated morphological awareness intervention as a tool for improving literacy. *Language, Speech, and Hearing Services in Schools, 40,* 341–351.

Klein, E. S. (1996). Phonological/traditional approaches to articulation therapy: A retrospective group comparison. *Language, Speech, and Hearing Services in Schools, 27*(4), 314–323.

Koegel, L. K., Koegel, R. L., & Ingham, J. C. (1986). Programming rapid generalization of correct articulation through self-monitoring procedures. *Journal of Speech and Hearing Disorders, 51*(1), 24–32.

Kronvall, E. L., & Diehl, C. F. (1952). The relationship of auditory discrimination to articulatory defects of children with no known organic impairment. *Journal of Speech and Hearing Disorders, 19,* 335–338.

Kuhl, P. K. (2004). Early language acquisition: Cracking the speech code. *Nature Reviews: Neuroscience, 5,* 831–843.

Kuhl, P. K., Conboy, B. T., Coffey-Corina, S., Padden, D., Rivera-Gaxiola, M., & Nelson, T. (2008). Phonetic learning as a pathway to language: New data and Native Language Magnet Theory Expanded (NLM-e). *Philosophical Transactions of the Royal Society, 363,* 979–1000.

Kuhl, P. K., Williams, K. A., Lacerda, F., Stevens, K. N., & Lindblom, B. (1992). Linguistic experience alters phonetic perception in infants by 6 months of age. *Science, 255,* 606–608.

Labov, W., Ash, S., & Boberg, C. (2006). *The atlas of North American English: Phonetics, phonology and sound change.* Berlin, Germany: Moutin/de Gruyter.

Ladefoged, P., & Johnson, K. (2010). *A course in phonetics* (6th ed.). Boston, MA: Wadsworth Cengage Learning.

Langdon, H. W., & Cheng, L. L. (2002). *Collaborating with interpreters and translators. A guide for communication disorders professionals.* Eau Claire, WI: Thinking Publications.

Larrivee, L. S., & Catts, H. W. (1999). Early reading achievement in children with expressive phonological disorders. *American Journal of Speech-Language Pathology, 8,* 118–128.

Law, J., Boyle, J., Harris, F., Harkness, A., & Nye, C. (2000). Prevalence and natural history of primary speech and language delay: Findings from a systematic review of the literature. *International Journal of Language & Communication Disorders, 35*(2), 165–188.

Law, J., Reilly, S., & Snow, P. C. (2013). Child speech, language and communication need re-examined in a public health context: a new direction for the speech and language therapy profession. *International Journal of Language & Communication Disorders, 48*(5), 486–496.

Lennox, M., Garvis, S., & Westerveld, M. (2017). Listening to the voices of education professionals involved in implementing oral language and early literacy program in the classroom. *Australian Journal of Teacher Education, 42*(8, Article 2). http://dx.doi.org/10.14221/ajte.12017v14242n14228.14222

Levelt, W. J. M., Roelofs, A., & Meyer, A. S. (1999). A theory of lexical access in speech production. *Behavioral and Brain Sciences, 22,* 1–75.

Lewis, B. A., & Freebairn, L. A. (1993). A clinical tool for evaluating the familial basis of speech and language disorders. *American Journal of Speech-Language Pathology, 2,* 38–43.

Lewis, B. A., & Freebairn, L. (1992). Residual effects of preschool phonology disorders in grade school, adolescence, and adulthood.

Journal of Speech and Hearing Research, 35, 819–831.

Lewis, B. A., Freebairn, L. A., Hansen, A., Taylor, H. G., Iyengar, S., & Shriberg, L. D. (2004). Family pedigrees of children with suspected childhood apraxia of speech. *Journal of Communication Disorders, 37,* 157–175.

Lewis, B. A., Freebairn, L. A., Hansen, A. J., Iyengar, S. K., & Taylor, H. G. (2004). School-age follow-up children with childhood apraxia of speech. *Language, Speech, and Hearing Services in Schools, 35,* 122–140.

Lewis, B. A., Freebairn, L. A., & Taylor, H. G. (2000). Follow-up of children with early expressive phonology disorders. *Journal of Learning Disabilities, 33*(5), 433–444.

Lewis, B. A., Shriberg, L. D., Freebairn, L. A., Hansen, A. J., Stein, C. M., Taylor, H. G., & Iyengar, S. K. (2006). The genetic bases of speech sound disorders: Evidence from spoken and written language. *Journal of Speech, Language, and Hearing Research, 49,* 1294–1312.

Ling, D. (1976). *Speech and the hearing-impaired child: Theory and practice.* Washington, DC: Alexander Graham Bell Association for the Deaf.

Locke, J. L. (1980a). The inference of speech perception in the phonologically disordered child. Part I: A rationale, some criteria, the conventional tests. *Journal of Speech and Hearing Disorders, 45,* 431–444.

Locke, J. L. (1980b). The inference of speech perception in the phonologically disordered child. Part II: Some clinically novel procedures, their use, some findings. *Journal of Speech and Hearing Disorders, 45,* 445–468.

Lof, G. L. (1996). Factors associated with speech-sound stimulability. *Journal of Communication Disorders, 29,* 255–278.

Lohmeier, H. L., & Shriberg, L. D. (2011). *Reference data for the Syllable Repetition Task (SRT). Technical Report No. 17.* Phonology Project, Waisman Center, University of Wisconsin–Madison. Retrieved from http://www2.waisman.wisc.edu/phonology/techreports/TREP17.pdf

Lohvansuu, K., Hämäläinen, J. A., Ervast, L., Lyytinen, H., & Leppänen, P. H. T. (2018). Longitudinal interactions between brain and cognitive measures on reading development from 6 months to 14 years. *Neuropsychologia, 108,* 6–12.

Lonigan, C. J., Burgess, S. R., Anthony, J. L., & Barker, T. A. (1998). Development of phonological sensitivity in 2- to 5-year-old children. *Journal of Educational Psychology, 90*(2), 294–311.

Lonigan, C. J., & Whitehurst, G. J. (1998). Relative efficacy of a parent teacher involvement in a shared-reading intervention for preschool children from low-income backgrounds. *Early Childhood Research Quarterly, 13*(2), 263–290.

Lund, S. K., Quach, W., Weissling, K., McKelvey, M., & Dietz, A. (2017). Assessment with children who need augmentative and alternative communication (AAC): Clinical decisions of AAC specialists. *Language, Speech, and Hearing Services in Schools, 48*(1), 56–68.

Lundeborg, I., & McAllister, A. (2007). Treatment with a combination of intra-oral sensory stimulation and electropalatography in a child with severe developmental dyspraxia. *Logopedics Phoniatrics, 32,* 71–79.

Maas, E. (2016). Speech and nonspeech: What are we talking about? *International Journal of Speech-Language Pathology, 9*(4), 345–359.

Maas, E., Robin, D. A., Austermann Hula, S. N., Freedman, S. E., Wulf, G., Ballard, K. J., & Schmidt, R. A. (2008). Principles of motor learning in treatment of motor speech disorders. *American Journal of Speech-Language Pathology, 17,* 277–298.

Maassen, B., Groenen, P., & Crul, T. (2003). Auditory and phonetic perception of vowels in children with apraxic speech disorders. *Clinical Linguistics & Phonetics, 17,* 447–467.

MacLean, M., Bryant, P., & Bradley, L. (1987). Rhymes, nursery rhymes, and reading in early childhood. *Merrill-Palmer Quarterly, 33,* 255–282.

Marshall, C., & Chiat, S. (2003). A foot domain account of prosodically-conditioned substitutions. *Clinical Linguistics & Phonetics, 17*(8), 645–657.

Masterson, J. J., & Apel, K. (2010). Linking characteristics discovered in spelling assessment to intervention goals and methods. *Learning Disability Quarterly, 33*(3), 185–198.

May, L., Byers-Heinlein, K., Gervain, J., & Werker, J. F. (2011). Language and the newborn brain: Does prenatal language experience shape the neonate neural response to speech? *Frontiers in Psychology, 2,* Article 222. doi:10.3389/fpsyg.2011.00222

McAllister Byun, T. (2017). Efficacy of visual–acoustic biofeedback intervention for residual rhotic errors: a single-subject randomization study. *Journal of Speech, Language, and Hearing Research, 60*(5), 1175–1193.

McBride-Chang, C. (1995). What is phonological awareness? *Journal of Educational Psychology, 87*, 179–192.

McCandliss, B., Beck, I. L., Sandak, R., & Perfetti, C. A. (2003). Focusing attention on decoding for children with poor reading skills: Design and preliminary tests of the word building intervention. *Scientific Studies of Reading, 7*(1), 75–104.

McCauley, R. J., & Swisher, L. (1984). Use and misuse of norm-referenced test in clinical assessment: A hypothetical case. *Journal of Speech and Hearing Disorders, 49*, 338–348.

McCormack, J., McLeod, S., Harrison, L. J., & McAllister, L. (2010). The impact of speech impairment in early childhood: Investigating parents' and speech-language pathologists' perspectives using the ICF-CY. *Journal of Communication Disorders, 43*, 378–396.

McCune, L., & Vihman, M. M. (2001). Early phonetic and lexical development: A productivity approach. *Journal of Speech, Language, and Hearing Research, 44*, 670–684.

McCune, L., Vihman, M. M., Roug-Hellichus, L., Bordenave Delery, D., & Gogate, L. (1996). Grunt communication in human infants (*homo sapiens*). *Journal of Comparative Psychology, 110*, 27–37.

McGrath, L. M., Pennington, B. F., Willcutt, E. G., Boada, R., Shriberg, L. D., & Smith, S. D. (2007). Gene × environment interactions in speech sound disorder predict language and preliteracy outcomes. *Development and Psychopathology, 19*, 1047–1072.

McKercher, M., McFarlane, L., & Schneider, P. (1995). Phonological treatment dismissal: Optimal criteria. *Journal of Speech-Language Pathology and Audiology, 19*, 115–123.

McLeod, S., & Baker, E. (2014). Speech-language pathologists' practices regarding assessment, analysis, target selection, intervention, and service delivery for children with speech sound disorders. *Clinical Linguistics and Phonetics, 28*, 508–531.

McLeod, S., Crowe, K., & Shahaeian, A. (2015). Intelligibility in context scale: Normative and validation data for English-speaking preschoolers. *Language, Speech, and Hearing Services in Schools, 46*(3), 266–276.

McLeod, S., & Harrison, L. J. (2009). Epidemiology of speech and language impairment in a nationally representative sample of 4- to 5-year-old children. *Journal of Speech, Language, and Hearing Research, 52*, 1213–1229.

McLeod, S., & McCormack, J. (2007). Application of the ICF and ICF-children and youth in children with speech impairment. *Seminars in Speech and Language, 28*, 254–264.

McLeod, S., & Singh, S. (2009). *Speech sounds: A pictorial guide to typical and atypical speech.* San Diego, CA: Plural.

McLeod, S., & Threats, T. T. (2008). The ICF-CY and children with communication disabilities. *International Journal of Speech-Language Pathology, 10*, 92–109.

McNeill, B. C., & Hesketh, A. (2010). Developmental complexity of the stimuli included in mispronunciation detection tasks. *International Journal of Language & Communication Disorders, 45*(1), 72–82.

McNeill, B. C., Wolter, J., & Gillon, G. T. (2017). A comparison of the metalinguistic performance and spelling development of children with inconsistent speech sound disorder and their age-matched and reading-matched peers. *American Journal of Speech-Language Pathology, 26*(2), 456–468.

McNutt, J. C. (1977). Oral sensory and motor behaviors of children with /s/ or /r/ misarticulations. *Journal of Speech and Hearing Research, 20*, 694–704.

McReynolds, L. V., & Bennett, S. (1972). Distinctive feature generalization in articulation training. *Journal of Speech and Hearing Disorders, 37*, 462–470.

Metsala, J. L. (1999). Young children's phonological awareness and nonword repetition as a function of vocabulary development. *Journal of Educational Psychology, 91*(1), 3–19.

Metsala, J. L., & Walley, A. C. (1998). Spoken vocabulary growth and the segmental restructuring of lexical representations: Precursors to phonemic awareness and early reading ability. In J. L. Metsala & L. C. Ehri (Eds.), *Word recognition in beginning reading* (pp. 89–120). Mahwah, NJ: Erlbaum.

Miccio, A. W. (2002). Clinical problem solving: Assessment of phonological disorders. *American Journal of Speech-Language Pathology, 11*, 221–220.

Miccio, A. W., Elbert, M., & Forrest, K. (1999). The relationship between stimulability and phonological acquisition in children with normally eveloping and disordered phonologies. *American Journal of Speech-Language Pathology, 8*, 347–363.

Miller, G. A., & Nicely, P. E. (1955). An analysis of perceptual confusions among some English consonants. *Journal of the Acoustical Society of America, 27*, 338–352.

Miller, J., & Chapman, R. (1981). Research note: The relation between age and mean length of utterance in morphemes. *Journal of Speech, Language, and Hearing Research, 24*, 154–161.

Miller, N. (2013). Measuring up to speech intelligibility. *International Journal of Language & Communication Disorders, 48*, 601–612.

Mol, S. E., Bus, A. G., & De Jong, M. T. (2009). Interactive book reading in early education: A tool to stimulate print knowledge as well as oral language. *Review of Educational Research, 79*, 979–1007.

Montgomery, J. K., & Bonderman, I. R. (1989). Serving preschool children with severe phonological disorders. *Language, Speech & Hearing Services in Schools, 20*(1), 76–84.

Moon, C., Cooper, R. P., & Fifer, W. P. (1993). Two-day-olds prefer their native language. *Infant Behavior and Development, 16*(4), 495–500.

Moore, M. W., Fiez, J. A., & Tompkins, C. A. (2017). Consonant age-of-acquisition effects in nonword repetition are not articulatory in nature. *Journal of Speech, Language, and Hearing Research, 60*(11), 3198–3212.

Morgan, A., Ttofari Eecen, K., Pezic, A., Brommeyer, K., Mei, C., Eadie, P., . . . Dodd, B. (2017). Who to refer for speech therapy at 4 years of age versus who to "watch and wait"? *Journal of Pediatrics, 185*, 200–204.e1.

Morley, M. (1957). *The development and disorders of speech in childhood*. Edinburgh, UK: Churchill Livingstone.

Morrison, J. A., & Shriberg, L. D. (1992). Articulation testing versus conversational speech sampling. *Journal of Speech and Hearing Research, 35*, 259–273.

Munson, B., Baylis, A., Krause, M., & Yim, D-S. (2006, June 30–July 2). *Representation and access in phonological impairment*. Paper presented at the 10th Conference on Laboratory Phonology, Paris, France.

Munson, B., Edwards, J., & Beckman, M. E. (2005). Phonological knowledge in typical and atypical speech-sound development. *Topics in Language Disorders, 25*(3), 190–206.

Munson, B., Kurtz, B. A., & Windsor, J. (2005). The Influence of vocabulary size, phonotactic probability, and wordlikeness on nonword repetitions of children with and without specific language impairment. *Journal of Speech, Language, and Hearing Research, 48*(5), 1033–1047.

Murdoch, B. E., Attard, M. D., Ozanne, A., & Stokes, P. D. (1995). Impaired tongue strength and endurance in developmental verbal dyspraxia: A phsyiological analysis. *European Journal of Disorders of Communication, 30*, 51–64.

Murray, E., McCabe, P., & Ballard, K. J. (2014). A systematic review of treatment outcomes for children with childhood apraxia of speech. *American Journal of Speech-Language Pathology, 23*(3), 486–504.

Murray, E., McCabe, P., & Ballard, K. J. (2015). A randomized controlled trial for children with childhood apraxia of speech comparing Rapid Syllable Transition Treatment and the Nuffield Dyspraxia Programme–Third Edition. *Journal of Speech, Language, and Hearing Research, 58*(3), 669–686.

Murray, E., McCabe, P., Heard, R., & Ballard, K. J. (2015). Differential diagnosis of children with suspected childhood apraxia of speech. *Journal of Speech, Language, and Hearing Research, 58*(1), 43–60.

Namasivayam, A. K., Pukonen, M., Goshulak, D., Hard, J., Rudzicz, F., Rietveld, T., . . . van Lieshout, P. (2015). Treatment intensity and childhood apraxia of speech. *International Journal of Language & Communication Disorders, 50*, 529–546.

Nathan, L., Stackhouse, J., Goulandris, N., & Snowling, M. J. (2004a). The development of early literacy skills among children with speech difficulties: A test of the "critical age hypothesis." *Journal of Speech, Language, and Hearing Research, 47*, 377–391.

Nathan, L., Stackhouse, J., Goulandris, N., & Snowling, M. J. (2004b). Educational consequences of developmental speech disorder: Key Stage I national curriculum assessment results in English and mathematics. *British Journal of Educational Psychology, 74*, 173–186.

Nazzi, T., Bertoncini, J., & Mehler, J. (1998). Language discrimination by newborns: Toward an understanding of the role of rhythm. *Jour-*

nal of Experimental Psychology: Human Perception and Performance, 24(3), 756–766.

Nelson, N., Plante, E., Helm-Estabrooks, N., & Hotz, G. (2015). *Test of Integrated Language and Literacy Skills (TILLS)*. Baltimore, MD: Brookes.

Ng, K. Y. M., To, C. K. S., & McLeod, S. (2014). Validation of the Intelligibility in Context Scale as a screening tool for preschoolers in Hong Kong. *Clinical Linguistics & Phonetics, 28*, 316–328.

Nittrouer, S. (2001). Challenging the notion of innate phonetic boundaries. *Journal of the Acoustical Society of America, 110*(3), 1598–1605.

Nittrouer, S., & Burton, L. T. (2005). The role of early language experience in the development of speech perception and phonological processing abilities: Evidence from 5-year-olds with histories of otitis media with effusion and low socioeconomic status. *Journal of Communication Disorders, 38*, 29–63.

O'Grady, W., & Dobrovolsky, M. (1997). *Contemporary linguistics* (3rd ed.). New York, NY: St. Martin's Press.

Ohala, J. J. (1999). The relation between phonetics and phonology. In W. J. Hardcastle & J. Laver (Eds.), *The handbook of the phonetic sciences*. Blackwell Reference Online. Retrieved from <http://www.blackwellreference.com/subscriber/tocnode?id=g9780631214786_chunk_g978063121478622>

Oller, D. K. (1980). The emergence of the sounds of speech in infancy. In G. H. Yeni-Komshian, J. Kavanagh, & C. A. Ferguson (Eds.), *Child phonology. Volume I: Production* (pp. 93–112). New York, NY: Academic Press.

Oller, D. K. (2000). *The emergence of the speech capacity*. Mahwah, NJ: Erlbaum.

Oller, D. K., Eilers, R. E., & Basinger, D. (2001). Intuitive identification of infant vocal sounds by parents. *Developmental Science, 4*(1), 49–60.

Oller, D. K., Eilers, R. E., Neal, A. R., & Schwartz, H. K. (1999). Precursors to speech in infancy: The prediction of speech and language disorders. *Journal of Communication Disorders, 32*, 223–245.

Olswang, L. B., & Bain, B. A. (1991). When to recommend intervention. *Language, Speech, and Hearing Services in Schools, 22*(4), 255–263.

Olswang, L. B., & Bain, B. (1994). Data collection: Monitoring children's treatment progress. *American Journal of Speech-Language Pathology, 3*, 55–66.

Osberger, M. J., Robbins, A. M., Todd, S. L., & Riley, A. I. (1994). Speech intelligibility of children with cochlear implants. *Volta Review, 96*, 69–180.

Pamplona, M. C., Ysunza, A., & Espinoza, J. (1999). A comparative trial of two modalities of speech intervention for compensatory articulation in cleft palate children: Phonological approach versus articulatory approach. *International Journal of Pediatric Otorhinolaryngology, 49*, 21–26.

Parker, M. D., & Brorson, K. (2005). A comparative study between mean length of utterance in morphemes (MLUm) and mean length of utterance in words (MLUs). *First Language, 25*(3), 365–376.

Pennington, B. F., & Bishop, D. V. M. (2009). Relations among speech, language, and reading disorders. *Annual Review of Psychology, 60*(1), 283–306.

Peterson, R. L., Pennington, B. F., Shriberg, L. D., & Boada, R. (2009). What influences literacy outcome in children with speech sound disorder? *Journal of Speech, Language, and Hearing Research, 52*, 1175–1188.

Piasta, S. B. (2016). Current understandings of what works to support the development of emergent literacy in early childhood classrooms. *Child Development Perspectives, 10*(4), 234–239.

Piasta, S. B., Connor, C. M., Fishman, B. J., & Morrison, F. J. (2009). Teachers' knowledge of literacy concepts, classroom practices, and student reading growth. *Scientific Studies of Reading, 13*(3), 224–248.

Pierrehumbert, J. (2003). Phonetic diversity, statistical learning, and acquisition of phonology. *Language and Speech, 46*, 115–154.

Pindzola, R. H., Jenkins, M. M., & Lokken, K. J. (1989). Speaking rates of young children. *Language, Speech, and Hearing Services in Schools, 20*, 133–138.

Plante, E., & Vance, R. (1994). Selection of preschool language tests: A data-based approach. *Language, Speech, and Hearing Services in Schools, 25*, 15–24.

Polka, L., & Werker, J. F. (1994). Developmental changes in perception of nonnative vowel contrasts. *Journal of Experimental Psychology: Human Perception and Performance, 20*(2), 421–435.

Porkorni, J. L., Worthington, C. K., & Jamison, P. J. (2004). Phonological awareness intervention:

Comparison of Fast ForWord, Earobics, and LiPS. *Journal of Educational Research, 97*(3), 147–157.

Powell, J., & McReynolds, L. (1969). A procedure for testing position generalization from articulation training. *Journal of Speech and Hearing Research, 12*(3), 629–645.

Preston, J. L., Brick, N., & Landi, N. (2013). Ultrasound biofeedback treatment for persisting childhood apraxia of speech. *American Journal of Speech-Language Pathology, 22*(4), 627–643.

Preston, J. L., & Edwards, M. L. (2007). Phonological processing skills of adolescents with residual speech sound errors. *Language, Speech, and Hearing Services in Schools, 38*, 297–308.

Preston, J. L., Felsenfeld, S., Frost, S. J., Mencl, W. E., Fulbright, R. K., Grigorenko, E. L., . . . Pugh, K. R. (2012). Functional brain activation differences in school-age children with speech sound errors: Speech and print processing. *Journal of Speech, Language, and Hearing Research, 55*, 1068–1082.

Preston, J. L., McAllister Byun, T., Boyce, S. E., Hamilton, S., Tiede, M., Phillips, E., . . . Whalen, D. H. (2017). Ultrasound images of the tongue: A tutorial for assessment and remediation of speech sound errors. *Journal of Visualized Experiments: JoVE*(119), 55123. doi:10.3791/55123

Preston, J. L., McCabe, P., Rivera-Campos, A., Whittle, J. L., Landry, E., & Maas, E. (2014). Ultrasound visual feedback treatment and practice variability for residual speech sound errors. *Journal of Speech, Language, and Hearing Research, 57*(6), 2102–2115.

Preston, J. L., Molfese, P. J., Mencl, W. E., Frost, S. J., Hoeft, F., Fulbright, R. K., . . . Pugh, K. R. (2014). Structural brain differences in school-age children with residual speech sound errors. *Brain and Language, 128*(1), 25–33.

Proctor-Williams, K., & Fey, M. E. (2007). Recast density and acquisition of novel irregular past tense verbs. *Journal of Speech, Language, and Hearing Research, 50*(4), 1029–1047.

Puranik, C. S., Petcher, Y., Al Otaiba, S., Catts, H. W., & Lonigan, C. J. (2008). Development of oral reading fluency in children with speech or language impairments: A growth curve analysis. *Journal of Learning Disabilities, 41*, 545–560.

Raitano, N. A., Pennington, B. F., Tunick, B. F., Boada, R., & Shriberg, L. D. (2004). Pre-

literacy skills of subgroups of children with speech sound disorders. *Journal of Child Psychology and Psychiatry, 45*(4), 821–835.

Ramus, F., Marshall, C., Rosen, S., & Van der Lely, H. K. J. (2013). Phonological deficits in specific language impairment and developmental dyslexia: A multidimensional model. *Brain, 136* 630–645.

Raphael, L.J. & Bell-Berti, F. (1975). Tongue musculature and the feature of tension in English vowels. *Phonetica, 32*, 61–73.

Redle, E., Vannest, J., Maloney, T., Tsevat, R. K., Eikenberry, S., Lewis, B., . . . Holland, S. K. (2015). Functional MRI evidence for fine motor praxis dysfunction in children with persistent speech disorders. *Brain Research, 1597*, 47–56.

Reese, E., & Cox, A. (1999). Quality of adult book reading affects children's emergent literacy. *Developmental Psychology, 35*(1), 20–28.

Rice, M. L., Smolik, F., Perpich, D., Thompson, T., Rytting, N., & Blossom, M. (2010). Mean length of uutterance levels in 6-month intervals for children 3 to 9 years with and without language impairments. *Journal of Speech, Language, and Hearing Research, 53*(2), 333–349.

Robbins, J., & Klee, T. (1987). Clinical assessment of oropharyngeal motor development in young children. *Journal of Speech and Hearing Disorders, 52*, 271–277.

Roberts, J., Hunter, L., Gravel, J., Rosenfeld, R., Berman, S., Haggard, M., . . . Wallace, I. (2004). Otitis media, hearing loss, and language learning: Controversies and current research. *Journal of Developmental & Behavioral Pediatrics, 25*, 110–122.

Robin, D. A., Somodi, C. B., & Luschei, E. S. (1991). Measurement of tongue strength and endurance in normal and articulation disordered subjects. In C. A. Moore, K. M. Yorkston, & D. R. Beukelman (Eds.), *Dysarthria and apraxia of speech: Perspectives on management*. Baltimore, MD: Brookes.

Romski, M., Sevcik, R. A., Adamson, L. B., Cheslock, M., Smith, A., Barker, R. M., & Bakeman, R. (2010). Randomized comparison of augmented and nonaugmented language interventions for toddlers with developmental delays and their parents. *Journal of Speech, Language, and Hearing Research, 53*(2), 350–364.

Roulstone, S., Miller, L. L., Wren, Y., & Peters, T. J. (2009). The natural history of speech impairment of 8-year-old children in the Avon Longitudinal Study of parents and children: Error rates at 2 and 5 years. *International Journal of Speech-Language Pathology, 11,* 381–391.

Rudolph, J. M., & Wendt, O. (2014). The efficacy of the cycles approach: A multiple baseline design. *Journal of Communication Disorders, 47,* 1–16.

Ruscello, D. M., Tekieli, M. E., & Van Sickels, J. E. (1985). Speech production before and after orthognathic surgery: A review. *Oral Surgery, Oral Medicine, Oral Pathology, 59*(1), 10–14.

Rvachew, S. (1994). Speech perception training can facilitate sound production learning. *Journal of Speech and Hearing Research, 37,* 347–357.

Rvachew, S. (2005). Stimulability and treatment success. *Topics in Language Disorders. Clinical Perspectives on Speech Sound Disorders, 25*(3), 207–219.

Rvachew, S. (2007). Phonological processing and reading in children with speech sound disorders. *American Journal of Speech-Language Pathology, 16,* 260–270.

Rvachew, S., & Andrews, E. (2002). The influence of syllable position on children's production of consonants. *Clinical Linguistics & Phonetics, 16*(3), 183–198.

Rvachew, S., & Brosseau-Lapré, F. (2010). Speech perception intervention. In L. Williams, S. McLeod, & R. McCauley (Eds.), *Treatment of speech sound disorders in children* (pp. 295–314). Baltimore, MD: Brookes.

Rvachew, S., & Brosseau-Lapré, F. (2018). *Developmental phonological disorders: Foundations of clinical practice* (2nd ed.). San Diego, CA: Plural.

Rvachew, S., & Brosseau-Lapré, F. (2015). A randomized trial of twelve week interventions for the treatment of developmental phonological disorder in francophone children. *American Journal of Speech-Language Pathology, 24,* 637–658.

Rvachew, S., Chiang, P., & Evans, N. (2007). Characteristics of speech errors produced by children with and without delayed phonological awareness skills. *Language, Speech, and Hearing Services in Schools, 38,* 60–71.

Rvachew, S., & Grawburg, M. (2006). Correlates of phonological awareness in preschoolers with speech sound disorders. *Journal of Speech, Language, and Hearing Research, 49,* 74–87.

Rvachew, S., & Grawburg, M. (2008). Reflections on phonological working memory, letter knowledge and phonological awareness: A reply to Hartmann (2008). *Journal of Speech, Language, and Hearing Research, 51,* 1219–1226.

Rvachew, S., & Jamieson, D. G. (1989). Perception of voiceless fricatives by children with a functional articulation disorder. *Journal of Speech and Hearing Disorders, 54,* 193–208.

Rvachew, S., & Matthews, T. (2017a). Demonstrating treatment efficacy using the single subject randomization design: A tutorial and demonstration. *Journal of Communication Disorders, 67,* 1–13.

Rvachew, S., & Matthews, T. (2017b). Using the Syllable Repetition Task to reveal underlying speech processes in childhood apraxia of speech: A tutorial. *Canadian Journal of Speech-Language Pathology and Audiology, 41*(1), 106–126.

Rvachew, S., Mattock, K., Clayards, M., Chiang, P., & Brosseau-Lapré, F. (2011). Perceptual considerations in multilingual adult and child speech acquisition In S. McLeod & B. A. Goldstein (Eds.), *Multilingual aspects of speech sound disorders in children* (pp. 58–68). Bristol, UK: Multilingual Matters.

Rvachew, S., & Nowak, M. (2001). The effect of target selection strategy on sound production learning. *Journal of Speech, Language, and Hearing Research, 44,* 610–623.

Rvachew, S., Ohberg, A., Grawburg, M., & Heyding, J. (2003). Phonological awareness and phonemic perception in 4-year-old children with delayed expressive phonology skills. *American Journal of Speech-Language Pathology, 12,* 463–471.

Rvachew, S., & Rafaat, S. (2014). Report on benchmark wait times for pediatric speech sound disorders. *Canadian Journal of Speech-Language Pathology and Audiology, 38*(1), 82–96.

Rvachew, S., Rafaat, S., & Martin, M. (1999). Stimulability, speech perception and the treatment of phonological disorders. *American Journal of Speech-Language Pathology, 8,* 33–34.

Sacks, S., Flipsen, P., & Neils-Strunjas, J. (2013). Effectiveness of systematic articulation training programming accessing computers (SATPAC) approach to remediate dentalized and interdental /s, z/: A preliminary study. *Perceptual and Motor Skills, 117*(2), 559–577.

Sasisekaran, J. (2014). Exploring the link between stuttering and phonology: A review and implications for treatment. *Seminars in Speech and Language, 32*(2), 95–113.

Schneider, P., Hayward, D., & Vis Dubé, R. (2007). Storytelling from pictures using the Edmonton Narrative Norms Instrument. *Journal of Speech-Language Pathology and Audiology, 30*(4), 224–238.

Schooling, T. L. (2003). Lessons from the National Outcomes Measurement System (NOMS). *Seminars in Speech and Language, 24*(3), 245–256.

Schuele, C. M., & Boudreau, D. (2008). Phonological awareness intervention: Beyond the basics. *Language, Speech, and Hearing Services in Schools, 39*, 3–20.

Schwanenflugel, P. J., Hamilton, A., Neuharth-Pritchett, S., Restrepo, M. A., Bradley, B. A., & Webb, M. (2010). PAVEd for success: An evaluation of a comprehensive program for four-year-old children. *Journal of Literacy Research, 42*, 227–275.

Secord, W. E., Boyce, S. E., Donahue, J. S., Fox, R. A., & Shine, R. E. (2007). *Eliciting sounds: Techniques and strategies for clinicians* (2nd ed.). Boston, MA: Cengage Learning.

Semel, E., Wiig, E. H., & Secord, W. (2004). *Clinical Evaluation of Language Fundamentals—Preschool, Second Edition (CELF-P2).* San Antonio, TX: Pearson.

Semel, E., Wiig, E. H., & Secord, W. (2013). *Clinical Evaluation of Language Fundamentals—Fifth Edition (CELF-5).* San Antonio, TX: Pearson.

Shattuck-Hufnagel, S., & Turk, A. E. (1996). A prosody tutorial for investigators of auditory sentence processing. *Journal of Psycholinguistic Research, 25*, 193–247.

Shine, R. E. (1989). Articulatory production training: A sensory motor approach. In N. A. Creaghead, P. W. Newman, & W. A. Secord (Eds.), *Assessment and remediation of articulatory and phonological disorders* (2nd ed.). New York, NY: Macmillan.

Shriberg, L. D. (1975). A response evocation program for /r/. *Journal of Speech and Hearing Disorders, 40*, 92–105.

Shriberg, L. D. (1994). Five subtypes of developmental phonological disorders. *Clinics in Communication Disorders, 4*, 38–53.

Shriberg, L. D., Austin, D., Lewis, B. A., McSweeny, J. L., & Wilson, D. L. (1997). The Speech Disorders Classification System (SDCS): Extensions and lifespan reference data. *Journal of Speech, Language, and Hearing Research, 40*(4), 723–740.

Shriberg, L. D., Fourakis, M., Hall, S. D., Karlsson, H. B., Lohmeier, H. L., McSweeny, J. L., . . . Wilson, D. L. (2010). Extensions to the Speech Disorders Classification System (SDCS). *Clinical Linguistics & Phonetics, 24*, 795–824.

Shriberg, L. D., & Kent, R. D. (2013). *Clinical phonetics* (4th ed.). Boston, MA: Allyn & Bacon.

Shriberg, L. D., & Kwiatkowski, J. (1980). *Natural process analysis: A procedure for phonological analysis of continuous speech samples.* New York, NY: Macmillan.

Shriberg, L. D., & Kwiatkowski, J. (1982). Phonological disorders III: A procedure for assessing severity of involvement. *Journal of Speech and Hearing Disorders, 47*, 256–270.

Shriberg, L. D., & Kwiatkowski, J. (1985). Continuous speech sampling for phonologic analyses of speech-delayed children. *Journal of Speech and Hearing Disorders, 50*, 323–334.

Shriberg, L. D., & Kwiatkowski, J. (1994). Developmental phonological disorders II: Short-term speech-sound normalization. *Journal of Speech and Hearing Research, 37*, 1127–1126.

Shriberg, L. D., Lohmeier, H. L., Campbell, T. F., Dollaghan, C. A., Green, J. R., & Moore, C. A. (2009). A nonword repetition task for speakers with misarticulations: The syllable repetition task. *Journal of Speech, Language, and Hearing Research, 52*, 1189–1212.

Shriberg, L. D., Lohmeier, H. L., Strand, E. A., & Jakielski, K. J. (2012). Encoding, memorial and transcoding deficits in Childhood Apraxia of Speech. *Clinical Linguistics & Phonetics, 26*, 445–482.

Shriberg, L. D., Tomblin, J. B., & McSweeny, J. L. (1999). Prevalence of speech delay in 6-year-old children and comorbidity with language impairment. *Journal of Speech, Language, and Hearing Research, 42*(6), 1461–1481.

Shuster, L. I. (1998). The perception of correctly and incorrectly produced /r/. *Journal of Speech, Language, and Hearing Research, 41*, 941–950.

Shuster, L. I., Ruscello, D. M., & Toth, A. R. (1995). The use of visual feedback to elicit correct /r/. *American Journal of Speech-Language Pathology, 4*(2), 37–44.

Singh, S., & Becker, G. M. (1972). A comparison of four feature systems using data from three psychophysical methods. *Journal of Speech and Hearing Research, 15*, 821–830.

Skahan, S. M., Watson, M., & Lof, G. L. (2007). Speech-language pathologists' assessment practices for children with suspected speech sound disorders: Results of a national survey. *American Journal of Speech-Language Pathology, 16*, 246–259.

Smit, A. B., Hand, L., Freilinger, J. J., Bernthal, J. E., & Bird, A. (1990). The Iowa articulation norms project and its Nebraska replication. *Journal of Speech and Hearing Disorders, 55,* 779–798.

Snow, P. C., Eadie, P. A., Connell, J., Dalheim, B., McCusker, H. J., & Munro, J. K. (2014). Oral language supports early literacy: A pilot cluster randomized trial in disadvantaged schools. *International Journal of Speech-Language Pathology, 16*(5), 495–506.

So, L. K. H., & Dodd, B. (1994). Phonologically disordered Cantonese-speaking children. *Clinical Linguistics & Phonetics, 18,* 235–255.

Sommers, R. K. (1962). Factors in the effectiveness of mothers trained to aid in speech correction. *Journal of Speech and Hearing Disorders, 27,* 178–186.

Sommers, R. K., Cockerille, C. E., Paul, C. D., Bowser, D. C., Fichter, G. R., Fenton, A. K., & Copetas, F. G. (1961). Effects of speech therapy and speech improvement upon articulation and reading. *Journal of Speech and Hearing Disorders, 26*(1), 27–38.

Sommers, R. K., Cox, S., & West, C. (1972). Articulatory effectiveness, stimulability, and children's performances on perceptual and memory tasks. *Journal of Speech and Hearing Research, 15,* 579–589.

Sommers, R. K., Furlong, A. K., Rhodes, F. E., Fichter, G. R., Bowser, D. C., Copetas, F. G., & Saunders, Z. G. (1964). Effects of maternal attitudes upon improvements in articulation when mothers are trained to assist in speech correction. *Journal of Speech and Hearing Disorders, 29,* 126–132.

Sparks, E., & Deacon, S. H. (2013). Morphological awareness and vocabulary acquisition: A longitudinal examination of their relationship in English-speaking children. *Applied Psycholinguistics, 36*(2), 299–321.

Spaulding, T. J., Plante, E., & Farinella, K. A. (2006). Eligibility criteria for language impairment: Is the low end of normal always appropriate? *Language, Speech, and Hearing Services in Schools, 37,* 61–72.

St. Louis, K. O., & Ruscello, D. M. (2000). *Oral Speech Mechanism Screening Evaluation* (3rd ed.). Austin, TX: Pro-Ed.

Stackhouse, J., & Wells, B. (1993). Psycholinguistic assessment of developmental speech disorders. *European Journal of Disorders of Communication, 28,* 331–348.

Stark, R. E., Rose, S. N., & Benson, P. J. (1978). Classification of infant vocalization. *British Journal of Disorders of Communication, 13,* 41–47.

Statistics Canada. (2012). *Linguistics characteristics of Canadians, language, 2011 census of population.* https://www12.statcan.gc.ca/census-recensement/2011/as-sa/98-314-x/98-314x2011001-eng.cfm

Stoel-Gammon, C., & Dunn, C. (1985). *Normal and disordered phonology in children.* Baltimore, MD: University Park Press.

Stokes, S. F., & Griffiths, R. (2010). The use of facilitative vowel contexts in the treatment of post-alveolar fronting: a case study. *International Journal of Language & Communication Disorders, 45,* 368–380.

Stokes, S. F., & Klee, T. (2009). The diagnostic accuracy of a new test of early nonword repetition for differentiating late talking and typically developing children. *Journal of Speech, Language, and Hearing Research, 52,* 872–882.

Strand, E. A., & Debertine, P. (2000). The efficacy of integral stimulation intervention with developmental apraxia of speech. *Journal of Medical Speech-Language Pathology, 8*(4), 295–300.

Strand, E. A., & Skinder, A. (1999). Treatment of developmental apraxia of speech: Integral stimulation methods. In A. Caruso & E. A. Strand (Eds.), *Clinical management of motor speech disorders in children* (pp. 109–148). New York, NY: Thieme.

Thomas-Stonell, N. L., Oddson, B., Robertson, B., & Rosenbaum, P. L. (2010). Development of the FOCUS (Focus on the Outcomes of Communication Under Six), a communication outcome measure for preschool children. *Developmental Medicine and Child Neurology, 52,* 47–53.

Thomas-Stonell, N., Oddson, B., Robertson, B., Walker, J., & Rosenbaum, P. (2012). *The FOCUS©: Focus on the Outcomes of Communication Under Six.* Toronto, ON: Holland Bloorview Kids Rehabilitation Hospital.

Thoonen, G., Maassen, B., Gabreels, F., & Schreuder, R. (1999). Validity of maximum performance tasks to diagnose motor speech disorders in children. *Clinical Linguistics & Phonetics, 13,* 1–23.

Tomblin, J. B., Records, N. L., & Zhang, J. (1996). A system for the diagnosis of specific language impairment in kindergarten children. *Journal of Speech and Hearing Research, 39,* 1284–1294.

Tsao, F., Huei-Mei, L., & Kuhl, P. K. (2004). Speech perception in infancy predicts language development in the second year of life: A longitudinal study. *Child Development, 75*(4), 1067–1084.

Tsao, F., Liu, H., & Kuhl, P. K. (2006). Perception of native and non-native affricate-fricative contrasts: Cross-language tests on adults and infants. *Journal of the Acoustical Society of America, 120,* 2285–2294.

Tyler, A. A. (1996). Assessing stimulability in toddlers. *Journal of Communication Disorders, 29,* 279–297.

Tyler, A. A., Edwards, M. L., & Saxman, J. H. (1987). Clinical application of two phonologically based treatment procedures. *Journal of Speech and Hearing Research, 52,* 393–409.

Tyler, A. A., & Tolbert, L. C. (2002). Speech-language assessment in the clinical setting. *American Journal of Speech-Language Pathology, 11*(3), 215–220.

Van Riper, C. (1978). *Speech correction: Principles and methods.* Upper Saddle River, NJ: Prentice-Hall.

Vance, M., Rosen, S., & Coleman, M. (2009). Assessing speech perception in young children and relationships with language skills. *International Journal of Audiology, 48*(10), 708–717.

Vargha-Khadem, F., Watkins, K., Alcock, K., Fletcher, P., & Passingham, R. (1995). Praxic and nonverbal cognitive deficits in a large family with a genetically transmitted speech and language disorder. *Proceedings of the National Academy of Sciences, 92,* 930–933.

Velleman, S. L. (2002). Phonotactic therapy. *Seminars in Speech and Language, 23,* 43–55.

Velleman, S. L., & Strand, K. (1994). Developmental verbal dyspraxia. In J. E. B. Bernthal & N. W. Bankson (Eds.), *Child phonology: Characteristics, assessment, and intervention* (pp. 110–139). New York, NY: Theime.

Vernon-Feagans, L. (1999). Impact of otitis media on speech, language, cognition and behavior. In R. M. Rosenfeld & C. D. Bluestone (Eds.), *Evidence-based otitis media.* Hamilton, ON: Decker.

Vihman, M. M., Macken, M. A., Miller, R., Simmons, H., & Miller, J. (1985). From babbling to speech: A re-assessment of the continuity issue. *Language, 61*(2), 397–445.

Vorperian, H. K., Kent, R. D., Gentry, L. R., & Yandell, B. S. (1999). Magentic resonance imaging procedures to study the concurrent anatomic development of vocal tract structures: preliminary results. *International Journal of Pediatric Otorhinolaryngology, 49,* 197–206.

Wagner, R., Toregesen, J., & Rashotte, C. (1999). *Comprehensive Test of Phonological Processing.* Austin, TX: Pro-Ed.

Waldman, F. R., Singh, S., & Hayden, M. E. (1978). A comparison of speech-sound production and discrimination in children with functional articulation disorders. *Language and Speech, 21,* 205–230.

Walley, A. C., Metsala, J. L., & Garlock, V. M. (2003). Spoken vocabulary growth: Its role in the development of phoneme awareness and reading ability. *Reading and Writing: An Interdisciplinary Journal, 16,* 5–20.

Warren, S. F., Fey, M. E., & Yoder, P. J. (2007). Differential treatment intensity research: A missing link to creating optimally effective communication interventions. *Mental Retardation and Developmental Disabilities Research Reviews, 13,* 70–77.

Washington, K. N., McDonald, M. M., McLeod, S., Crowe, K., & Devonish, H. (2017). Validation of the Intelligibility in Context Scale for Jamaican Creole-speaking preschoolers. *American Journal of Speech-Language Pathology, 26,* 750–761.

Wasik, B. A., Bond, M. A., & Hindman, A. (2006). The effects of a language and literacy intervention on Head Start children and teachers. *Journal of Educational Psychology, 98*(1), 63–74.

Webster, P. E., Plante, A. S., & Couvillion, M. (1997). Phonologic impairment and prereading: Update on a longitudinal study. *Journal of Learning Disabilities, 30*(4), 365–376.

Weiner, F. (1981). Treatment of phonological disability using the method of meaningful minimal contrasts: Two case studies. *Journal of Speech and Hearing Disorders, 46,* 97–103.

Weismer, S. E., & Hesketh, L. J. (1996). Lexical learning by children with specific language impairment: Effects of linguistic input presented at varying speaking rates. *Journal of Speech, Language, and Hearing Research, 39,* 177–190.

Weizman, Z. O., & Snow, C. E. (2001). Lexical input as related to children's vocabulary acquisition: Effects of sophisticated exposure and support for meaning. *Developmental Psychology, 37*(2), 265–279.

Werker, J. F., Fennell, C. T., Corcoran, K. M., & Stager, C. L. (2002). Infants' ability to learn phonetically similar words: Effects of age and vocabulary size. *Infancy, 3*(1), 1–30.

Werker, J. F., & Lalonde, C. E. (1988). Cross-language speech perception: Initial capabilities and developmental change. *Developmental Psychology, 24*(5), 672–683.

Werker, J. F., & Tees, R. C. (1983). Developmental changes across childhood in the perception of non-native speech sounds. *Canadian Journal of Psychology, 37*(2), 278–286.

Werker, J. F., & Tees, R. C. (1984). Cross-language speech perception: Evidence for perceptual reorganization during the first year of life. *Infant Behavior and Development, 7*(1), 49–63.

Whitehurst, G. J., Epstein, J. N., Angell, A. L., Payne, A. C., Crone, D. A., & Fischel, J. E. (1994). A picture book reading intervention in day care and home for children from low-income families. *Developmental Psychology, 30*, 679–689.

Whitehurst, G. J., Falco, F., Lonigan, C. J., Fischel, J. E., DeBaryshe, B. D., Valdez-Menchaca, M. C., & Caulfield, M. (1988). Accelerating language development through picture book reading. *Developmental Psychology, 24*, 552–558.

Whitehurst, G. J., Zevenburger, A. A., Crone, D. A., Schultz, M. D., Velting, O. N., & Fischel, J. E. (1999). Outcomes of an emergent literacy intervention from Head Start through second grade. *Journal of Educational Psychology, 91*(2), 261–272.

Wilcox, K., & Morris, S. (1999). *Children's Speech Intelligibility Measure.* San Antonio, TX: Psychological Corporation.

Wilcox, M. J., Gray, S. L., Guimond, A. B., & Lafferty, A. E. (2011). Efficacy of the TELL language and literacy curriculum for preschoolers with developmental speech and/or language impairments. *Early Childhood Research Quarterly, 26*, 278–294.

Williams, A. L. (2010). Multiple oppositions intervention. In A. L. Williams, S. McLeod, & R. J. McCauley (Eds.), *Interventions for speech sound disorders in children* (pp. 73–93). Baltimore, MD: Brookes.

Williams, A. L. (2012). Intensity in phonological intervention: Is there a prescribed amount? *International Journal of Speech-Language Pathology, 14*(5), 456–461.

Williams, N., & Chiat, S. (1993). Processing deficits in children with phonological disorder and delay: A comparison of responses to a series of output tasks. *Clinical Linguistics & Phonetics, 7*, 145–160.

Williams, P. (2009). The Nuffield Centre Dyspraxia Programme Third Edition (NDP3). In C. Bowen (Ed.), *Children's speech sound disorders* (pp. 269–275). Chichester, UK: Wiley-Blackwell.

Williams, P., & Stephens, H. (2010). The Nuffield Centre Dyspraxia Programme. In A. L. Williams, S. McLeod, & R. J. McCauley (Eds.), *Interventions of speech sound disorders in children* (pp. 159–177). Baltimore, MD: Brookes.

Wise, B. W., Ring, J., & Olson, R. K. (1999). Training phonological awareness with and without explicit attention to articulation. *Journal of Experimental Child Psychology, 72*, 271–304.

Wolter, J. A., & Dilworth, V. (2013). The effects of a multilinguistic morphological awareness approach for improving language and literacy. *Journal of Learning Disabilities, 47*(1), 76–85.

Wolter, J. A., Wood, A., & D'zatko, K. W. (2009). The influence of morphological awareness on the literacy develoment of first-grade children. *Language, Speech, and Hearing Services in Schools, 40*, 286–298.

World Health Organization. (2001). *International Classification of Functioning, Disability and Health (ICF).* Geneva, Switzerland: WHO.

World Health Organization. (2006). *World Health Organization Constitution.* Geneva, Switzerland: WHO.

World Health Organization. (2007). *International Classification of Functioning, Disability and Health for Children and Youth (ICF-CY).* Geneva, Switzerland: WHO.

Wright, A. A. (2017). *Profiling developmental speech sound disorders: Differences, deficits and outcomes* (Ph.D. thesis). University of Limerick, Limerick, Ireland.

Wulf, G., Schmidt, R. A., & Deubel, H. (1993). Reduced feedback frequency enhances generalized motor program learning but not parameterization learning. *Journal of Experimental Psychology: Learning, Memory, and Cognition, 19*(5), 1134–1150.

Yavas, M., & Goldstein, B. A. (1998). Phonological assessment and treatment of bilingual speakers. *American Journal of Speech-Language Pathology, 7*, 49–60.

Yont, K. M., Snow, C. E., & Vernon-Feagans, L. (2003). Is chronic otitis media associated with differences in parental input at 12 months of age? An analysis of joint attention and directives. *Applied Psycholinguistics, 24,* 581–602.

Zevenbergen, A. A., Whitehurst, G. J., & Zevenbergen, J. A. (2003). Effects of a shared-reading intervention on the inclusion of evaluative devices in narratives of children from low-income families. *Applied Developmental Psychology, 24,* 1–15.

Zhang, X., & Tomblin, J. B. (2000). The association of intervention receipt with speech-language profiles and social-demographic variables. *American Journal of Speech-Language Pathology, 9*(4), 345–357.

Zuk, J., Iuzzini-Seigel, J., Cabbage, K., Green, J. R., & Hogan, T. P. (2018). Poor speech perception is not a core deficit of childhood apraxia of speech: Preliminary findings. *Journal of Speech, Language, and Hearing Research,* 1–10.

INDEX

A

Accuracy
  of identification, 80–81
  measures of, 90–92
  of speech, 49, 56–59, 104, 108, 122–123, 134, 145–146
Acoustic
  analysis, 21, 134, 172
  cues, 20–22, 26
  phonetics, 2, 39
Acoustic-phonetic
  information, 22, 68
  representation, 3, 20, 49, 112, 183–185, 187, 193, 226–227
Activity limitations
  assessment of, 156–157
  participation restrictions and, 153, 157, 160
Affricates, 6, 7, 9, 12, 28, 37, 39, 174, 182, 239, 240
Age
  of acquisition of consonant clusters, 59–60, 70
  of acquisition of consonants, 58–60, 74
  of suppression, 65–66
Alignment, 99, 100
Allophones, 26–27, 32, 45, 75
Alphabetic principle, 253, 256–257, 260
Alveolar
  fricative, 13
  ridge, 8–9, 23, 35, 100, 139, 219
  sounds, 8, 11, 36, 100, 139, 172, 245, 252
Ambisyllabic consonants, 31–33, 67, 240, 248
Amount of intervention, 163, 165
Amplitude, 20–21, 26, 39, 68

Analysis
  independent, 53–55
  relational, 57
  speech sample, 16–18
Ankyloglossia, 100
Aperiodic, 20–21
Approximants, 6–9
Apraxia of speech, 126–127, 129, 131, 134, 136, 148–149
  assessment, 252
  intervention, 162, 200, 259, 261
Articulation, 3
  accuracy, 157–158
  disorder, 126–128, 130, 145, 148, 252
  tests, 14, 92–94, 96, 154
  therapy, traditional, 216–217, 226, 230, 234–235, 261
  visual analysis, of, 18
Articulators, 2–7, 15, 18, 97, 101, 116, 200, 203, 206, 211, 218–219, 230
Articulatory
  complexity, 61, 74
  knowledge, 1, 16, 18, 20
  phonetics, 2–4, 11, 39, 219
Articulatory-phonetic representations, 3, 200
Aspiration, 7, 22, 31, 126, 221, 249
Assessment
  of articulation/phonology, and, 91–96
  dynamic, and, 82, 85, 175, 205
  of hearing, 87, 89–90, 105
  of intelligibility, 106–109
  of oral-motor structure and function, 96–102
  of phonological processing, and, 111–116
  predictive, and, 158–159
  of stimulability, 96

Assimilation, 4–6, 36–39, 65–66, 68–69, 245
Asymmetry, 97
Atypical errors, 18, 41, 61–62, 65, 77, 122, 126–131, 140, 146, 148, 153, 156, 158, 237, 248, 252
Auditory
  bombardment, 190–191, 198, 208, 245, 247–248, 262
  discrimination, 23, 25–26, 45, 112, 137, 190, 223, 250
  input, 3, 20, 22, 26, 32, 43–46, 52–54, 61, 63, 68–69
  processing, 87, 112, 115, 123
Auditory Processing Disorder (APD), 116
Augmentative and alternative communication (AAC), 201, 228
Automaticity, 204, 208, 212

B

Babble, 50–53, 89, 184, 200, 203
  marginal, 51–52
  reduplicated, 51, 53, 203, 205
  canonical, 51–52, 76
Baseline data, 82
Basic goals, 166–169, 174, 178, 182
Below normal limits, 83–85
Bilabial, 8, 10–12, 15–16, 32, 54
Bilateral, 97
Bilingualism, 118–119
Biofeedback, 221
Birth history, 88–89
Bite, 99–100
Block treatment, 163, 166, 174
Blocked practice schedule, 206, 208
Bottom-up factors, 44
Branching onset, 70–73
Broad transcription, 15–16, 39, 54–55

C

Canonical
  babbling, 51–52, 57, 76
  syllables, 52
Capacity, 79, 85, 89, 138, 197
Caseload, 66–68, 139, 145, 159, 161–162, 180
Cases, 42, 67, 79, 82
Casual-correlates, 123
Categorical perception, 1, 22, 24–26, 39

Category boundary, 25, 45
Central auditory processing disorder, 265
Chaining, 221, 242–243, 247
Challenge point framework, 207, 229
Childhood Apraxia of Speech (CAS), 101, 127, 131, 136, 200, 252, 259, 261
  assessment, 101, 126
  intervention, 200
Chronological mismatch, 156
Citation-form tests, standardized single-word, 93
Classification of Functioning, Disability and Health, 153, 156
Cleft palate, 155
Client-centered approach, 161
Cluster
  acquisition of, 59, 70–71, 73–74
  reduction, 37–38, 65–67, 70, 72–73, 78, 255
  simplification of, 36–39, 63, 65–67, 70–73, 181–182
Coalescence, 68–69, 71–73, 78
Co-articulation, 3–5, 18, 39, 92, 204
Cognates, 7, 11, 14, 26
Collapse of contrast, 125, 172
Complementary distribution, 27
Completion prompts, 104, 186, 194
Complex onsets, 28–31, 70, 74, 167, 170, 239–240
Complexity approach to target selection, 209
Computer-based
  ear training, 256
  speech perception interventions, 262
Connected speech, 59, 103, 127, 130, 143, 148, 157
Consistent Atypical Phonological Disorder, 126–128, 131, 148, 158, 248
Consonants, 5–7
  age of acquisition of, 57–59, 62
  assessment of, 47, 58, 67
  deletion, final, 36–38, 65, 67, 244
  mastery of, 58–61, 70, 74, 168–169, 171, 216
Consonants, phonetic inventory of, 16, 243
Constant practice, 209–210, 214
Constraints, 28, 53, 67, 68
Contextual
  facilitation, 217–219, 228

factors, 88, 90, 109, 156–157
Continuous speech sample, 87, 92, 102–104, 108, 116
Contrasts
  discrimination of phonetic, 42
  perception of, 26, 43–45, 125, 137, 173
  phonetic, 42–43, 45, 48, 63, 75, 141, 173, 243, 248, 252
  voicing, 42, 173, 205, 245, 248
Coordinated speech movements, 101
Core vocabulary approach, 237, 240, 243, 246, 261, 263
Covert contrast, 126, 172, 174, 249
Craniofacial anomalies, 201
Criterion-referenced assessments , 85
Cross-sectional, 130
CROWD acronym, 194, 196
Cued articulation, 242
Cultural competence, 79–80, 118–119
Cumulative intervention intensity, 151, 162, 164–165, 182
Customary production, 41, 58–59, 61, 74, 77, 169, 206
Cycles
  approach, 244, 246, 248, 261
  goal attack strategy, 235
Cyclical goal attack strategy, 169, 174

D

De novo, 135
Decoding, 145, 253– 254, 256, 260
Default features, 35–36, 38, 73
Delayed phonological development, 244, 251
Delinking, 71–73
Dental
  fricatives, 64, 100
  occlusions, 100
Dentition, 97, 99, 159
Developmental
  errors, 61, 66
  history, 88–89, 182
  order, 170, 172, 174, 233, 249
  trajectory, 41, 123–124, 132, 155, 234
Developmental Language Disorder, 115, 138, 144–145
Developmental Psychosocial Involvement, 131–133, 136, 149

Developmentally stable, 126
Diadochokinetic rates, 101, 244
Diagnosis, 121–124, 126–127, 129–130, 136
  differential, 111, 121, 126–127, 130, 148
Diagnostic, speech assessment, 81
Dialect, 13, 15, 38, 80, 83, 113, 117–119
Dialogic reading, 184, 194–198, 256–257, 262–263
Diphthong, 6–7, 14, 28–29, 205, 211, 214
Discharged planning, 81, 90–91, 160–161, 163
Discrimination task, 25, 26, 112, 137
Distal cause, 121, 132, 136
Distancing prompts, 196
Distinctive feature, 21, 32, 39, 248, 252, 256
Distortion errors, 56, 64, 92, 94–95, 125, 127, 130, 134, 143–144, 159, 216
Distributed practice, 162, 166, 210
Disyllabic, 168, 208, 210
Dodd's linguistic classification system, 126–131, 136, 148
Dorsal sounds, 34–36, 239, 252
Dose, 157, 161–166, 185, 209
  form, 162, 164
  frequency, 151, 162–165
Drill
  play, 162, 176, 213, 222–225, 241, 247–248
  practice, 184–185, 213, 222–223, 242
Drooping, 97–98
Dynamic
  assessment, 85, 96
  stability, 205, 212, 216, 229
Dysarthria, 131, 134, 136, 141, 157, 200
Dyslexia, 254
Dyspraxia, 101, 127, 129, 134, 204

E

Ear training, 183–184, 189–193, 198, 216–217, 227–230, 246–247, 262
Ecological validity , 16, 103
Educational history, 89
Electropalatography (EPG), 9, 18–19, 139–140, 212
Elision tasks, 49
Emergent literacy, 168, 197, 253, 257–261
Environmental factors, 87–90, 156–157, 160
Epenthesis, 71, 73, 78
Epidemiology, 141–142, 147

Error detection, 190–193, 197, 208, 216–217
Etiology, 97, 132
Evidence-based practice, 175, 181
Expand goal, 173–175, 188
Expansion stage, 51–52, 57, 76, 202
Expressive language, 103, 110
Extend goal, 173–174, 188

F

Facial characteristics, 97
Facilitators, contextual barriers and, 156
Familial aggregation, 135
Family pedigree, 135
Faucial pillars, 100
Feedback, 165, 194, 212–213
    auditory, 245, 247
    knowledge of performance, and, 199,
        209, 212, 214, 218–219, 222–223
    knowledge of results, and, 199, 209,
        212–214, 222–223
    performance accuracy, and, 85
    precise, 177
    sensory, 52, 202–203, 212, 216
    summative, 213, 223
    ultrasound, visual, 19
    verbal, 161–162, 205
    visual, 217–219
Final consonant deletion, 36–38, 65, 67, 244
Five-way scoring, 92, 94–96, 116
Flow charts, decision, 157–158
Fluency, 103, 145, 147, 160
Focus on the Outcomes of Communication
    Under Six, 109–110, 156
Focused stimulation, 183–191, 261–262
Formants, 20–21, 221
Frenulum, 100
Fricatives, 6–8, 16, 34,
    stopping of, 37–38
Fronting,
    palatal, 37–38, 65
    velar, 36–37, 63, 65–67
Fully resonant vowel (FRV), 51–52
Functional load, 62–63, 170, 172–174

G

Generalization
    response, 178–179, 181

    stimulus, 151, 178, 181, 226–227
Glaspey Dynamic Assessment of
    Phonology (GDAP), 96
Glides, 6, 8, 28–29, 54–55
Gliding, 38, 63, 65–66, 127–128
Glottal, 10–12, 54, 65–66
Glottal stop, 10, 16, 31, 36
Goal attack strategies, 169–170, 173–174,
    182, 216, 221, 228, 235
Goals, selecting treatment, 92, 102, 110, 152,
    166, 171–173, 182

H

Harmony processes, 63
Health, as defined by World Health
    Organization, 156
Hearing
    acuity, 90
    impairment, 131, 142, 201–205
Heterogeneous, 122
Hierarchy, phonological, 47
Homophone, 248–249
Horizontal goal attack strategy, 169,
    173–174, 235

I

ICY-CY approach, 156
Identification, 22–26, 38, 49, 53, 80–81, 108,
    112–113, 137, 190–193, 208, 240–241,
    247
Imitation, 188–189, 201, 210, 214–215, 218,
    235, 240, 247
Implicit, 47–48
Implicit, phonological awareness, 42,
    46–47, 50, 75, 244
Incisors, 100, 219
Inconsistent Phonological Disorder, 106,
    126–131, 158, 236–237, 240, 243, 252
Independent analysis, 53–55
Infant
    ability to segment stress patterns, 44–45
    babble, 50–53, 200, 203
    directed speech, 186, 201–202, 229
    perception of prosodic units in, 43, 133
    preference for speech input, 44
    stages of speech development, 45, 50–51,
        56–57

Inflections, 260
Informal measurement tools, 82–83
Input
  frequency, 61, 63, 74, 170, 172
  functional load, and, 63, 170
  varied, concentrated, focused, 184
Input-oriented approaches to intervention, 183–184, 197
  dialogic reading and, 184, 194–197
  ear training and, 184, 189–193
  focused stimulation and, 184–189
Instructional objective, 175–177, 181–182, 214–215
Integral stimulus hierarchy, 209–211, 214, 219, 230
Integrative stage, 53, 57, 76
Intelligibility, 56, 106–109, 132–133, 152, 157, 164, 170, 173, 180, 189, 253
  assessment of, 87, 92, 103, 106–108,
Intermediate goals, 167–169, 173–174, 244, 263–264
International Classification of Functioning Disability and Health (ICF), 153, 156, 182
International Phonetic Alphabet (IPA), 11–16, 20, 26, 32, 96, 102
Intervention
  agents, 164
  desirable amount of, 161–164
  input oriented approaches to, 183–198
  output-oriented approaches to, 199–231
  parents as agents of, 164–165, 178, 180, 187, 194, 201, 204, 243, 263
Intonation, 30, 45, 191
Iowa-Nebraska norms, 59
Isolation, 30, 44, 96, 112, 114, 190, 193, 203–204, 217, 221, 256

J

Jargon, 53

K

Knowledge
  articulatory, 16, 18, 20
  metaphonological, 252–254, 261
  perceptual, 20, 26, 45–46, 48, 68, 70 , 113, 137, 141, 171–174, 248, 250, 261
  of performance feedback, 212, 214, 218–219, 222–223, 227
  phonological, 53, 57, 71, 103, 126, 165, 170–175, 233–235, 244–245, 252–254
  of results, 212–214, 222–223

L

Labiodental, 8, 11, 34
  fricative, 34
Language
  exposure, 88
  impairment, 110–111, 132–137, 186, 196, 259
  skills, 75, 90, 103, 110–111, 137, 145, 182, 189, 194, 196, 256–257, 259
  speech sound disorder and, 147
Language
  general, 42–43, 48, 50, 75
  general, phonetic perception, 42–43, 75
  specific, 36, 41–45, 48, 50, 75
  specific phonetic perception, 41–43, 50, 75
Lateral
  bracing, 139, 140
  fricative, 12, 16
  lisp, 62, 130, 140, 161, 191
Lesson plan, 175, 213–215, 233, 246, 248, 257
Lexical
  contrast, 56, 63, 234
  representations, 45, 57, 236
  stress, 30, 135
Lexicon, 56, 63, 111–112, 123, 138, 184, 226, 235–236
Lingual frenum, 100
Linguistic classification system, 130
Lips, 3–8, 10–11, 14–15, 97–99, 101
Liquid
  gliding, 38, 63, 66, 244
  simplification, 36–39, 65, 66, 78
Liquids, 6, 8, 28–29, 38, 66, 77, 128, 159, 182, 217, 245
Literacy difficulties, 159
Live voice, 49, 113, 137
Longitudinal, 74, 130, 143
Long-term goals, 166
Long-term normalization, 123, 130, 134, 140, 149
Low perceptual prominence, 68

M

Maintenance, 199, 206–207, 216–217,
    226–228, 231
Malocclusions, 98, 99
Manner of articulation, 5–6, 8, 15, 17, 39, 42,
    54, 259
Marginal babbling, 51–52
Massed, 210
Mastery, 41, 58–59, 61, 70, 74, 77, 153, 156,
    168–171, 216, 226, 235
Maximum
    performance tasks, 98, 101, 136
    phonation duration, 101
    repetition rate, 101
Mean length of utterance, 110, 185, 238
Meaningful minimal pairs, 248–249,
    251–252
Medical
    approach, 153, 155, 157, 160
    history, 88–89
Metalinguistic
    awareness, 252
    knowledge, 47
Metaphon approach, 251, 254, 256
Metaphonological knowledge, 233, 252,
    254, 261
Minimal pair, 27, 32, 39, 46, 62, 125, 170,
    191, 233, 248–251, 262
Minimize pressure to speak, 201
Misalignment, 100
Mispronunciation
    detection task, 46
    identification task, 112–113
Modeling, 185, 189, 202, 219
Molar, normal occlusion, 99–100
Molars, 100
Monitoring treatment progress, 92, 181
Monosyllabic, 208, 210
Morphological awareness, 259–261
Morphology, 110–111, 144
Motor equivalence, 18, 219
MSD (Motor Speech Disorders), 101, 131,
    134–136, 139, 149, 158, 204
    apraxia of speech, 101, 126–129, 131,
        134–136, 141, 148–149, 162, 252, 259,
        261
    dysarthria, 131, 134, 136, 141, 157, 200

not otherwise specified, 131, 134
Multilinear analysis, 237, 239, 246
Mutually exclusive, 126, 136

N

Narrow transcription, 15–16, 27, 39
Nasal
    airflow, 6, 50
    cavity, 3–6
    sounds, stops, 7–9, 29, 32, 35–36, 38, 42,
        54–55
Nasopharynx, 5–7
National Outcome Measurement System
    (NOMS), 163, 164
Natural
    classes, 32, 36, 38–39, 64, 74, 235, 246, 248
    history, 123, 142
    phonological processes, 36, 38, 67, 237,
        246
Near minimal pairs, 27
Neurodevelopmental disorder, 121, 123,
    144
Neutralization, 64, 68–69, 78
Nondevelopmental,
    errors, 61
    Speech Disorder, Shriberg's framework
        for research in and, 36–38, 131–132,
        135–136
Nonlinear phonology, 32, 34, 68, 70
    rules in, *see also* Multilinear phonology,
        34, 70
Nonsense syllable, 203–206, 211, 235
Nonword, 115, 138, 145, 256–257, 260
    repetition, 115, 138–139, 141
    Nonword Repetition Task (NRT),
        114–115
Normal curve, 83
Normative data, 56, 58–59, 97, 102, 110, 154
    for phonological processes, 56, 63–67, 114
    phonological development, 58, 154
    preschool age children, 58, 63
Normative sample, 83–85, 94, 97
Norm-referenced
    approach, 152–154, 157, 160
    test, 83, 85, 114, 118, 152–153, 156–157
Norms, 38, 58–59, 61, 63, 66, 74, 171
Nouns, segmented, 92, 103

O

Obligatory, 10, 28, 39, 65, 80, 90
Obstruents, 38, 67
Occlusions
    dental, 99
    molar, 100
Open-ended prompts, 104, 194, 196
Optimum challenge point, 199
Oral
    apraxia, 101, 127, 129
    mechanism, 96, 135
    movements, 101, 229
    peripheral examination, 96–98, 101, 105,
        116, 123, 129, 139, 141
    structure, 97, 99, 116
Oral-motor function
    dentition, 122–123
    facial characteristics, 122–123
    maximum performance tasks, 122–123
    palatal/pharyngeal areas, 122–123
    standardized measures for, 122–123
    tongue, 122–123
Orthograph, 13, 17, 257, 259–261
Orthographic representations, 13, 17, 257,
    259–261
Otitis media, 119, 132, 136, 142, 149
    with effusion (OME), 131–132, 136, 149
Output-oriented approaches, 189, 199–233

P

Paired stimuli, 219
Palatal fronting, 37–38
Palate and pharyngeal, 3, 5, 7–9, 11, 18–19,
    98–101, 139–140, 155
Parallel talk, 186, 198
Parent training programs, 164–165
Parents, as intervention agents, 164–166,
    180, 187, 194, 204, 223, 251
Participation restrictions, 109–110, 153,
    156–157, 159–160
    activity limitations and, 156–157
Pediatric, 131, 135, 163
PEER sequence, 196
Percent Consonants Correct (PCC), 56, 157,
    237
Percentile rank, 84–85, 92, 152– 153, 160

Perception
    of prosodic units in infancy, 45
    skills, phonetic structure and, 45–46, 50
Perceptual
    encoding, complexity in, 132–134, 139
    knowledge, 20–24, 45–48, 68, 70, 113, 137,
        171–174, 246–248, 250, 261
    sensitivity, to phonetic contrast, 43
Periodic, 20
Perseverate, 136, 149
Personal factors, 87–90, 109, 156–157
Pharyngeal, oral-motor function and, 97
Phonation stage, 50
Phone, 2
Phoneme, 2
Phoneme awareness, 47, 50, 53, 58, 60, 64,
    67, 92, 112–114
Phonemes
    allophonic variants of, 27
    development order, 28, 61, 66, 70, 134
    establishing correct articulation
        procedure, 28, 32, 96
    implicit awareness of, 32, 41, 47, 49, 105
    input frequency/functional load, 34, 36,
        44, 46, 56, 170
    stabilization of new, 57, 67, 73, 139
Phonemic
    disorder, 125
    paraphasias, 64, 129, 148
Phonetic
    disorder, 125, 126
    encoding, 2
    inventory, 16, 17, 243
    knowledge, 45, 126, 233
    placement, 172, 217–220, 228, 242, 246,
        247, 251
    repertoire, 14, 16, 54, 57, 74, 96, 189, 205,
        237
    representations, 3, 52, 183, 189
Phonetics, 2
Phonics, 260
Phonological approaches
    to intervention, 165
    word-based phonology, 236–243
Phonological awareness, 46–47, 114, 138
Phonological
    delay, 128–130
    disorders, 166

Phonological *(continued)*
    generalization, 178–179
    hierarchy, 28–34, 47
    memory, 114–116
    patterns, 65– 66, 244
    planning deficit, 129, 139, 145, 236, 238
    processes, 36–39, 63–67
    processing, 111–112, 116
    representations, 67, 138
    structure, 70, 112
Phonological knowledge, 53, 57, 67, 71, 103,
        126, 138, 165, 170–173, 184, 233–235
    allophonic rules, 26, 27, 32, 249
    covert contrast, 126, 172, 249
    independent vs. relational descriptions,
        53–55, 57
    inventory constraints, 96
    neutralization rules, 64, 68, 69, 78
    perceptual, 42, 112, 113, 115, 116, 137, 172
    phoneme and the phonemic repertoire,
        16–20, 41, 54–57
    phonotactic constraints, 27–30, 39
    productive, and, 261
    segmental, and, 167, 234
    in toddlers and infants, 53, 57, 67, 71,
        103, 126
    underlying, 54, 67–74, 112, 172–174, 234
Phonology
    natural, 36, 38, 67, 237, 246
    word-based, 63, 236
Phonotactic, 27, 39
    constraints, 28
    repertoire, 54, 55
Place
    of articulation, 5, 7, 8, 11, 15, 25, 32, 38,
        42, 54, 185
    node, 34, 73
Planning deficits, 139, 145
Plosives, 6, 7, 32
Post-alveolar, 8, 9, 11, 38
Practice
    performance, 207–210, 222–223
    schedule, 206, 208, 209, 214
Pragmatics, 110
Predictive assessment, 158–159
Preschool, normative data and, 46
Prevalence, 141
Primary prevention, 142

Primitive articulation stage, 51
Probe, 177–178, 181, 215, 244, 247, 251
Prognosis, 89
Progress monitoring plan, 160, 165, 175,
        181
Prosodic bootstrapping hypothesis, 45
Prosodic units, acquisition of, 67
Prosodic units, perception of in infancy, 45
Protrusion of the lips, 99
Proximal cause, 132, 134, 136, 141
Pseudopalate, 18
Psycholinguistic approach, 136, 137, 141

Q

Quasiresonant vowels (QRVs), 50, 51

R

Random practice schedule, 208
Randomized control trials, 193, 197, 223
Raspberries, 51–52
Raw score, 92
Reading Disability, 114, 132, 145, 147, 160,
        253, 258
Recall prompts, 196
Recast, 105, 186, 187
Receptive language skills, 111
Reciprocal, 45, 46, 52, 111
Reduplicated babbles, 53
Reduplication, 52, 63, 68, 69
Referral, 80, 81, 82, 86, 87, 90, 99, 111
Reflexive sounds, 50
Registers, 15, 103, 117
Relational analysis, 57
Repetition rate, monosyllabic, 101, 136, 141,
        238
Repetition tasks, multisyllable, 101, 139,
        141, 238
Representative sample, 91
Residual Speech Errors, 134
Resonance, 6–7, 18, 52, 100, 103, 136, 200,
        202
Response generalization, 178–179, 181
Response-to-Intervention (RTI), 166
Retraction of the lips, 99
Retroflex, 8, 12, 221
Rhotic, 6, 8, 10, 14, 38, 134, 136, 216

Root morphemes, 260
Rule-governed, 234

S

Sagittal profiles, 9
School age children, normative data and, 49, 109, 114
Scopes of practice, 122, 165
Secondary prevention, 142
Segmental, tiers, 12
Segmentation, 44, 114, 240, 255
Self-monitoring, 208, 217, 223, 227, 254, 256
Sensitivity, 43–44, 81, 109–110
Sensorimotor approach, 203–204, 206–207, 213, 216–217, 234, 243
Sensory feedback, 52, 202, 203, 212, 216, 219
Sequential bilingualism, 118–119
Service delivery model, 161, 165–166, 256
Short-term normalization, 123, 131–132, 146
Shriberg's framework for research in, 36–38, 56, 103, 121–124, 131–139, 149
Sibilants
 age acquisition of, 58–60
 coronal, 64
 dental distortion of, 159, 168
 distortions, 64, 65, 134, 136, 159, 168
 lateralized, 159
 misarticulated, 64–65, 134, 136, 159, 168
Signal-to-noise ratio, 49
Simultaneous, 118–119
SOAP note, 177
Sonority Sequencing Principle, 29, 70, 73, 74
Specific goals, 167–169, 171, 173–178, 194, 222, 244–246
Specificity, 81, 236
Specified, 34, 36, 73, 131, 134, 136, 154, 165, 173
Spectrogram, 21–22, 39, 221
Speech
 assessment of, 80–82, 90, 114, 118, 193
 accuracy, 49, 56–59, 104, 108, 122–123, 134, 145–146
 development, 42, 46
 infant-directed, 186, 201–202
 screening, 80

Speech Delay (SD), 132–136, 143–144, 146, 149, 154–156, 158–160, 166, 180, 201, 248
 genetic, and, 131–132
 otitis media with effusion, and, 132
 psychosocial involvement, and, 132–133
 versus speech disorder, 155–156
Speech Disorders Classification System (SCSD), 131, 136
Speech errors
 residual, 134
 as SSD subcategory, 92, 118
Speech input, 20, 22, 32, 44–46, 68, 111, 128, 133, 138, 184–186, 190–191, 193, 197
Speech motor control, 67, 101, 139, 201, 206, 207
Speech perception, 112
 development, 42–43, 46
 nonword repetition and, 115
 skills, 26, 45, 46, 171, 194
Spelling intervention, 259, 261
Spondees, 30
Stabilize goal, 173–174, 188
Standard score, 84, 92, 152, 157
Standardized tests, 82–83, 85, 152, 154, 156–157, 159
 scoring, 96, 154
 single-word citation-form tests, 93
Static assessments, 85, 86
Statistical learning, 44
Stimulability, 96, 116, 170–172, 174, 246
Stimulation, 202, 209–214, 216–219, 222, 228
 focused, 184–191, 261–262
 integral, 210–211, 214, 219
Stimulus generalization, 178, 226
Stopping, 37–38, 64–67, 106, 127–128, 154, 182
 of fricatives, 37, 64, 128
Stress patterns, 30–31, 39, 45–46, 68, 75, 145, 167, 205–206
Strident, 25–26, 245
Stuttering, 143–145, 147
Submucous cleft, 100
Substitution, 63, 67
Successive approximation, 217–218, 220–221, 228
Suffixes, 260

Summative, 213, 222–223
Supernumerary, 99
Suprasegemental characteristics of speech, 11–12, 30, 118
Surface characteristics of the speech errors, 122
Syllable
    deletion, 38, 66–69, 255
    structure processes, 63, 67
    weak, 38, 66–69, 254
    weakening, 68, 69
Syllable Repetition Task (SRT), 115, 129, 135, 138–139, 237–238
Symmetrical, 97, 100
Syntax, 110–111, 144

T

Target selection, 173, 246
Target words, 63, 91–92, 106, 109, 137, 183–187, 189, 236, 240, 243, 247, 262–264
Task
    ABX and, 25
    analysis, 177, 220
    categorical perception, and, 1, 22, 24–26, 39
    discrimination, and, 1, 23, 25–26, 39, 45, 112, 137, 190, 223, 250
    identification, and, 1, 22–23, 25–26, 38–39, 49, 53, 80–81, 108, 112–113, 137, 190–193, 216, 247
    oddity, 25, 47
Teeth, malocclusion, 98–99
Telegraphic speech, 187, 198
Templates, 45, 54, 56, 57, 236, 257
Terminal objective, 176–177
Tertiary, 90, 155
    prevention, 142
Token economy, 222
Tongue, 3–9, 11–12, 14–15, 18–19, 23, 35–36, 50–52, 97–101, 134, 137, 139, 140–141, 176, 202, 206, 218–221, 225, 241
Tonsils, 100
Top-down factors, 44
Total intervention duration, 151, 162–164, 167
Tracking treatment progress, 175

Transfer, 178–179, 181, 199, 213, 216–217, 226–228, 231, 234–235, 246
Treatment
    decisions, protocol for, 152, 157, 173
    effectiveness, 164–165, 180
    efficacy, 180, 184
    goals, 67, 81, 92, 110, 151, 163, 166, 168, 171–173, 175, 177, 182–183, 234–236, 239, 244
    planning, 61, 66–67, 81, 86–88, 90–92, 105, 111, 151–180, 249
    progress, monitoring, 32, 181
    schedule, intensity of, 162–163
    session, cycles approach demonstration, 244, 246, 248, 261
    session, traditional approach, 190, 199, 216–217, 228, 230, 262
Trochaic stress pattern, 30–31, 39, 45
Trochee, 30, 69
Two-way scoring, 92, 94–96, 116, 244

U

Ultrasound, 18–19, 140, 212, 218, 221
Underlying
    phonological knowledge, representation, 67, 70, 171–172, 174, 194, 234, 244
    speech processes, 122–124, 126, 130, 132, 137, 141
Underspecification, 34, 36
Undifferentiated, 51
    lingual gestures, 140–141
Unilateral, 97
Unintelligible speech, 110, 244, 246
Universal, 43, 67, 75
Universally applicable, 126
Unstimulable, 96, 172, 185, 217
Unstressed syllable deletion, 37–38
Unusual prosody, 127, 130, 135, 139, 148
Use strengths to support needs, 173

V

Van Riper's approach, 228, 230
Variability, 23, 32, 46, 58, 67, 70, 74, 105–106, 117, 165, 173, 205, 207–210, 230
Variable practice, 209–210, 214, 222
Variegated babbles, 53

Velar, 9–12, 16, 19, 36, 39, 54, 62–63, 65–66, 98, 128, 130, 169, 252
   fronting, 63, 182, 244–246, 248, 255–256
Verbal dyspraxia, 101, 127, 129, 134
Vertical goal attack strategy, 169, 216, 221, 228, 235
Visual
  analysis of articulation, 18
  feedback, 19, 205, 217–218, 221, 228
Vocal
  development, 16, 41, 50–51, 57, 202
  tract, 3, 5–11, 14, 18, 20, 35, 50–52, 61, 134, 139, 202
Voiced, 5–7, 12, 22, 26, 29, 52, 54, 135, 177, 248
  cognates, 11, 26
Voiceless, 5–7, 10, 12, 22, 26, 29, 32, 135
  cognates, 11, 26
  fricative, 29
Voice-onset-time (VOT), 22, 249
Voicing contrasts, 42, 205, 245
Vowel space, 200
Vowels, 3–8, 11–16, 20–21, 23, 27–32, 38–39, 46, 51, 94, 103, 217, 228, 234, 256, 260
Vowels, accuracy of production of, 46, 49
Vowels, production of, 211, 214, 215

Vowels, development in infancy, 42, 51–52, 54

W

Warm-up, prepractice, 208, 212–214, 222, 227, 230, 235
Waveform display, 21, 39
Weak syllables, 41, 68, 78, 254
Whole word measures, 56, 57
Whole word templates, 57
Within-phoneme inconsistency, 105–106
Within-word inconsistency, 106, 135, 236
Word learning, in infancy, 45
Word templates, 54, 234, 237
Word-based phonology, 54
Words, acoustic-phonetic representations for, 49, 184–185, 187, 189, 198–199
Words, determining syllable structure of, 27–28, 30
Words, minimum pair, 46, 62, 125, 191, 233
Words, perceptual representations for, 46
Words, target, 38, 46, 55, 63, 91–92, 106, 109, 112, 137, 183–191, 236, 240–243, 247, 249, 261–264
World Health Organization (WHO), 156